THE EFFECTS OF AUTISM ON THE FAMILY

CURRENT ISSUES IN AUTISM
Series Editors: Eric Schopler and Gary B. Mesibov

University of North Carolina School of Medicine
Chapel Hill, North Carolina

AUTISM IN ADOLESCENTS AND ADULTS
Edited by Eric Schopler and Gary B. Mesibov

THE EFFECTS OF AUTISM ON THE FAMILY
Edited by Eric Schopler and Gary B. Mesibov

THE EFFECTS
OF AUTISM
ON THE FAMILY

Edited by

Eric Schopler

and

Gary B. Mesibov

University of North Carolina School of Medicine
Chapel Hill, North Carolina

PLENUM PRESS • NEW YORK AND LONDON

Library of Congress Cataloging in Publication Data

Main entry under title:

The Effects of autism on the family.

(Current issues in autism)
Includes bibliographical references and index.
1. Autistic children—Rehabilitation—Congresses. 2. Autistic children—Family rela-
tionships—Congresses. 3. Behavior therapy—Congresses. I. Schopler, Eric. II.
Mesibov, Gary, 1945–   . III. Title. IV. Series.
RJ506.A9E4   1984   362.2   84-8414
ISBN 0-306-41533-X

This limited facsimile edition has been issued
for the purpose of keeping this title available
to the scientific community.

©1984 Plenum Press, New York
A Division of Plenum Publishing Corporation
233 Spring Street, New York, N.Y. 10013

Printed in the United States of America

Contributors

MARY S. AKERLEY • 10609 Glenwild Road, Silver Spring, Maryland 20901

LORIAN BAKER • UCLA Neuropsychiatric Institute, Room C8-871, 760 Westwood Plaza, Los Angeles, California 90024

ANNE BASHFORD • Southeastern TEACCH Center, 1516 Market Street, Wilmington, North Carolina 28401

JAMES C. BERNIER • Child Development Center, Rhode Island Hospital, 593 Eddy Street, Providence, Rhode Island 02902

MARIE M. BRISTOL • Carolina Institute for Research on Early Education of the Handicapped, Frank Porter Graham Child Development Center, University of North Carolina, Chapel Hill, North Carolina 27514

JOHN C. BURKE • Department of Speech, University of California, Santa Barbara, California 93106

DENNIS P. CANTWELL • UCLA Neuropsychiatric Institute, Room C8-871, 760 Westwood Plaza, Los Angeles, California 90024

BARBARA COYNE CUTLER • School of Education, Division of Counseling, Reading, Language Development and Special Education, Boston University, Boston, Massachusetts 02215

ROBERT FROMBERG • 5411 Tralee Place, Raleigh, North Carolina 27609

SANDRA L. HARRIS • Graduate School of Applied and Professional Psychology, Rutgers University, Piscataway, and Douglass Developmental Disabilities Center, New Brunswick, New Jersey 08903

ROBERT L. KOEGEL • Social Process Research Institute, University of California, Santa Barbara, California 93106

DAVID J. KOLKO • Western Psychiatric Institute and Clinic, School of Medicine, Department of Psychiatry, Division of Child and Adolescent Psychiatry, University of Pittsburgh, Pittsburgh, Pennsylvania 15213

MARTIN A. KOZLOFF • Department of Sociology, Boston University, 100 Cummington Street, Boston, Massachusetts 02215

LEE M. MARCUS • Piedmont TEACCH Center, 504 South Wing, Division of Health Affairs, University of North Carolina School of Medicine, Department of Psychiatry, Chapel Hill, North Carolina 27514

SUSAN M. McHALE • College of Human Development, Pennsylvania State University, State College, Pennsylvania 16802

GARY B. MESIBOV • Division TEACCH, 310 Medical School Wing E, 222H, University of North Carolina, Chapel Hill, North Carolina 27514

DEBRA L. MILLS • Psychology Department, University of California, San Diego, La Jolla, California 92093

MICHAEL D. POWERS • Graduate School of Applied and Professional Psychology, Rutgers University, Piscataway, and Douglass Developmental Disabilities Center, New Brunswick, New Jersey 08903

SIGFRIED M. PUESCHEL • Child Development Center, Rhode Island Hospital, 593 Eddy Street, Providence, Rhode Island 02902

ERIC SCHOPLER • Division TEACCH, 310 Medical School Wing E, 222H, University of North Carolina, Chapel Hill, North Carolina 27514

LAURA SCHREIBMAN • Psychology Department, University of California, San Diego, La Jolla, California 92093

VICTORIA SHEA • Division for Disorders of Development and Learning, Biological Sciences Research Center, 220H, University of North Carolina, Chapel Hill, North Carolina 27514

R. HAL SHIGLEY • Eastern TEACCH Center, Stratford Arms Apts., #30-B, 1900 South Charles Street, Greenville, North Carolina 27834

RUTH CHRIST SULLIVAN • Autism Services Center, 101 Richmond Street, Huntington, West Virginia 25702

JAMES E. SURRATT • Burlington City Schools, P.O. Box 938, Burlington, North Carolina 27215

RUNE J. SIMEONSSON • Frank Porter Graham Child Development Center, University of North Carolina, Chapel Hill, North Carolina 27514

JERRY L. SLOAN • Southeastern TEACCH Center, 1516 Market Street, Wilmington, North Carolina 28401

FRANK WARREN • Community Services for Autistic Adults and Children, 751 Twinbrook Parkway, Rockville, Maryland 20851

EDWARD ZIGLER • Department of Psychology, Yale University, Box 11A Yale Station, New Haven, Connecticut 06520

Preface

As the oldest statewide program serving autistic people in the United States, North Carolina's Division TEACCH (Treatment and Education of Autistic and related Communication handicapped CHildren) has had a major impact on services for these people and their families. As we move into our second decade, we are frequently questioned about all aspects of our procedures, techniques, and program. Of all the questions that are asked, however, the one that comes up most frequently and seems to set our program apart from others concerns the ways in which we work with families. To help answer this question we identified what we have found to be the major components in our parent–professional relationships, and we elaborate on these with the most current research information, clinical insights, and community knowledge available through the expertise of our distinguished contributors. Our purpose was to collect the most recent information and to organize the resulting volume along the outlines of the parent–professional relationship found most important in the TEACCH program. Thus, the four main sections of the book include these four major ways professionals work with parents: as their advocates, their trainers, their trainees, and their reciprocal emotional support source. To the extent this effort was successful, we acknowledge that it is easier to organize book chapters along these dimensions than it is to provide their implementation in the field.

This volume grew out of the annual TEACCH conference held in Chapel Hill during May 1982, which focused on the effects of autism on the family. As with the other books in this series, however, this volume is not simply the conference proceedings. Additional contributions were solicited in order to present a more comprehensive elaboration of the conference theme.

To the parents of autistic people with whom we work and to the University of North Carolina and the North Carolina General Assembly, who have supported their struggle, we dedicate our efforts.

E. S.
G. B. M.

Acknowledgments

It is our great pleasure to acknowledge the many sources of help we have had during various phases of this project. First, our thanks to Connie Brite and Lightning Brown, who helped organize and coordinate the conference that was the starting point for this book. We would also like to acknowledge the able secretarial and typing assistance we received from Cindy Fesmire, Raymina Y. Mays, and Evy Nilsen. The invaluable editorial assistance of Judy Davis has been instrumental in strengthening individual chapters, coordinating our efforts, and making sure this project proceeded on schedule. As always, the members of the resourceful and competent TEACCH staff have provided many insights that are reflected in our work.

Finally, and most important, most of what we have learned and put in this book has been brought to us by the courageous and resilient families of autistic people in North Carolina. We hope this will help them and others in continuing their important struggle.

E. S.
G. B. M.

Contents

Chapter 3

RESEARCH CONCERNING FAMILIES OF CHILDREN WITH
AUTISM   41

Dennis P. Cantwell and Lorian Baker

Chapter 4

HELPING AUTISTIC CHILDREN THROUGH THEIR PARENTS: THE
TEACCH MODEL   65

Eric Schopler, Gary B. Mesibov, R. Hal Shigley, and Anne Bashford

Part III: Parents as Advocates

Chapter 5

DEVELOPMENTAL CHANGES IN FAMILIES WITH AUTISTIC
CHILDREN: A PARENT'S PERSPECTIVE   85

Mary S. Akerley

Chapter 6

THE ROLE OF THE NATIONAL SOCIETY IN WORKING WITH FAMILIES   99

Frank Warren

Chapter 7

THE PROFESSIONAL'S ROLE AS ADVOCATE   117

Siegfried M. Pueschel and James C. Bernier

Chapter 8

ADVOCACY: EFFECTIVELY CHANGING THE SYSTEM   129

James E. Surratt

Part IV: Parents as Trainees

Chapter 9

PARENTS AS BEHAVIOR THERAPISTS FOR THEIR AUTISTIC
CHILDREN: CLINICAL AND EMPIRICAL CONSIDERATIONS   145

David J. Kolko

Chapter 10

A TRAINING PROGRAM FOR FAMILIES OF CHILDREN WITH
AUTISM: RESPONDING TO FAMILY NEEDS   163

Martin A. Kozloff

Chapter 11

TRAINING PARENT–CHILD INTERACTIONS   187

Laura Schreibman, Robert L. Koegel, Debra L. Mills, and John C. Burke

Chapter 12

BEHAVIOR THERAPISTS LOOK AT THE IMPACT OF AN AUTISTIC CHILD ON THE FAMILY SYSTEM   207

Sandra L. Harris and Michael D. Powers

Part V: Parents as Trainers

Chapter 13

MY GREAT TEACHERS   227

Eric Schopler

Chapter 14

PARENTS AS TRAINERS OF LEGISLATORS, OTHER PARENTS,
AND RESEARCHERS   233

Ruth Christ Sullivan

Chapter 15

THE PARENT AS TRAINER OF PROFESSIONALS: ATTITUDES AND
ACCEPTANCE   .   247

Barbara Coyne Cutler

Part VI: Emotional Support and Siblings

Chapter 16

EXPLAINING MENTAL RETARDATION AND AUTISM TO PARENTS 265

Victoria Shea

Chapter 17

FAMILY RESOURCES AND SUCCESSFUL ADAPTATION TO AUTISTIC CHILDREN   289

Marie M. Bristol

Chapter 18

COPING WITH BURNOUT   311

Lee M. Marcus

Chapter 19

CHILDREN WITH HANDICAPPED BROTHERS AND SISTERS   327

Susan M. McHale, Rune J. Simeonsson, and Jerry L. Sloan

Chapter 20

THE SIBLING'S CHANGING ROLES   343

Robert Fromberg

INDEX   355

Introduction

Professional Attitudes toward Parents

A Forty-Year Progress Report

ERIC SCHOPLER and GARY B. MESIBOV

Our understanding of autism, its causes and treatments, is still far from complete, although much has been learned about the syndrome Kanner first identified 40 years ago. There is no single aspect of our knowledge developed during this period that is more far-reaching and important to the effective and humane treatment of autistic people than the change in attitude toward their parents.

An introduction to this volume on the current knowledge of families with autistic children must place the attitudinal changes toward such families in historical perspective. The change from regarding parents as the primary cause of their child's disorder to regarding them as cotherapists, advocates, developmental agents, and the primary cure for the problems of autism occurred during a relatively brief period (Schopler, 1971). There are still regions in which these changes are not recognized. But the transition in the literature, led by empirical research (Rutter and Schopler, 1978) and increasingly translated into practice, is a dramatic one—almost 180 degrees over four decades. It is an exciting chronicle to which those of us involved with the North Carolina TEACCH (Treatment and Education of Autistic and related Communication handicapped CHildren) program have made an important contribution over the years (Runck, 1979).

The discussion of such changes is not an easy task. Attitudes are illusive and difficult to measure, and the experiences of individual parents are still too variable. However, there appear to be four major elements contributing to the changed attitudes toward parents of autistic children: (1) changes in the definition

ERIC SCHOPLER and GARY B. MESIBOV • Division TEACCH, University of North Carolina, Chapel Hill, North Carolina 27514 of autism, produced by empirical research in the published literature; (2) a shift in the focus of service providers and clinicians, who sometimes contribute to the research literature and social policy and sometimes develop their own procedures without reference to empirical research; (3) the parents of autistic children themselves and their own attitudes, which are at least partly formed by the technical information they obtain from professionals; and (4) community understanding of the disorder and the resulting social policy. This chapter includes a review of these elements and how they have changed over the past four decades.

CHANGES IN THE DEFINITION OF AUTISM

At the risk of repetition from our first volume in this series, *Autism in Adolescents and Adults* (Schopler and Mesibov, 1983), the reader is reminded that Kanner's definition of autism is alive and well. His is a unique diagnostic category in that it has lasted longer than the many other diagnostic labels referring to similar children. The reason for this viability is that Kanner's definition was primarily based on clinical and behavioral descriptions, readily investigated by empirical research. Most of the other labels, on the other hand, depended mainly on theory, especially psychoanalytic theory, and have now faded into disuse.

Some aspects of the Kanner syndrome have been changed by empirical research, while other aspects have remained the same, supported by subsequent research. Parts of the definition that are still used include (1) lack of human relatedness from the beginning of life, (2) disordered language, and (3) insistence on repetitive behaviors, with upset when such behaviors or routines are interrupted. These are still considered the primary features of autism. Their empirical support has been documented in Rutter's (1978) admirable review of research. A fourth feature of the syndrome, not mentioned by Kanner, is distortion and impairment of perceptual processes (O'Conner and Hermelin, 1975; Ornitz and Ritvo, 1968; Schopler, 1965). The inclusion of this feature in the definition of autism developed by the National Society for Children and Adults with Autism (NSAC) (NSAC, 1978; Schopler, 1978) has been supported by subsequent diagnostic data (Schopler, Reichler, DeVellis, and Daly, 1980).

Other aspects of the Kanner definition have been modified by subsequent research, including the following five issues: single underlying disease process, peak skills and mental retardation, autism versus childhood schizophrenia, parent psychogenesis, and socioeconomic status.

Single Underlying Disease Process

Kanner (1943) believed that the autism syndrome represented a unitary underlying, possibly psychogenic disease process. This was widely interpreted as meaning that the child's symptoms were caused by parental pathology. Since that time, we have learned that the disorder is primarily the result of various brain abnormalities from the prenatal and perinatal period.

Lotter (1978) found that more than 25% of autistic children in his study developed seizures when they were between 15 and 29 years of age. These children were not epileptic, nor had brain damage been considered at intake. Hauser, DeLong, and Rosman (1975) found evidence that the language impairment in autism may involve asymmetrical bilateral temporal lobe disease. Autism has also been associated with conditions such as maternal rubella during pregnancy (Chess, 1977), metabolic conditions such as Celiac's disease (Coleman, 1978), tuberous sclerosis, and, occasionally, Down's syndrome (Wakabayashi, 1979). Genetic factors were demonstrated in Folstein and Rutter's (1978) twin study. More recently, fragile-X syndrome was identified in four autistic boys (Brown, Jenkins, Friedman, Brooks, Wisniewski, Raguthu, and French, 1982), and genetic implications were inferred from the disproportionate three or four males to one female ratio (Lord, Schopler, and Revicki, 1982; Tsai, Stewart, and August, 1981). None of the mechanisms identified above are claimed to operate in all autistic children. The evidence indicates, however, that a number of different biologic factors acting singly or in combination are most likely to produce the autism syndrome.

Peak Skills and Mental Retardation

From the outset, Kanner reported that autistic children showed certain peak skills of mental functioning, including unusual abilities of musical pitch, rote memory, and number manipulation. Kanner (1943) interpreted these observations as meaning that these children actually had normal intellectual potential, and that their poor functioning was simply the result of their inability to form social relationships, an inability attributed to parents' inadequate child-rearing practices. However, when mental functions in these children were studied systematically, a number of specific and general cognitive deficits were identified (Hermelin and O'Connor, 1970).

Virtually all studies, including a large sample of more than 300 autistic children, reported that over 50% of the children had IQ scores of less than 50 (Ando and Yoshimura, 1979; Barry and James, 1978; Campbell, Hardesty, and Burdock, 1978; DeMyer, Barton, Alpern, Kimberlin, Allen, Yang, and Steele, 1974; Lockyer and Rutter, 1970; Schopler and Dalldorf, 1980). Thus, there is no longer any reasonable doubt that autism and mental retardation can and do coexist. Recognition of this coexistence was delayed by the belief held during the early Kanner era that autistic children were "untestable." This belief was disproven by Alpern (1967; Alpern and Kimberlin, 1970) when he showed that some children who failed or would not respond to age-appropriate test items would respond correctly when they were asked test items that were easier or at earlier levels of development. When a test was developed that took such developmental considerations into account, autistic children were no longer untestable (Schopler and Reichler, 1979). As the myth of untestability was deflated, so was the myth that autistic children were essentially normal children who had withdrawn from unfavorable learning conditions.

With increasing acceptance that autism and mental retardation could coexist came the acceptance that autism is a "developmental disorder" rather than an "emotional disturbance." Concurrently, assessment of so-called untestable autistic children is now being carried out in the context of behavior therapy (Koegel, Rincover, and Egel, 1982), functional analysis within the natural environment (Brown, Nietupski, and Hamre-Nietupski, 1976), and language training (Schuler and Bormann, Note 1).

Autism versus Childhood Schizophrenia

Kanner had defined autism as the earliest form of chilhood schizophrenia. Consequently, many clinicians did not attempt to differentiate the two designations (Bender, 1947; Goldfarb, 1961), or they used the two terms synonymously (Creak, 1961). With the development of more systematic studies, important differences were reported between psychotic children with early age of onset and those with late onset after pubescence (Makita, 1966; Vrono, 1974). Kolvin (1971a, 1971b) and his colleagues found a markedly bipolar distribution according to age of onset, with one peak at infancy and another at adolescence. Their early-onset group showed fewer incidents of thought disorder, a higher frequency of repetitive behaviors, and more abnormal body movements than the late-onset group. Kolvin's data were consistent with Rutter's (1970) follow-up studies, showing that in contrast to schizophrenic children, autistic children rarely developed delusions or hallucinations when they reached adulthood. The evidence is compelling that autistic children are different from schizophrenic children by a number of characteristics, including age of onset, and there is no significant support for considering autism to be the earliest form of childhood schizophrenia.

The confirmation of these distinctions between autism and childhood schizophrenia have been instrumental in moving autism from the category of emotionally disturbed to the category of developmentally disordered. There was sufficient professional consensus on these changes that the *Journal of Autism and Childhood Schizophrenia,* founded by Leo Kanner, changed its title in 1979 to the *Journal of Autism and Developmental Disorders.* Because of the widely held belief among our mental health professionals that emotional disturbances have their origins primarily in early child–parent relationships, the shifting of autism to the developmental-disorder category also had the effect of reversing the parent-blaming attitudes of professionals. However, the most important shift came directly from the family literature.

Parental Psychogenesis

Kanner reported that parents of autistic children were unique in that they were highly educated and professionally successful. Out of Kanner's first series of 11 autistic children, 8 out of 11 parents were represented in *Who's Who in America* or in *American Men of Science*. These upper-middle-class parents were described as emotionally cold and obsessive about the details of their own lives. Thus, they seemed to mirror the potential for autism realized in their children through childrearing practices characterized in the literature as undemonstrative, introverted, obsessive, symbiotic, overprotective, cold, and administered by "refrigerator mothers."

Theories on the nature of family factors in the genesis of autism are many but can usually be grouped under three general headings: (1) severe stress during the child's early life, (2) deviant parental personality characteristics, and (3) deviant parent–child interactions. We will not attempt to discuss the growing number of studies examining these family factors because this was already done by Cantwell, Baker, and Rutter (1978) and will be brought up to date in Chapter 3 by Cantwell and Baker. The results of these studies are cumulative and unambiguous in showing no empirical support for the assertions of parental pathology as a primary cause of autism. On the other hand, they confirm the observation that parents of autistic children are no more or less normal than the rest of us, with the notable exception that they have a handicapped child in their family.

Socioeconomic Status

Beginning with Kanner's (1943) original publication, autistic children have frequently been reported as coming from upper-class families. While this finding is related to the parental pathology theory, it is different in that it was based on objective measures of family socioeconomic status (SES). Since all of Kanner's original series of 11 children came from highly educated, affluent families, the groundwork was laid for incorporation of this observation into the definition. Although not all studies reported this finding, a recent survey by Schopler, Andrews, and Strupp (1979) found that 12 out of 18 studies with large subject samples reported a predominance of high SES families with autistic children.

In that study, based on a statewide sample of 264 autistic children, we found 61% of the autistic children in families of lower SES and only 22% in families of higher SES. This difference in SES predominance from the majority of the studies could be due to differences in diagnostic criteria, but this explanation did not account for the disproportionate numbers of studies that might also use different diagnostic emphases and yet report more children from high SES families. We examined the possibility that a number of selection factors may be operating, and found support in our data for the following four factors selecting for high SES families.

1. Age of onset before 30 months is widely accepted as a primary feature of autism (Eisenberg and Kanner, 1956; Rutter, 1978). During the first 2 years of the child's life, abnormalities in relating to adults and in speech development are more subtle and difficult to recognize than they will be at a later age. We hypothesized that parents with more education and more resources for consultation may be expected to identify onset of symptoms earlier than parents with less education and lower SES. When comparing parents who noticed something wrong with their children before 24 months with parents noting concerns at a later time, it was found that a significantly greater number of high SES families observed early indicators.

2. The second significant selection factor confirmed was that parents who traveled a greater distance for treatment, as from other states or countries, would have more special knowledge, funds for travel, and higher SES than parents who came for treatment within the state.

3. Availability of services was the third selection factor. Because public services for autistic children were not available until recently, McDermott, Harrison, Schrager, Lindy, and Killins (1967) reported that many autistic children in Michigan were deliberately diagnosed and masqueraded as mentally retarded in order to find special public school placements for them. We confirmed this selection factor by finding that children referred to our program when it was the specially funded Child Research Project included significantly more higher SES families than when the program was adopted and funded by the state as a public program, thereby becoming available to families of all SES levels.

4. The fourth selection factor was a detailed child history. A number of studies (Creak and Ini, 1960; Lotter, 1978; Prior, Gajzago, and Knox, 1976; Schain and Yannet, 1960) have excluded children from their sample because of incomplete history data. Bender and Grugett (1956) also noted the diagnostic difficulties encountered by researchers and clinicians when dealing with children from lower SES families. We compared parents who described a typical day on our parent questionnaire with little detail (3 lines or less) with parents who wrote a page or more. We found that the higher SES families included significantly more detail than the lower SES families.

We did not expect that these four selection factors accounted for all the studies reporting disproportionately high SES families with autistic children.

There are no doubt many other factors. Subsequent studies also reported autistic children from low SES families (Gillberg and Schaumann, 1982; Tsai, Stewart, Faust, and Shook, 1982). Confirmation of an additional selection factor came from Wing's (1980) epidemiological study, in which fathers belonging to the British National Society for Autistic Children were mainly from higher SES backgrounds. Otherwise, Wing also found more low SES families. The data on selection factors support the conclusion that when studies control for selection factors, they do not show more autistic children from high than from low SES families.

In summary, the past four decades of research have produced some significant changes in the definition of autism. The assumption of an underlying unitary disease process has been replaced by evidence for multiple etiologies capable of giving expression to the autism syndrome. Peak skills occur in a small percentage of autistic children and are not a primary feature in a disorder that coexists with mental retardation. Autism is distinct from childhood schizophrenia according to age of onset and the primary symptom characteristics. Most important to the improved welfare of such children, treatment now includes behavior modification and special education; psychopathology in upper-middle-class parents is no longer considered the primary explanation for the autism syndrome. Moreover, parents, not just their autistic children, are increasingly recognized as victims of this disorder.

SERVICE PROVIDERS AND CLINICIANS

The second major change in attitudes toward parents of autistic children comes from the changed perspective in the attitudes of service providers and clinicans. During the Kanner era, when autism was considered a form of emotional or social withdrawal, the treatment of choice for autistic children was play therapy (Axline, 1947; Ekstein and Friedman, 1966), designed for ventilation of the extreme stress assumed to be generated by the family. While the child was seen in play therapy, his parents were seen by another member of the clinical team, usually a social worker. The purpose of these therapy sessions was usually to provide new insights aimed at changing parental personalities so as to enable the child to overcome his autism. Even more common was the position advocated by Bettelheim (1967) that the only potential for the child's improvement was to remove him from his family in a "parentectomy." In order to qualify for these treatment modalities, parents were required to acknowledge guilt for their child-rearing inadequacies and to pay the high fees required by many mental health professionals. Parents of autistic children submitted to this treatment because not much else was available to them. Autistic children were usually excluded from public schools, and since the disorder appeared to strike mainly upper-middle-class families, parents felt they were simply paying the bills for their own mistakes.

The change from the psychoanalytic orientation was promoted by the application of behavioral principles through operant conditioning. The effective demonstration of a technology for increasing desirable behavior and decreasing undesirable behavior took some of the steam out of the expectations for personality reorganization from long-term psychotherapy. Many behaviorists, like Ferster (1961), believed that the autistic symptoms were the result of parents' failure to provide an appropriate reinforcement history. In that sense, behavioral theories were not so different from the psychodynamic theories of parental guilt. They were different, however, in that they were committed to the concept that behavior modification was a potentially scientific enterprise that parents and others could learn to use. One of the controversies to be sparked by the use of operant conditioning was the charge that the procedures were mechanistic and turned children into robots. In the case of autism, however, this was clearly a confusion between cause and effect. Autistic children were, after all, showing inappropriate, repetitive, and mechanical behaviors before they were referred for treatment and while they lived in the same family structures that enabled their siblings to grow up normally.

Our own research on the effects of structure (Schopler, Brehm, Kinsbourne, and Reichler, 1971) showed that autistic children need more learning structure than was usually provided by play therapy. Moreover, that need varied with the child's level of development. Children at lower levels of development needed external structure more than did children at higher levels who had certain concepts and skills already internalized. We found that with the younger children, the most appropriately individualized education programs and behavior modification procedures could best be developed by working with parents as cotherapists (Schopler and Reichler, 1971).

CHANGES IN ATTITUDES OF PARENTS

The way in which parents of autistic children have seen themselves in their parenting role has also changed over the years. Our summary of these changes is based largely on clinical reports from parents during the past 20 years. During the Kanner era, when autism was just being recognized, few professionals could offer advice to allay parental concerns. This tended to increase self-blame. For example, when a child says a few words, but then stops and seems to withdraw, parents often think it was because of something they did or said. Moreover, the presence of an autistic child frequently inhibited the family's social life or church attendance. Their embarrassment and shame, coupled with their inability to explain their child's strange behavior, made many parents withdraw increasingly from social activity. School systems did not provide appropriate education and excluded children from attendance. Well-meaning relatives offered advice that often took the form of yet another criticism. When parents sought the help of mental health professionals, the confused and perplexed reactions of parents to their autistic child were easily turned around and presented as the primary cause of the autistic syndrome. The resulting demoralization made such parents ready and even willing victims for scapegoating (Schopler, 1971).

This scapegoating process could also be understood in terms of the incongruent roles between professionals and parents. The professional role required special knowledge and information on the cause and treatment of the condition. Although this knowledge was not always available, pressure on clinicians to produce such information was great. The parental social role, on the other hand, required the need to have explanations about their handicapped child. So both parents and professionals accepted the parental-blame theories. However, the cost to parents in inappropriate treatment efforts and demoralization was great. Unlike parents of other handicapped children, they were unable to form a parent group until the psychogenic theory was challenged.

This trend was reversed in the mid-1960s when Rimland (1964), the father of an autistic child, published a scholarly review of the literature criticizing the psychogenic theory. This book won an award in psychology, sustaining Rimland's prestige and creating the leadership necessary for establishing the National Society for Autistic Children (NSAC). This organization grew rapidly and became effective in promoting research and services for the disorder that had invaded its members' families. Members offered each other helpful coping suggestions, which were rarely forthcoming from professionals.

One mother reported that she took along NSAC leaflets containing the definition of autism whenever she took her autistic son to the store. She now had a way of handling hostile stares and comments when her boy took to snatching cans from other shoppers' baskets. Instead of being embarrassed by questions such as "What's wrong with your undisciplined child?" she now simply handed out the leaflet defining autism.

By the 1980s parents' self-image had undergone some basic changes. Rather than seeing themselves as the primary causes of their children's autism, they now saw themselves as cotherapists, as their child's developmental agent and special advocate.

COMMUNITY UNDERSTANDING AND SOCIAL POLICY

Social attitudes are sometimes defined by what neighbors and relatives think, but today social consensus, when it occurs, is mostly produced by the news media in their various forms. During the Kanner era, the public knew little about autism and many professionals were unfamiliar with the term. The idea that mental illness was caused by poor child-rearing attitudes and practices was widely accepted in this country, as was the belief that the unhappiness caused by such problems would be cured or alleviated with psychoanalytic information and treatment. These public views reached fad proportions in this country. They also shaped and contributed to public misunderstanding of autism.

Today, the public's understanding of autism has increased greatly. It was promoted by publications written by parents of autistic children including Greenfield (1972), Kysar (1968), May (1958), Park (1982), and others. Research on autism was discussed in the public press and included on television programs, such as "Marcus Welby," during prime time.

The relationship between research findings and public press coverage is highly unreliable. Stories that sell newspapers and fix the gaze of television viewers do not always coincide with research interests and findings. In the case of autism, however, the relationship between research publications and public press has been surprisingly good, if not uniformly accurate. By 1975 autism was included in the Developmental Disabilities Act, and by 1977 Public Law 94-142 mandated public school education for all handicapped children, including the autistic, thanks to a better informed public.

In summary, we have traced some of the special and far-reaching changes in our understanding of and attitudes toward parents of autistic children, changes that have not always produced more effective treatment. We have also tried to summarize some of the evidence of this change from journal sources, research data, clinical work, parents' perceptions, and social attitudes. Each of these elements has contributed to the change from parents' being seen as the primary cause of their child's disorder to being the child's cotherapist and primary cure agent. There can be no doubt that this change in attitudes toward parents has been instrumental in providing better care and more humane treatment of autistic people of all ages, with the most cost-effective being the treatment and maintenance of autistic children in their own homes, schools, and communities.

OVERVIEW OF THE VOLUME

It is with a sense of breathlessness that we have tried to review in this brief space the extent of the changes in attitudes about parents of autistic children. It has helped us to regain our perspective by remembering the broader social context in which changes have been taking place, at an equally rapid rate.

During this time, there has been an increased emphasis in our society on individual rights and what in political jargon are called single-issue campaigns. Our society has reached a point where many different minority groups are demanding rights denied to them in the past, rights that are sometimes perceived as an unfair imposition by other members of society. Even though the nature of these claims from different minority groups varies greatly, they have shaped our recent conservative political climate.

However, parents of autistic children are different in some important respects from parents of children with other handicaps. Handicaps like blindness, deafness, mental retardation, or cerebral palsy are more visible and obvious than autism—easier to explain. Parents of such children have had less difficulty in obtaining social and political support, while parents of autistic children have had to play a more active role in educating both professionals and the public. Even more important, parents of other handicapped children were not usually first falsely blamed for their child's handicap. It is therefore not surprising that parents of autistic children have been especially motivated and enthusiastic about setting the record straight and lobbying for appropriate social support. It can be that precisely this unique historical position makes parents of autistic children more vulnerable to a negative reaction for what may be seen as excessive demands.

In reviewing the parental attitude literature and thinking about the parent–professional relationship within our program over the past 15 years, it appears that both have evolved toward the behavioral model of parents as trainees with professional trainers. However, both the literature and our experience suggest that this is too simple to be sufficient for all aspects of the parent–professional relationship needed for teaching these most complicated children. Therefore, our North Carolina TEACCH program applies four concepts of parent–staff relationships: (1) parent–staff collaboration for child advocacy within the community, (2) parents as trainees and staff as trainers, (3) parents as trainers and staff as trainees, and (4) parent–staff emotional support interaction. We have found that these parent–professional relationships are essential in any attempt to provide optimum service to autistic persons and their families. For this reason we have used these four categories as the guiding organization of this volume by grouping chapters according to these kinds of parent–professional relationships.

Before describing these four kinds of parent–professional interactions, the volume begins with an overview section, which places this work in a larger context. Zigler discusses the role of all handicapped children and their families in American society. His long and varied experiences make his observations especially relevant and important. Cantwell and Baker follow with an extensive review of the research literature on families and autism, highlighting what we have learned and what methodological issues still need resolution. Finally, Schopler, Mesibov, Shigley, and Bashford explain how our TEACCH program has used all four kinds of parent–professional relationships to deliver a comprehensive network of statewide services for over a decade.

The chapters in Part III explore the theme of parents as advocates from three different points of view. Mary Akerley presents a crisp account of the changing needs of an autistic child and his family as the child grows up. Although she advocates from a parent's perspective, her views are informed by her knowledge of public policy and law. Frank Warren approaches the families' advocacy for their children through the parent organization, NSAC, now named the National Society for Children and Adults with Autism, which he heads as the executive director. His chapter draws on his experience administering the parents' organization at a national level; at a deeper level, he draws on his knowledge as the father of a son with autism. Jim Surratt, also the father of an autistic son, takes a pragmatic approach to advocacy. Surratt's cogent analysis of working within the system should be of help to both parents and professionals. Pueschel and Bernier, on the other hand, have seen advocacy problems as professionals responsible for an agency providing services and diagnostic evaluations.

Part IV includes chapters that speak to parents functioning as trainees in their relationships with professionals. Kolko privides a useful review of the research literature on training parents, while the other three chapters in this section report from direct experience. Kozloff's training program has demonstrated the viability of parent training for nearly a decade, while Schreibman, Koegel, Mills, and Burke demonstrate how parents can be more effective trainers than professionals. Harris and Powers grapple with the limits of parents as trainees in the context of overall family needs and pressures.

The chapters in Part V pertain to the parent–professional relationship in which parents function as trainers. In his chapter, Schopler recounts a professional's experience of being trained by parents. Sullivan's chapter is based on her rich experience as trainer of clinicians, researchers, other parents, and legislators, while Cutler describes her personal experiences in the painful transition from being a parent of an autistic child to being a professional.

Part VI deals with the very important emotional reciprocity between parents and professionals. Shea delineates how professionals can turn the interpretation of the child's diagnostic evaluation into the most constructive parent experience possible. Bristol reviews factors in the family support system that can provide resources instrumental to family adaptation, and Marcus identifies factors that can lead to discouragement in helping handicapped people—for both parents and professionals. The final two chapters discuss the most frequently neglected aspect in the emotional support network—the siblings. McHale, in her chapter with Simeonsson and Sloan, reviews the limited literature and her own experiences with siblings, while Fromberg gives a moving account of his own experience with an autistic brother after the deaths of their parents.

In short, through our organization of this book, we have tried to show the various ways in which parents and professionals relate to one another and how this has evolved over the past four decades. Beginning with the Kanner era, when parents were regarded as patients requiring treatment and seen as the major cause of their children's autism, dramatic changes have occurred in the way parents are viewed and the roles they assume. At present, parents are seen by professionals as important collaborators in the treatment and education of their autistic children, and parent–professional relationships include training, advocacy, and emotional support. The remainder of this book will focus on these current roles and how they have affected current perspectives and practices in the area of autism.

REFERENCE NOTE

1. Schuler, A. L., and Bormann, C. *The interaction of communicative and cognitive development in childhood autism.* Unpublished manuscript, San Francisco State University, 1980.

REFERENCES

Alpern, G. D. Measurement of "untestable" autistic children. *Journal of Abnormal Psychology,* 1967, *72,* 478–496.

Alpern, G. D., and Kimberlin, C. C. Short intelligent test ranging from infancy levels through childhood levels for use with the retarded. *American Journal of Mental Deficiency,* 1970, *75,* 65–71.

Ando, H., and Yoshimura, I. Effects of age on communication skill levels and prevalence of maladaptive behaviors in autistic and mentally retarded children. *Journal of Autism and Developmental Disorders,* 1979, *9,* 83–94.

Axline, V. M. *Play therapy.* Houghton Mifflin, 1947.

Barry, R. J., and James, A. L. Handedness in autistics, retardates, and normals of a wide range. *Journal of Autism and Childhood Schizophrenia,* 1978, *8,* 315–323.

Bender, L. Childhood schizophrenia clinical study of one hundred schizophrenic children. *American Journal of Orthopsychiatry,* 1947, *17,* 40–56.

Bender, L., and Grugett, A. E. A study of certain epidemiological problems in a group of children with childhood schizophrenia. *American Journal of Orthopsychiatry,* 1956, *26,* 131–145.

Bettelheim, B. *The empty fortress—Infantile autism and the birth of the self.* New York: Free Press, 1967.

Brown, L., Nietupski, J., and Hamre-Nietupski, S. The criterion of ultimate functioning and public school services for severely handicapped students. In M. A. Thomas (Ed.), *Hey don't forget about me: Education's investment in the severely, profoundly and multiply handicapped.* Reston, Va.: Council for Exceptional Children, 1976.

Brown, W. T., Jenkins, E. L., Friedman, E., Brooks, J., Wisniewski, K., Raguthu, S., and French, J. H. Association of fragile-X syndrome with autism. *Lancet,* 1982, *1,* 100.

Campbell, M., Hardesty, A. S., and Burdock, E. I. Demographic and perinatal profile of 105 autistic children: A preliminary report. *Psychopharmacology Bulletin,* 1978, *14,* 36–79.

Cantwell, D. P., Baker, L., and Rutter, M. Family factors. In M. Rutter and E. Schopler (Eds.), *Autism: A reappraisal of concepts and treatment.* New York: Plenum, 1978.

Chess, S. Follow-up report on autism in congential rubella. *Journal of Autism and Childhood Schizophrenia,* 1977, *1,* 69–81.

Coleman, M. A report on the autistic syndrome. In M. Rutter and E. Schopler (Eds.), *Autism: A reappraisal of concepts and treatment.* New York: Plenum, 1978.

Creak, M. Schizophrenia syndrome in childhood: Progress report of a working party. *Cerebral Palsy Bulletin*, 1961, *3*, 501–504.

Creak, M., and Ini, S. Families of psychotic children. *Journal of Child Psychology and Psychiatry*, 1960, *1*, 156–175.

DeMyer, M. K., Barton, S., Alpern, G. D., Kimberlin, C., Allen, J., Yang, E., and Steele, R. The measured intelligence of autistic children. *Journal of Autism and Childhood Schizophrenia*, 1974, *4*, 42–60.

Eisenberg, L., and Kanner, L. Early infantile autism 1943–55. *American Journal of Orthopsychiatry*, 1956, *26*, 556–566.

Ekstein, R., and Friedman, S. The function of acting out, play action, and play acting in the psychotherapeutic process. In R. Ekstein (Ed.), *Children of time and space, of action and impulse*. New York: Appleton-Century-Crofts, 1966.

Ferster, C. B. Positive reinforcement and behavioral deficits of autistic children. *Child Development*, 1961, *32*, 437–456.

Folstein, S., and Rutter, M. A twin study of individuals with infantile autism. In M. Rutter and E. Schopler (Eds.), *Autism: A reappraisal of concepts and treatment*. New York: Plenum, 1978.

Gillberg, C., and Schaumann, H. Social class and infantile autism. *Journal of Autism and Developmental Disorders*, 1982, *12*, 223–228.

Goldfarb, W. *Childhood schizophrenia*. Cambridge, Mass.: Harvard University Press, 1961.

Greenfield, J. *A child called Noah: A family journey*. New York: Holt, Rinehart & Winston, 1972.

Hauser, S. L., DeLong, G. R., and Rosman, N. P. Pneumographic findings in the infantile autism syndrome: A corelation with temporal lobe disease. *Brain*, 1975, *98*, 667–688.

Hermelin, B., and O'Connor, N. *Psychological experiments with autistic children*. Oxford: Pergamon Press, 1970.

Kanner, L. Autistic disturbances of affective contact. *Nervous child*, 1943, *2*, 217–250.

Koegel, R. L., Rincover, A., and Egel, A. L. *Educating and understanding autistic children*. San Diego: College Hill Press, 1982.

Kolvin, I. Psychoses in childhood: A comparative study. In M. Rutter (Ed.), *Infantile autism: Concepts, characteristics, and treatment*. Edinburgh: Churchill-Livingstone, 1971. (a)

Kolvin, I. Studies in the childhood psychoses: I. Diagnostic criteria and classification. *British Journal of Psychiatry*, 1971, *118*, 381–384. (b)

Kysar, J. The two camps in child psychiatry: A report from a psychiatrist-father of an autistic and retarded child. *American Journal of Psychiatry*, 1968, *125*, 103.

Lockyer, L., and Rutter, M. A five- to fifteen-year follow-up study of infantile psychosis. IV. Patterns of cognitive ability. *British Journal of Psychiatry*, 1970, *9*, 152–163.

Lord, C., Schopler, E., and Revicki, D. Sex differences in autism. *Journal of Autism and Developmental Disorders*, 1982, *12*, 317–330.

Lotter, V. Follow-up studies. In M. Rutter and E. Schopler (Eds.), *Autism: A reappraisal of concepts and treatment*. New York: Plenum, 1978.

Makita, K. The age of onset of childhood schizophrenia. *Folia Psychiatrica et Neurologica Japonica*, 1966, *20*, 111–121.

May, J. M. *A physician looks at psychiatry*. New York: John Day, 1958.

McDermott, J. F., Harrison, D. I., Schrager, J., Lindy, J., and Killins, E. Social class and mental illness in children—The question of childhood psychosis. *American Journal of Orthopsychiatry*, 1967, *37*, 548–557.

National Society for Autistic Children. National Society for Autistic Children definition of the syndrome of autism. *Journal of Autism and Childhood Schizophrenia*, 1978, *8*, 162–167.

O'Conner, N., and Hermelin, B. Modality specific spatial coordinates. *Perception and Psychophysics*, 1975, *17*, 213–216.

Ornitz, E. M., and Ritvo, E. R. Perceptual inconstancy in early infantile autism. *Archives of General Psychiatry*, 1968, *18*, 76–98.

Park, C. C. *The siege*. Boston: Little, Brown, 1982.

Prior, M. R., Gajzago, C. C., and Knox, D. T. An epidemiological study of autistic and psychotic children in the four eastern states of Australia. *Australian and New Zealand Journal of Psychiatry*, 1976, *10*, 173–184.

Rimland, B. *Infantile autism*. New York: Appleton-Century-Crofts, 1964.

Runck, B. Basic training for parents of psychotic children. In E. Corfman (Ed.), *Families today*. Rockville, Md.: NIMH, Division of Scientific and Public Information, 1979.

Rutter, M. Autistic children: Infancy to adulthood. *Seminars in Psychiatry*, 1970, *2*, 435–450.

Rutter, M. Diagnosis and definition of childhood autism. *Journal of Autism and Childhood Schizophrenia*, 1978, *8*, 139–161.

Rutter, M., and Schopler, E. (Eds.). *Autism: A reappraisal of concepts and treatment*. New York: Plenum, 1978.

Schain, R. J., and Yannet, H. Infantile autism: An analysis of 50 cases and a consideration of certain relevant neurophysiologic concepts. *Journal of Pediatrics*, 1960, *57*, 560–567.

Schopler, E. Early infantile autism and receptor processes. *Archives of General Psychiatry*, 1965, *13*, 327–335.

Schopler, E. Parents of psychotic children as scapegoats. *Journal of Contemporary Psychotherapy*, 1971, *4*, 17–22.

Schopler, E. Discussion (NSAC definition of the syndrome of autism). *Journal of Autism and Childhood Schizophrenia*, 1978, *8*, 167–169.

Schopler, E., Andrews, C. E., and Strupp, K. Do autistic children come from upper-middle-class parents? *Journal of Autism and Developmental Disorders*, 1979, *9*, 139–151.

Schopler, E., Brehm, S. S., Kinsbourne, M., and Reichler, R. J. Effect of treatment structure on development in autistic children. *Archives of General Psychiatry*, 1971, *24*, 416–421.

Schopler, E., and Dalldorf, J. Autism: Definition, diagnosis, and management. *Hospital Practice*, 1980, *15*(6), 64–73.

Schopler, E., and Mesibov, G. B. *Autism in adolescents and adults* (Current Issues in Autism, Vol. 1). New York: Plenum, 1983.

Schopler, E., and Reichler, R. J. Parents as cotherapists in the treatment of psychotic children. *Journal of Autism and Childhood Schizophrenia*, 1971, *1*, 87–102.

Schopler, E., and Reichler, R. J. *Individualized assessment and treatment for autistic and developmentally disabled children, Vol. I: Psychoeducational profile*. Baltimore, Md.: University Park Press, 1979.

Schopler, E., Reichler, R. J., DeVellis, R. F., and Daly, K. Toward objective classification of childhood autism: Childhood Autism Rating Scale (CARS). *Journal of Autism and Developmental Disorders*, 1980, *10*, 91–103.

Tsai, L., Stewart, M. A., and August, G. Implication of sex differences in the familial transmission of infantile autism. *Journal of Autism and Developmental Disorders*, 1981, *11*, 165–173.

Tsai, L., Stewart, M. A., Faust, M., and Shook, S. Social class distribution of fathers of children enrolled in the Iowa autism program. *Journal of Autism and Developmental Disorders*, 1982, *12*, 211–221.

Vrono, M. Schizophrenia in childhood and adolescence. *International Journal of Mental Health*, 1974, *2*, 7–116.

Wakabayashi, S. A case of infantile autism associated with Down's syndrome. *Journal of Autism and Developmental Disorders*, 1979, *9*, 31–36.

Wing, L. Childhood autism and social class: A question of selection? *British Journal of Psychiatry*, 1980, *137*, 410–417.

II

Overview

Handicapped Children and Their Families

EDWARD ZIGLER

In the field of work with handicapped children, professionals have always been under great pressure. In the work with the children themselves, there is the sense of responsibility to the lives and well-being of youngsters afflicted with serious disabilities, and the call to compassion that accompanies this as well. The parents of a handicapped child are also a factor; they themselves are pressured and also have a call on the professionals, sometimes in very legitimate terms, sometimes overwhelmingly so. The fact that social policy in the United States is neither mobilized toward nor adequately committed to comprehensively dealing with the lives of children, handicapped or otherwise, makes this field an even more difficult one in which to be engaged.

Such a situation overall generates a very potent demand for answers to the problems of the handicapped and creates a special vulnerability to looking for generalized or one-track methods for resolving the particular problems of what is, after all, a complex and unique entity—the individual human being that the handicapped child, like any child, is. Certainly the constant bombardment with research results that are heralded as the latest breakthrough and the effects of social policy as regards handicapped children—and especially these two in combination—conduce to the tendency to adopt now one orientation and then another, each one hailed at first as a solution and then dropped when it is found not to be wholly satisfactory.

The historical account suggests that there has been a great deal of progress in the treatment of handicapped children. A look at the history of social programs and treatment modalities in the United States, however, also points up that too

EDWARD ZIGLER • Department of Psychology, Yale University, New Haven, Connecticut 06520.

many of these are based on unrealistic expectations and social fads with a usual life-span of about one decade. This is true in the treatment of mentally retarded, for instance. At the turn of the century, the idea in ascendancy was that, given the right training experience, retarded children would be made "normal." When it was perceived that this did not, in fact, make the retarded normal, the attempt at training was quickly abandoned, and the state training schools became human warehouses.

Some years later the importance of special training was rediscovered, and special education was promoted as the solution; by the 1960s school psychologists were claiming that special-class placement was important, regardless of the outcome, in order to prevent the adverse effects of competition with nonretarded children (Quay, 1963, p. 672). In less than another decade, however, special education became suspect on the grounds that it is inherently stigmatizing. Under the banner of normalization, "deinstitutionalization" and "mainstreaming" have become the slogans for treating developmentally disabled children.

Any massive change in social policy or treatment applied across the board is unlikely to have entirely positive effects on individual children or groups of children. It is not reasonable to expect, in the first place, that it should. Professionals in the field of child development and the treatment of the handicapped must develop the sensitivity to be on their guard against wholesale advertisements of what will work in any case or set of cases. The entire area of children's welfare in all its aspects is already an ideological battleground. What is going to become increasingly necessary is to assess ideas, theories, and movements; to distinguish what is nonsense from what can be used with genuinely fruitful results and to ascertain how these results can be brought about; and to cultivate the inner strength and the knowledgeability that will guarantee that these evaluative efforts will be an integral aspect of the commitment to working with handicapped children and their families.

THE SYSTEMS APPROACH

Those who are concerned with and work with handicapped children are working within a multifaceted, multilevel complex of situations, which involves systems within systems, some interlocking, some overlapping, some encased one within another—all interacting with and affecting the others. A great deal of ambiguity is the result, yet these complexities mean that we must not merely tolerate but recognize and actively incorporate them into our working perspective and strategy. Twenty-five years ago there were only two elements in our conception of how to approach the problems in this field—the handicapped child we were working with and the curriculum or intervention being designed for that child. Such a simple approach is no longer possible. By now many professionals must realize that in our work with handicapped children and in our conceptualization of the problems involved we must adopt a systems approach. By adopting this approach we can elicit for the children and families we are working with, and for ourselves, a coherence within the ambiguity that surrounds us.

To begin with, there are two basic systems within which the child functions. The child is part of a family, which is an important system in its own right, with its own needs and functioning, which we must try to understand, both for its impact on the child and for the child's on it. The child also attends a treatment center or a school or resides in an institution, which is another system and which has its own modes of operating.

The family as a system does not exist in isolation. The family has its own character, which sociologists have studied; it has needs and functions that both do and do not focus on the handicapped child that is one of its members, and it is itself a part of the community, in which it may or may not have supports and contacts. Nor does the treatment center function in isolation: It serves a particular population, also exists in a community, and responds to numerous demands made upon it from many and various directions.

From the start, then, the child is functioning in two quite different systems. This gives the professionals and the parents the particular task of looking at these two systems from the viewpoint of the child so that the child can be helped to obtain a sense of continuity as he or she moves from one to the other. This is a vital necessity no matter how good the family or the center is for the child. The child needs a sense of belonging within each one and a sense of continuity between them in order to function at his maximum capacity. It is the job of both parents and professionals to address this issue and mediate it for the child.

The plethora of professionals who work with a handicapped child—psychologists, social workers, occupational therapists, medical doctors—are themselves parts of different systems. They function on one level as a part of their work situation and on another as members of their own professions, each of which has its own special language, practices, and approaches.

Finally, all of these interacting systems are themselves embedded in and dependent on government and other institutions at the federal, state, and local levels. At the local level, numerous authorities and systems come into play. The intricacies of these systems and of their operations is formidable, and all of them have an impact on the child.

If everything functioned ideally and as theorists try to explain it, these systems and interactions would constitute a collection of synergistic support systems. The fact is that these various systems are not synergistic. They interact in complex ways and are often at serious odds with one another. Such discrepancies not only affect the individual lives of the children we are working with, they also affect those working with and caring for them—both the parents and the professionals. There are day-to-day problems, issues for consideration over the duration of whole lives, and questions of morale involved as well.

Related to this is the question of the moral community. It is through the social relationship that values are transmitted. The moral community in behalf of children must finally include the entire society in which we live, for it is the broader society that gives parents a message of how important children are by the decisions it makes and by how it spends its money.

The community of people who work with handicapped children is a visible community that operates from the philosophy that children are valuable, that children need help, and that adults who care enough and who are properly trained can provide that help. The way in which we professionals function in our work with children and in our dealings with the larger community in their behalf is a primary means of conveying the message that children are worth helping and that they deserve our fullest attention and concern.

If a child is valuable and is worth helping, it is the whole of a child who is worth our time, not merely the rehabilitation of the handicap. It is the entire personality of the child as well as the handicap that must be considered in the effort to help and the whole of the child's familial and social and educational environment must be addressed too. No one aspect of a child's life can reflect that child, and no one level of response on our part is sufficient.

The normalization movement in this country, as discussed below, is a case in point. Many children will benefit from a program whose thrust is normalization; others will not and, by being put into a situation that does not sufficiently suit them, may in fact suffer setbacks and further developmental delay than they may already be experiencing as a result of their handicap. Neither normalization nor, on the other hand, institutionalization—nor indeed any other particular program—can be regarded as a wholesale remedy for the needs of handicapped children. Yet the problems of the individual child and of the group we call handicapped, together with the social and economic pressures involved, encourage the tendency to hope for an answer that will cover all contingencies.

Instead, we are badly in need of a fundamental perspective that can encompass the wide range of individual variations and at the same time remain a viable and unified base from which these variations can be approached. Emanating from the research in child development of the last two decades are principles that might give us some direction and allow us to maintain our sanity in the midst of so much confusion.

These will be discussed in detail in the section on principles of child development. To put it simply, the substance and overview of the research is that children's growth is continuous and that children benefit from a consistency between the stages of their lives and the social and educational institutions in their lives, and, concomitantly, that children are themselves, as they ought to be to us, whole beings whose feelings, thoughts, concerns, and motivations are of supreme importance in their well-being and functioning as children and as adults. The optimal development of the human being must be our concern in dealing with children. Since handicapped children are particularly at risk when their needs are too narrowly interpreted, it is appropriate for us to consider these needs and our approaches to them in light of known, accepted, and basic principles of child development.

Normalization—An Oversimplified Response

A discussion of the important factors in a handicapped child's life cannot be understood without reference to the predominant ideology in the United States in the treatment of the handicapped—normalization. Normalization can be seen as the effort to bring an individual as close to the cultural norm in behavior and performance as is feasible. This concept has been widely accepted as desirable and, in the forms of "deinstitutionalization" and "mainstreaming" is the thrust of most recent programs for the handicapped.

This was not always the case. In the not-so-distant past, professionals were nearly unanimous in advising parents to institutionalize their severely handicapped children. Now professionals are essentially telling parents that if they put the child in an institution, they are not succeeding as parents. I do not believe it is the responsibility of professionals to tell parents what to do with their child. Values change. It is the responsibility of society to provide a wide range of choices for the care of handicapped children. It is the job of professionals to give information and spell out the alternatives to the parents, and it is for the parents themselves, after being informed of what is available, to decide, without professionals passing judgment on them for their decision.

Institutions will always be needed. Leaders in this field like Harvey Stevens and George Tarjan have shown how to make them habitable. At the same time, there are many children who will do well at home, depending on the family situation and the availability of services to the parents and to the child.

Public Law 94-142. With the passage of Public Law 94-142, the Education for All Handicapped Children Act of 1975, parents of school-age handicapped children may have the necessary leverage to hold the state accountable for some of the support services needed to raise a seriously handicapped child at home. The handicapped have gained legitimate access to a major public system and a potential service network where previously they had none. Perhaps the most revolutionary aspect of the legislation is its mandate for parent participation in developing an "individualized education program" for each handicapped child (Public Law 94-142, 1975). This provision, if properly implemented, is a step toward parental entitlement to be envied by many parents of normal children.

The law, however, may be inherently flawed, and the end result of its implementation may be the constriction of parental options and actual disservice to the child. In the first place, handicapped children are being placed in schools that do not have the in-service training to deliver a program that is suited to their needs. The law's admonition that handicapped children be educated to the maximum extent feasible in regular classes is easily mishandled by the failure to provide sufficient special classes or by discouraging the use of high-quality private services.

This law is demanding an enormous amount from schools and providing for very little of the cost. PL 94-142 in the end pays only 9% of the actual cost of delivering the program mandated by the law (Washington Report, 1978). Is it realistic to expect already financially pressed school systems to serve all handicapped children with this kind of money? By contrast, Head Start receives nearly 80% of its expenditure for special services from the federal government. Assuming the schools really do comply with the federal mandate, school officials may well come under financial pressure to interpret the least restrictive alternative as the least expensive one. In extreme cases it will be seen as the state's interest to simply refuse the federal contribution and ignore the mandate of the law.

Mainstreaming. The second problem with PL 94-142 is that children as a group are heterogeneous, and the variability is as great among handicapped children as among members of any other group. Given the diversity of disabilities and of personality, there are no panaceas for promoting the full development of handicapped children. Thus, we share the concern of Sarason and Doris (1978) that the schools are perceiving mainstreaming primarily in terms of nonretarded handicapped children—that is, those with learning disabilities, emotional disturbances, and physical handicaps. As a result, mentally retarded children may be neglected under this new policy. It is also of concern that the Education for All Handicapped Children Act requires all children to receive a "free appropriate public education" without specification of the criteria for determining what is "appropriate." PL 94-142 was conceived in the tradition of civil rights advocacy, with proponents rightly protesting the mislabeling and unnecessary placement of large numbers of minority children in special education classes. But while a nonretarded black child may well benefit from his removal from a special class, will the civil rights of a retarded child, or a deaf child, necessarily be advanced by placement in a large class of normal children? For some children, "mainstreaming" represents a denial of the right to be different or to have special needs met.

It is not my intent to oppose mainstreaming, but to call for some objective criteria by which to evaluate services for handicapped children. Unless the criteria are specified, the measure of evaluation is likely to become IQ tests and academic skills, rather than the optimum development of the human being.

Social competence should be the ultimate criterion for monitoring the effectiveness of mainstreaming (see Zigler and Trickett, 1978). In academic areas, mainstreamed retarded children appear to do as well as children in special classes, although there is little evidence that mainstreaming is more effective (Gruen, Ottinger, and Ollendick, 1974). But the expectation that mainstreamed retarded children would be less stigmatized than children in special classes has not been borne out (Goodman, Gottlieb, and Harrison, 1972; Gottlieb and Budoff, 1973). Clearly, more research is needed to determine which children, with which handicaps, are most likely to benefit from mainstreaming, and how best to promote their acceptance by the children's normal peers.

Help for Raising Handicapped Children at Home. Most important, whatever the outcome of the implementation of PL 94-142, educational services can only go so far in helping parents to raise their severely handicapped children at home. Social and public policy in general in the United States, however, continues to be oriented toward the institutionalization of these children. It is in a child's best interest to experience continuity between the care he or she receives from parents and that from other adult caregivers; handicapped children, like all children, are best raised by their parents, when at all possible, not by "experts." Yet many jurisdictions still provide financial incentives for parents to institutionalize severely handicapped children. For instance, those who need special and expensive schooling or medical care must frequently become wards of state before they can obtain such services (Keniston and The Carnegie Council on Children, 1977).

What sort of community support services are needed to help families with handicapped children? There is no question that homemaker services could help keep many children out of institutions. Yet the United States lags far behind other Western industrialized nations in the development of home-help services. The United Kingdom has one homemaker-health aide for every 667 persons, Denmark one for every 760, and the Netherlands one for every 380. The rate in the United States is one for every 7000 persons (Kahn and Kamerman, 1975). In this respect, our nation's social policy seems to be penny-wise and pound-foolish. The United States should also expand daytime care facilities to help relieve the burden of full-time care of severely handicapped children.

While deinstitutionalization and mainstreaming can have many positive effects on handicapped children, these policies will be empty slogans, with many unfortunate side effects, if policymakers are allowed to lose sight of sound developmental principles. Instead of following blindly along with the idea of deinstitutionalization, we must develop the kinds of family support services that make that option feasible. We need to remove the remaining financial incentives to institutionalize children. In addition, we should stop equating the Education for All Handicapped Children Act with mainstreaming—a word that does not even appear in the legislation. Instead, we should view the law as a tool to entitle handicapped children to services from which they have previously been excluded. Mainstreaming should be an option, not an excuse for denying children access to special services. Nor can deinstitutionalization and mainstreaming become excuses for forgetting the some 200,000 children who remain in state institutions. And finally, no public system, such as the schools, should be expected to absorb the full cost involved with handicapping conditions. This is a problem whose prevention and amelioration properly rests with us all.

PRINCIPLES OF CHILD DEVELOPMENT

Partnership with Parents and the Principle of Continuity

The principle of continuity is one of the most basic in child development. A child benefits when he has a sense of the continuity both between the stages of his own life and among the social institutions in his life. From this follows the centrality and importance of professionals developing and maintaining a true partnership with parents in the treatment of the handicapped child. This means a democratic partnership based on a common commitment and the trust that develops between people who recognize that they share a mutual commitment.

When we work with the parents in this way, we are creating a partnership with the most important people in a child's life. The parents are the child's first teachers, and the family is the predominant influence on the child. The strength of the parents for professionals has been underestimated. They are the most cost-effective lever there is to help in the optimization of the child's development. Any program for a handicapped child that does not have a strong parent component—that is, certain elements of the child's treatment are carried out at the treatment center and certain other elements are carried out at home—is for all practical purposes bankrupt. The principle of continuity in child development demands that the work of professionals dovetail in some positive way with the time the child spends with the parents and vice versa, or the work of each can easily be undone. There must be a clear and explicit partnership between parents and professionals in the programming for the child.

This does not mean an extracurricular type of involvement on the part of the parents. Fund-raising activities, conferences on a child's progress, parents' visiting days, and the like, are certainly positive aspects of a treatment center's outreach to parents, but such activities do not add up to that direct involvement that is so vital in the treatment and development of the handicapped child. What professionals and parents alike must do is develop concrete mechanisms for forging the kind of partnership that is needed. These mechanisms might include, for instance, retreats where they are given a chance to get to know each other, as people and as co-workers in a mutual endeavor; ongoing seminars and training sessions for the parents; parent self-help groups led by professionals.

The nature of such a partnership as that I am describing here is trust; its development takes two simple but profoundly effective elements. The first is listening. Most professionals in any area of the human services are trained to listen, and listening makes so much difference to everyone involved. But how many professionals really take the time to listen? Time, then, is the second element in the development of trust, and I believe that any professional who deals with handicapped children who cannot take the time to listen, even if he or she knows how, is in the wrong business.

To emphasize the importance of listening and the time it takes may seem paradoxical when there is already so much work to be done and so little time to accomplish it during a day. Real listening, however, is actually a very powerful tool in any treatment plan. Listening is social in nature, but it fosters at the same time a flow of information exchange between and among those involved. Parents who are given a chance can offer feedback, information, and insight about their child that can be extremely valuable to our work and likewise we can better share with the parents our expertise and observations so that the parents can cooperate more fully and more effectively than if they are simply carrying out a set of instructions. On the other side of the coin, the fact that listening *is* social in nature in itself helps to elicit the sense of personal trust in both parties that is necessary for an effective collaboration.

The fruits of such a full partnership between parents and professionals are of inestimable benefit to the child, who obtains the sense that those people who are working for him are a contiguous unit instead of merely communicating *at* each other, or even not at all—the principle of continuity again.

There is another benefit that those who have established such a partnership with parents can attest to and that those who have not yet done so may not recognize, and that is the sense of community that develops—in this case a community that, unlike the larger society around us, does value the child.

Working with handicapped children is not easy for the professionals, and it is hard indeed for the parents who so often lack the extended family and the community roots that used to be a support for families in difficult times. Many working in this field also feel very isolated and unsupported in our efforts. We all need support systems. To develop a firm sense of partnership with parents is one way in which we can counteract this isolation and support ourselves more effectively in this work.

The kind of alliance between parents and professionals described here not only is useful in the direct treatment of the child and for enhancing the effectiveness of the working process but is part of the sound base that is needed for effective advocacy in behalf of children. Building a strong community of those who are concerned for the welfare of the handicapped starts with those most immediately involved in their lives. Money is vital, more research is vital—without these we cannot function; but the force of positive interaction among those engaged in any enterprise may be one of the least appreciated tools we as human beings have.

Parent Self-Help Groups. Another aspect of the ways in which professionals can be helpful to parents concerns parent self-help groups. Parents can be of tremendous help to each other, and parent self-help groups are a big contribution in this regard. Professionals do have a contribution to make to these groups, however. One phenomenon that surfaces in self-help groups is the hostility many parents feel for professionals, not only for M.D.s, but for social workers, psychologists, and others. Some of this hostility is understandable, although it's displaced, but at the same time, in self-help groups there can be the type of partnership between parents and professionals that I am recommending. There are times when parents can learn less from each other than from a professional who is there to direct the discussion, to tell parents why they and their children are at different points in development and progress, and why their experiences differ. Professionals can be of definite use in this way in such groups and should become aware that this is so.

Parent Education. A further and broader form of the partnership between parents and professionals is parent education. Professionals in all areas of concern with the growth and development of children ought by now to be in favor of instituting parent education in the schools, for all young people before they become parents. Such programs should include components on both normal and abnormal development, since it is not possible to understand abnormal development without a clear knowledge of what the normal steps in development are. Courses in parent education are already given in many places in Europe and ought to become an integral part of the curriculum in American schools.

Early Intervention and the Principle of Continuous Development

The second principle that must underlie work with handicapped children is that of early intervention. It has been recognized for a number of years that in the case of any handicapping condition, the earlier intervention takes place, the better, and that with numerous handicaps early intervention, even during just the first few months of life, can make a difference.

However, it is also quite clear that for nearly every handicap there is nothing that can be completely accomplished in the first few months, the first year, the first two years of life. The handicapped child, like all children, is in a process of continuous development. This is one of those principles of child development that has emerged from many decades of work on the developmental process and is generally agreed upon by developmentalists. Our own observations ought to tell us this as well; life in *all* its stages is continuous. The most enduring gains and the fullest development of handicapped children will be made if intervention on their behalf is rooted not just in good intentions but in basic principles of human development, and childhood programs must be launched on the basis of these same principles. The child, including the handicapped child, moves from stage to stage. Each stage is built on the stage that precedes it. At each stage there must be the program and the environmental nutrients that are appropriate to that stage and that dovetail with the program designed for the previous stage.

Commitment to the principle that life is continuous should lead us away from seeking magic periods in a child's life during which all that can be accomplished is going to be accomplished. There is no such magic period—all of the periods of growth and development are critical and have their own requirements and possibilities. In the social policy sphere, recognition of the principle of continuity of development demands that we offer special programs for high-risk children that meet the particular needs of the child in each stage of development. Since this is expensive, it is easy to think there's one magic period to work with. Early intervention is emphasized simply because in the early stages of development there is such rapid growth. Intervention when such rapid growth is taking place is vital so that bad habits won't be learned and have to be unlearned later, and good ones can be mastered early.

When should early intervention begin? Once we start viewing the child's development in its totality, we quickly learn that it is not enough to educate children or to provide them with compensatory services. We are going to have to develop an entirely new concept of intervention—and along with that an entirely new concept of social supports for families and an entirely different school.

First of all, for early intervention *per se,* we must recognize that behavioral development is intimately linked to physical well-being. Behavioral scientists must join with health and health education workers in the prevention of handicap, because no intervention program can fully compensate for deficiencies incurred *in utero.* The prenatal period deserves much more attention. It makes more sense to do everything possible for the prenatal child than to rely on special programs and look to childhood specialists for a "cure" after the child is born with brain damage. Those first few months *in utero* are part of the business of those concerned with children. Poor prenatal care and maternal malnutrition are major factors in the incidence of prematurity, mental retardation, and other birth defects (Begab, 1974; Clarke and Clarke, 1977). Yet at least one-third of pregnant women in the United States receive no prenatal care during the first trimester of pregnancy; many have never been told of the importance of health care during this critical period.

What is needed is not just a piece of legislation to address problems of the handicapped, or a short-lived program to improve the prenatal nutrition of a selected few pregnant mothers, but a new commitment, both public and private, to improve the national climate toward child rearing. The nation needs a support system for children and families, and among its components should be improved delivery of maternal and child health care, with an emphasis on preventive medicine rather than treatment after the fact; improved parent education; and the expansion of homemaker services and child care options.

As for a new system of supports for families in an entirely different school, I envision a time when the practicality of what has been said here will become so evident that children will be enrolled in school immediately upon conception. The American school, after all, is the one institution that almost every child enters. How can we use it to the child's greatest benefit? When the child is enrolled prenatally in this system, the school serves as a support system for the child and the parents. This school will see to it that the mother has proper prenatal care, that she learns why nutrition is important, that she learns about child development. Home visitors may be used as well. The mother learns how to screen her own child periodically, and if there are any problems, the child may be brought to the school for further evaluation.

The result is that by the time the child begins school, a firm partnership has developed between the parents and the school, and there would be much less of what we see now, which is that many parents who really need the school's help are exactly the ones with the greatest animosity toward the school.

The notion of this new school is not as farfetched as it may sound. There are a few scattered around the country—one in Brookline, Massachusetts, one in Little Rock, Arkansas—that have many of these features, and there must be others we do not yet know about already in operation. These kinds of services for the support of parents and children are very much needed. People are alienated from the institutions that can serve them. Society has become enormously complex. There are now over 200 federal programs for children, but where is the information referral service that directs parents to the appropriate resources for their child? Most parents of children who have any kind of special need must spend a very great amount of time and effort, and usually money as well, going from professional to professional and from agency to agency simply to obtain information about what is available and where it can be found. A central referral service, bolstered by the utilization of trained and informed home visitors, would be a great boon to these parents and their children.

The Child as a Whole Human Being—The Continuity of the Person

The principle that the child is a whole human being ought to be the foundation stone and directing force for all our efforts in behalf of children. A child—or an adult, for that matter—is not synonymous with the handicap he or she might have. It is easy to understand that a confusion between the child and the handicap—the child is a Downs, the child is a cerebral palsy—can take hold very pervasively when one is confronted with a seriously or even a mildly handicapped or retarded child. The particular needs for instruction and intervention tend to focus attention on the treatment of the handicapping condition, often to the exclusion of the child who has the handicap. It is just at this juncture, however, that we must reinforce what is surely intuitively true to us and reassert the principle that the child is a whole human being with needs, desires, concerns, and a unique personality that also requires attention and development.

For a good number of years in the field of child development and in work with deprived, retarded, and handicapped children there has been continuing dissension between those who emphasize the importance of cognition, intelligence, and achievement and those who de-emphasize them and put the emphasis instead on the motivational and emotional factors as the major determinant of the outcome for the child.

As I have said elsewhere before (Zigler, 1971; Zigler and Harter, 1969), what must be emphasized is that cognitive development and/or intelligence does not equal social competence. Why is there such concern with intelligence anyway? Is it that accurate a predictor of how someone behaves? Workers long thought that the institutionalized retarded child's prognosis could be determined by giving him an intelligence test. The view here was a simple and appealing one. If the child had a relatively high IQ, he would be socially competent if released from the insitution; if he had a low IQ, he would not. This is a clear example of the tendency to overemphasize the importance of intelligence. Several reviews (Goldstein, 1964; Tizard, 1958; Windle, 1962; Zigler and Harter, 1969) of follow-up studies directed at assessing the adjustment of the vast majority of the retarded (IQs between approximately 50 and 75) have generated the conclusion that there seems to be little relationship between intelligence and the ability to function successfully in our society. Even in children of normal intellect, the relation between intelligence and a variety of social competence indices is not terribly striking.

The point being made here is that full development involves much more than the cognitive system. Personality factors—the development of positive attitudes and motives—are as important as the development of the intellect or of particular accomplishments (see, e.g., Penrose, 1963; Sarason, 1953). The failure to appreciate how much a child's values, motives, and psychological orientation affect his social competence has led to a misunderstanding of what optimal child development is composed of. This misunderstanding in turn has led to our interacting with the child in an erroneous fashion. In this day of computers and the emphasis in psychology on cognition and intelligence testing, it's rare to find people who see a child as something more than a little computer that must be programmed.

In the case of retarded children in particular, for instance, the overly cognitive approach to their behavior is in part the result of the relative absence of a sound and extensive body of empirical work dealing with personality factors. The dearth of such work has invariably been noted by scholars faced with the task of reviewing those efforts that do deal with the personality functioning of the retarded (Gardner, 1969; Heber, 1964). Had such a body of work developed over the years, it would have unquestionably played an important moderating role in the overly cognitive approach.

Professionals who work with children need to learn that what's on the child's mind is as important as what's in it. There is invariably a personality constructed over the handicap, and it is this personality, this character structure, this motivational structure that really determines the prognosis and final outcome. The heterogeneity of outcome in any given condition is striking. Why do some children do well and other children, with exactly the same diagnosis and perhaps the same IQ, do so poorly? A good worker in this field will, of course, be concerned with what a child is capable of doing cognitively and rhetorically, but will be just as concerned with the appropriateness or inappropriateness of affect and the presence or lack of enthusiasm. If a child is in the process of withdrawing, what happens when that child gets older? It's much more important at that time to see that that child does not withdraw but stays in this world and engaged with it than it is to teach one more skill right then.

It is by now common knowledge that the early years are important for the intellectual development of the child. This is equally true in regard to the child's emotional and social development. The child has a strong and natural need for positive interaction with adults, and the real magic in human development resides in the quality of the social interactions between the child and his or her adult caretakers. If we appreciate the child's emotional needs and attempt to satisfy them, instead of focusing entirely on the task to be accomplished, the child 9 times out of 10 goes on to a better performance.

What is at stake here is an extremely important developmental dimension, namely, the child's normal move from dependence to independence. It would appear that such movement is impaired in children who do not receive a sufficient amount of positive interaction with adults and of their affection and attention. Such children, when faced with tasks to perform, are not motivated by the problems confronting them. Rather, they employ their interaction with adults to satisfy their hunger for attention, affection, and love (Zigler, 1971). As a result, it is difficult for these children to leave off dependency and become autonomous and independent to the full extent of their capabilities. Without such feelings of independence and of self-respect, as well as positive attitudes toward interactions with others, the child does not become a very good task-oriented person and becomes immune as well to many of the satisfactions of life that concern relations with others. Given this relationship between feelings of autonomy and problem solving, and between early experiences of interactions with adults and later social competence, it is important for people who work with handicapped children to see that the child develops feelings of autonomy and a healthy view of himself.

In the learning situation itself, we must view things from within the child's framework. I take exception to the prevailing view of the learning process which holds that the child's mind is like a computer and if the environment and the teaching methods are programmed in a certain way, learning can be forced into the child. Workers in this field need to understand and trust the nature of the child and his development.

A mystique has developed around the question "How do we make the child learn?" In my opinion, learning is the natural condition of the child, and that question should never have been raised at all. The child is a much more autonomous learner than adherents of a forced-programming approach would have us believe. Learning is an inherent feature of being a human being, and the child probably accomplishes some of the most significant learning in his everyday interaction with his environment. Learning for the child is thus a continuous process and not one limited to the formal instruction and intensely programmed remedial efforts that have recently captured our attention.

What are the alternatives? I am convinced that the child does most of his learning on his own and that often the way to maximize it is simply to leave the child alone. This does not mean abandoning him in a room full of toys or special equipment, because what is going to determine the growth of that child's personality is not play with inanimate objects but the nature and quality of his relationship with the important adults in his life. What it does mean is a sensitivity to and respect for the child's natural desire to explore and interact with his environment and for the child's needs and moods on any particular day. There are times when the child does need someone there and to be with him, and there are times when we need to back off because he is learning and growing when we are doing nothing at all—the child needs the opportunity for both. This approach requires restraint and patience, and it is not an easy one. Such sensitivity is an expertise in itself, however, and well worth cultivating, because when it does function properly the results are often quite amazing.

The meaningful question we can ask with regard to learning in children is why it is that some children do not learn. Approached in this way, the problem is not one of how you go about getting learning into nonlearners but rather one of determining the conditions that interfere with the natural process of learning and then removing them. This is a far cry from approaching the child with a view in which learning is an alien enterprise that must be forced upon an unwilling and recalcitrant organism. It is an approach, moreover, that requires a recognition of far more than the cognitive or performance deficits that a child may bring to the learning situation.

IMPLEMENTATION OF SOCIAL POLICY

The role of social policy and governmental commitment is a related issue. Dedicated people and organizations in the field of child development have been working for decades to improve the lives of children and families in America.

The struggle continues. The temper of our times—faltering economy, tense political and social conditions, and taxpayer resistance to the growing costs of government programs—means that we must intensify our efforts.

Public education to give the citizenry a sense of the problem, the development of a broad-based lobby or of coalitions working to support the formulation of policy, and the identification of leverage points in Congress and the executive branch where the pressure of that lobby can be brought to bear are the preconditions that are essential if we are to stimulate national political action in behalf of children. These are necessary, although by no means sufficient, elements in the policy process. National policy will never become responsive to children until adults learn to be more effective politically in their behalf. Our failure in past decades to improve the lives of children and families is not because we have not tried. We have failed because we have not acknowledged the importance of social and political structure within which we must operate.

A Sense of the Problem in the Public Mind

The average citizen is not aware that there is anything wrong with the status of children in America, and no society can attempt to correct a problem until there is a shared sense that a real problem exists to be solved. We are operating within a society that cherishes the myth that it is child-oriented and that everything that needs to be done for children is already being done. This myth is the single greatest impediment to our work in changing national policy with regard to children. Most Americans sincerely feel that our nation does care about children and never seriously question whether our social institutions and policy perform adequately in fulfilling children's needs. Very often they are not even receptive to hearing the facts.

One reason for this lack of awareness is the fact that families today function in isolation due to the major social, economic, and demographic changes that have split families off from their communities, their neighbors, and their own kin. These changes have resulted not only in serious psychological and emotional problems among people of all socioeconomic levels but also in general lack of concern and compassion for others.

A second problem has been our pattern as professionals and scholars. We place our data in the public pool of knowledge and trust that its implications will be recognized and put to work in practical settings. Our work and concern tend to remain within the professional sphere: We speak at professional conferences and make presentations to each other; we write articles on children and families in professional journals. Professionals need to expand their boundaries. For instance, no top national newspaper or television network covers social services on a regular basis (Lynn, 1980). What is worse, there are indications that journalists interested in covering these issues are discouraged from doing so (Lynn, 1980). We must learn to elicit regular media coverage of these issues. We should also launch our own public education efforts and attempt to disseminate research findings beyond the professional literature so that the immediacy of the problem becomes evident to both policymakers and the general public.

Broad-Based Lobby

The second requirement for the effort to politicize children's issues is the development of a broad-based lobby. This would provide a structure within which we could become involved in the policy process. Children do not vote and cannot be advocates for themselves, so they need representation. There are different options that may be taken in the creation of public policy or in the undertaking to change policy. The impetus may come from legislators, community organizers, social services professionals, or social scientists. Indeed, when policy is formulated or change does occur, it is usually the result of an interaction among a variety of such groups (see Lasswell, 1971). Impetus may also come in the form of citizen-advocacy groups engaged in lobbying tactics to bring about the involvement of different people for the purpose of policy change. Representation of children on a national scale would facilitate the interaction of key people working to develop social policy for handicapped children and their families, or the monitoring of the effects of other policies on child and family life. It would also provide a forum for scholars to pool their collective knowledge of child development for the benefit of policy-makers. In the decision-making process for the area of child and family policy there has been a serious imbalance in the representation of children by experts in this area in favor of individuals or groups opposing such policy.

Leverage Points in Government

As a third requirement for national action in behalf of children, we must have leverage points in government. In order to be successful, our lobbying efforts must be targeted and calculated to exert pressure at the right moments on key leverage points of the political system.

We must also identify appropriate congressional committees and subcommittees and attempt to advocate for children's issues through these. How many workers in this field know which committee in the House and which committee in the Senate handles the money for handicapped children? Those are the pressure points to contact. Advocates for children often overlook the work and power of these committees. However, the most important phase of the congressional process is the action taken by committees (Ebert-Flattau, 1980). The committee is the place where bills are given most intensive consideration and where people outside the Congress are given the opportunity to be heard. Assigning a bill to the appropriate committee determines the ultimate future of the bill (Ebert-Flattau, 1980), but this is difficult to achieve because there are often several committees seeking jurisdiction over a bill.

It is also crucial to identify key leverage points within the executive branch. The Administration for Children, Youth and Families, which succeeded the Office of Child Development, has dropped in stature in recent years, a factor directly affecting its power and its ability to get things done. We must work toward upgrading the agency and seeking closer ties to the president. With competition among differing groups for every dollar of the federal budget, not having a direct contact with the president means that children's issues suffer.

It is important to realize that what we are dealing with are political decisions. They are not etched in concrete and can be turned around, once our political muscle is greater than the political muscle of the people who are opposing us or suggesting some other alternative. It is difficult, but much can happen. Professionals and parents don't do enough just by forming a partnership with each other; they must take that partnership and use it as a lever to make the society move in directions they wish to see it move. Rather than continue to advocate in behalf of children from a defensive and minority standpoint, we should develop strategies to support our efforts and use our cumulative knowledge in child development as a powerful tool to bring about positive changes for this nation's children. A reexamination of our commitment to doing what is in the best interest of every child in America is the first step.

REFERENCES

Begab, M. The major dilemma of mental retardation: Shall we prevent it? (Some social implications in mental retardation). *American Journal of Mental Deficiency*, 1974, *78*, 519–529.

Clarke, A. D. B., and Clarke, A. M. Prospects for prevention and amelioration of mental retardation: A guest editorial. *American Journal of Mental Deficiency*, 1977, *81*, 523–533.

Ebert-Flattau, P. *A legislative guide*. Washington, D.C.: Association for the Advancement of Psychology, 1980.

Gardner, W. I. Personality characteristics of the mentally retarded: Review and critique. In H. J. Prehm, L. A. Hamerlynch, and J. E. Crosson (Eds.), *Behavioral research in mental retardation, Rehabilitation Research and Training Center in Mental Retardation* (No. 1). Eugene, Ore.: University of Oregon Press, 1968.

Goldstein, H. Social and occupation adjustment. In H. A. Stevens and R. Heber (Eds.), *Mental retardation: A review of research*. Chicago: University of Chicago Press, 1964.

Goodman, H., Gottlieb, J., and Harrison, R. H. Social acceptance of EMRs integrated into a nongraded elementary school. *American Journal of Mental Deficiency*, 1972, *76*, 412–417.

Gottlieb, J., and Budoff, M. Social acceptability of retarded children in nongraded schools differing in architecture. *American Journal of Mental Deficiency*, 1973, *78*, 15–19.

Gruen, G., Ottinger, D., and Ollendick, T. Probability learning in retarded children with differing histories of success and failure in school. *American Journal of Mental Deficiency,* 1974, *79,* 417–423.

Heber, R. F. Personality. In H. A. Stevens and R. Heber (Eds.), *Mental retardation: A review of research.* Chicago: University of Chicago Press, 1964. Pp. 143–174.

Kahn, A. J., and Kamerman, S. B. *Not for the poor alone: European social services.* Philadelphia: Temple University Press, 1975.

Keniston, K., and Carnegie Council on Children, The, *The American family under pressure.* New York: Harcourt Brace Jovanovich, 1977.

Lasswell, H. D. *A preview of the policy sciences.* New York: American Elsevier, 1971.

Lynn, J. Filed and forgotten: Why the press has taken up new issues. *Washington Journalism Review,* 1980, *2*(4), 32–37.

Penrose, L. S. *The biology of mental defect.* London: Sidgwick & Jackson, 1963.

Public Law 94–142, Education for all Handicapped Children Act, November 29, 1975.

Quay, L. C. Academic skills. In N. R. Ellis (Ed.), *Handbook of mental deficiency.* New York: McGraw-Hill, 1963.

Sarason, S. B. *Psychological problems in mental deficiency.* New York: Harper, 1953.

Sarason, S., & Doris, J. Mainstreaming: Dilemmas, opposition, opportunities. In M. C. Reynold (Ed.), *Futures of education for exceptional students: Emerging structures.* Minneapolis: National Support Systems Project, University of Minnesota, 1978.

Tizard, J. Longitudinal and follow-up studies. In A. M. Clarke and A. D. Clarke (Eds.), *Mental deficiency: The changing outlook.* New York: Free Press, 1958.

Washington report: School systems bitterly complain about education act problems. *Arise,* 1978, *1*(6), 4.

Windle, C. Prognosis of mental subnormals. *American Journal of Mental Deficiency,* 1962, *66*(Monogr. Suppl. 5).

Zigler, E. The retarded child as a whole person. In H. E. Adams and W. K. Boardman, III (Eds.), *Advances in experimental clinical psychology* (Vol. 1). New York: Pergamon Press, 1971.

Zigler, E., and Harter, S. Socialization of the mentally retarded. In D. A. Godlin and D. C. Glass (Eds.), *Handbook of socialization theory and research.* New York: Rand McNally, 1969.

Zigler, E., and Trickett, P. K. IQ, social competence, and evaluation of early childhood intervention programs. *American Psychologist,* 1978, *33*(9), 789–798.

Research Concerning Families of Children with Autism

DENNIS P. CANTWELL and LORIAN BAKER

INTRODUCTION

This chapter presents a selective review of the research on families of autistic individuals from infancy through adolescence.* To understand the significance of research dealing with the families of autistic children, one must understand certain basic facts about the role and structure of the family. It is known that the family serves a number of child development functions (including providing the child with emotional bonds, a secure base, life experinces, a network of communication, models of behavior and attitudes, and shaping of behavior through discipline and structure). It is also known that the success with which a family meets these functions is dependent upon a number of factors (including marital harmony, parental stability, patterns of childrearing, and family communication patterns). It is important to realize, however, that because of the complex structure of the family, it is unlikely that there can be any simple relationship between any one particular family factor and the subsequent behavior and development of a child. This is because the family is essentially a variety or network of relationships, which themselves are not unidirectional, which are changing over time, which are themselves influenced by outside factors, and which are, to some extent, self-regulating (Hinde, 1981).

The fact that the structure of the family is influenced by so many factors has

---

*A brief version of this chapter was presented at the TEACCH Conference, Chapel Hill, North Carolina, May 21, 1982.

DENNIS P. CANTWELL and LORIAN BAKER • UCLA Neuropsychiatric Institute, Los Angeles, California 90024 important implications for research. Transactional effects must be considered when examining the role of family factors on child development. It cannot be assumed that because a variable produces no discernible effect in the context of one variable it will not produce an effect in association with another variable. Nor can it be assumed that a given variable will not produce an effect at one developmental period if it does not produce an effect at an earlier or later period. Influences that are potentially significant may have varying degrees of effects, depending upon (1) whether or not they are associated with other factors at particular times, (2) whether individuals select actively from those influences they encounter or have "thresholds" for experiences, and (3) whether the influences are short-term or long-lasting.

The literature on family studies with autistic individuals is divided into four main areas: (1) the family as an "environmental" etiologic agent, (2) family and genetic aspects of autism, (3) the impact of the autistic individual on the family, and (4) the role of the family on the development of the child and the outcome of autism. The conclusions and practical significance of the research will be summarized for each of these areas.

RESEARCH ON THE FAMILY AS AN "ENVIRONMENTAL" ETIOLOGIC AGENT

By far the major thrust of family research relating to autism has been the investigation of the possible etiological effect of various family factors. A review of the literature from 1960 to the present time shows that over 150 papers address this topic. Three aspects of the family have been examined as possible etiological agents: (a) the occurrence of severe stress or trauma early in the life of the child, (b) the presence of parental psychiatric disorder or deviant personality characteristics, (c) the presence of deviant parent–child communication or interaction patterns. We have reviewed this literature in detail elsewhere (Cantwell, Baker, and Rutter, 1978) and will only briefly outline it here.

"Severe early stress" was frequently postulated as an etiological agent for infantile autism in the 1950s and early 1960s. Growing out of psychoanalytic theory, this school of thought proposed that separation from the parents (either physical or emotional) during the "critical periods" of ego formation resulted in the development of autism. Later variants of this hypothesis considered the possible role of miscellaneous traumas in the life of the child (such as the birth of a sibling, physical illness, parental divorce, family discord, death in the family, and psychosocial stress such as financial or housing problems). While the earliest literature provided some "support" for these hypotheses, the evidence was of a weak nature, consisting usually of retrospective reports of a highly biased nature. Later studies addressing themselves to this topic (DeMyer, Pontius, Norton, Barton, Allen, and Steele, 1972; Cox, Rutter, Neuman, and Bartak, 1975; Folstein and Rutter, 1978; Rutter, 1977) have, however, been quite consistent in finding that early stress cannot explain the development of infantile autism. In recent years, this hypothesis has not been considered seriously in any of the literature.

"Deviant personality" in the parents of autistic children was first mentioned by Kanner in 1943. Since then, various authors have postulated such aspects of personality as coldness, undemonstrativeness, introversion, obsessions, lack of empathy, overprotectiveness, and outright mental illness as possible etiological factors in the development of autism. Of the studies implicating parental pathology with childhood autism or psychosis (Alanen, 1960; Block, 1969; Eisenberg and Kanner, 1956; Goldfarb, Goldfarb, and Scholl, 1966; Goldfarb, Levy, and Meyers, 1966; Kanner, 1943; Kaufman, Frank, Heims, Herrick, and Willerm 1959; Klebanoff, 1959; Ogdon, Bass, Thomas, and Loroi, 1968; Rice, Kebecs, and Yahalom, 1966; Williams and Harper, 1973), the majority were written prior to 1970. Conversely, of the studies concluding that parental pathology does not play a role in the etiology of infantile autism (Allen, DeMyer, Norton, Pontius, and Yang, 1971; Block, 1969; Cantwell, Baker, and Rutter, 1977, 1978; Cox *et al.*, 1975; Creak and Ini, 1960; DeMyer, Alpern, Barton, DeMyer, Churchill, Hingtgen, Bryson, Pontius, and Kimberlin, 1972; DeMyer, Hingtgen, and Jackson, 1981; Kolvin, Ounsted, Richardson, and Garside, 1971; McAdoo and DeMyer, 1978; Netley, Lockyer, and Greenbaum, 1975; Rutter, Bartak, and Newman, 1971; Wolff and Morris, 1971), the majority were written after 1970. We feel that the literature does not support the hypothesis that parents of autistic children are excessively cold, introverted, undemonstrative, or mentally disordered. When the studies are closely examined, it can be seen that all of them with positive findings suffer from many methodological weaknesses.

"Deviant parent–child communication or interaction patterns" is the third aspect of family life that has been postulated as a factor in the development of infantile autism. The postulated "defects" in family interaction include aspects of general family functioning (such as lack of (1) adequate stimulation for the child, (2) clearly established family roles, (3) shared family pleasures, and (4) reinforcements for the child) as well as aspects of family communication in particular (such as "double bind," "parental perplexity" or ambiguity, lack of responses to the child's verbalizations, inadequate amount of communication, syntactic or semantic deficits, or overt "thought disorder"). The "deviant family interaction" hypothesis has received more recent attention than the other two etiological hypotheses, with papers both supporting (Fraknoi and Ruttenberg, 1971; Frank, Allen, Stein, and Myers, 1976; Massie, 1975; Ruttenberg, 1971; Tinberger and Tinberger, 1972) and refuting (Cantwell *et al.*, 1977, 1978, 1979; DeMyer, Pontius, Norton, Barton, Allen, and Steele, 1972; Lennox, Callias, and Rutter, 1977; Netley *et al.*, 1975; Wild, Shapiro, and Abelin, 1977; Zeven, 1973) the hypothesis.

Much of the research on parental communication/family interaction has suffered from methodological flaws, however. Each technique for assessing family functioning suffers from its own inadequcies: The examination of case records suffers from incompleteness and an uneven quality of information across patients and across time; parental interviews suffer from distortions and omissions, both unconscious and willful; observations and ratings of interactions suffer from observer bias (since the observer cannot be "blind" to the diagnosis of the child) and sensitivity to external variables such as the setting chosen for observation or the length of observation; data obtained by testing procedures is affected by the skill of the person administering and scoring the tests, by the standardization procedures of the tests, and by confounding by outside factors. The most common such flaws are inadequately obtained or analyzed language samples.

We have conducted a series of studies (Cantwell et al., 1978, 1979) on the family interaction patterns of "autistic families" that compared parents of children with autism to parents of children with developmental receptive dysphasia. None of the children in our studies suffered from complicating factors such as intellectual retardation, neurological impairment, or hearing loss, and the methodology employed in our studies included a variety of techniques: parental interviews, rating scales, direct observations, as well as blind ratings of taped language samples taken from lengthy parent–child interactions in the home. Separate analyses examined for possible social class, age, and language level effects.

Our studies revealed no significant differences between the parents of dysphasic children and the parents of autistic children in any of the following measures: (1) functional use of language, including amount of questions, answers, imitations, mitigated echoes, reductions, expansions, reinforcement, prompts, directions, statements or critical remarks, amount of language used; (2) complexity of language as revealed in mean sentence length, mean preverb length, and number of phrases; (3) grammaticality as measured by number of ungrammatical utterances, and corrections of the child's grammar; (4) amount of utterances made in flat or negative tones of voice; (5) disparity between tone of voice used and semantic content of utterances; (6) "clarity" of utterances; (7) amount of time spent in activities with the child, basic care of the child, outings with the child, and other activities; (8) intensivity of interaction between parent and child.

Practical Significance of Etiological Effect Research

Stress has not been found to be more frequent in the lives of autistic children than in the lives of any other handicapped children. Parents, when expressing concern over some early trauma that their autistic child may have suffered, should be told that such stresses do make life difficult, but that they do not cause autism.

The most recent research on parental personality has been quite consistent in providing no support for the early stereotype of the cold, unfriendly, "refrigerator" parent. Nonetheless, the popular media still maintain the myth of the cold parent to a certain degree. Articles in women's magazines emphasize the tremendous importance of maternal warmth in preventing major developmental disorders; popular novels mention in passing that lack of maternal love is said to cause autism; recent books and television programs have presented inspiring stories of how "good" parents are able to cure their children of autism by love and patience (Kaufman, 1981).

Parents of handicapped children suffer many difficulties that parents of normal children do not have to experience. It is sad that this parental burden has been increased by the media suggestions that they are somehow responsible for having caused, or having failed to cure, their child's condition due to inadequate love and commitment.

Professionals working with parents must emphasize the blamelessness of the parents for the child's condition. We feel that professionals who are familiar with the lack of research evidence for cold, unloving parents of autistic children should speak out against the media presentations that show this hypothesis as having some validity.

While we do not feel that familial communication factors are significant to the genesis of autism, we do acknowledge that such family factors may play a role in the course of autism after it has developed. We also believe that the research has not ruled out the possibility of some type of communication deficit existing in some parents of autistic children, and signaling a potential genetic (rather than an environmental etiological) factor.

We believe that more research on family interaction and communication patterns could provide invaluable information on the classification of various childhood psychoses, the course and prognosis of psychotic children based on family characteristics, the selection of treatment interventions for psychotic children, and the differentiation of genetic environmental factors in etiology of the childhood psychoses.

Practitioners dealing with parents of autistic children need first to make clear to the parents that deviant parental communications are a highly unlikely cause of the development of autism. Nonetheless, since the exact role of family communications is unclear, particularly as they affect the course of the disorder, parents must be encouraged to achieve the best possible communications with their children. We also feel that it is important that parents be encouraged to take part in research dealing with the more subtle and long-term effects of family interactions.

RESEARCH ON FAMILY-GENETIC FACTORS IN AUTISM

Although a variety of methods are possible for the investigation of genetic factors (including family studies, adoption studies, twin studies, high-risk longitudinal studies, and linkage studies), few of these methods have been employed to investigate the role of genetic factors in the development of infantile autism. Essentially all that exists in the literature at the present time are a few family studies and twin studies. Hanson and Gottesman (1976) have reviewed the literature and have found that the family studies do suggest an increased prevalence rate for autism among the close family relatives of autistic children, but a rate considerably lower than would be predicted on a strict genetic model.

Further evidence for a genetic role in autism is found in a Japanese study of over 600 children with childhood autism (Honjo and Wakabayashi, 1981). The researchers found that in this study, the incidence of autistic twins was 1.65%, more than 3.5 times higher than the rate of autism in the general population.

The twin study of Folstein and Rutter (1978) provides further strong evidence for genetic factors operating in the syndrome of autism. These researchers studied 21 same-sex twin pairs involving an autistic child aged 5 through 23 years. They found that, of 10 dizygotic twin pairs, none were concordant for autism, but of 11 monozygotic twin pairs, 4 were concordant for autism. Furthermore, concordance was found for other cognitive disabilities in 9 of the 11 monozygotic twin pairs and 1 of the dizygotic twin pairs. Analyses showed that biological hazards did not account for the presence of this cognitive concordance. Folstein and Rutter concluded that the size of the monozygotic–dizygotic difference coupled with the population frequency of autism indicated that the hereditary influences were not simply limited to autism *per se* but were concerned with a wide variety of cognitive abnormalities that usually involved disorders of spoken language.

A study by August, Stewart, and Tsai (1981) also suggests a family-genetic relationship between autism and other cognitive disabilities. Individual components of cognitive disability were assessed in siblings of 41 autistic probands and were compared with similar measures from a control group made up of siblings of probands who had Down's syndrome. The results indicated that there was a significant familial clustering of cognitive disabilities in the siblings of the autistic probands. These included disturbances in language, both expressive and receptive, specific learning disability, and varying degrees of mental retardation.

Recently, Ritvo and his colleagues at the UCLA Neuropsychiatric Institute (Ritvo and Ritvo, 1981) have begun a study of multiple-incidence families. They are exploring two nonmutually exclusive hypotheses: first, that there is a subgroup of autistic families in which specific genetic mechanisms are operative, and second, that there is a subgroup of families in which defects in immunogenetic defense systems make children more vulnerable to insults to the central nervous system. Ritvo and his colleagues are searching for autistic persons who have any relative with any type of mental, neurological, or developmental disability or serious medical condition. Between January 1980 and April 1981, 260 families were found, including 25 families with monzygotic twins (in which both twins were diagnosed as autistic) and 22 families with dizygotic twins (consisting of 13 autistic plus normal pairs, 7 autistic plus developmentally disordered pairs, and 2 pairs in which both twins were autistic). Other families found included 47 families with autistic siblings, 77 families with siblings who had developmental disorders, 79 families in which second-degree relatives had developmental disorders including 26 with autism, and 10 families in which a parent had a developmental disorder. Although these data are preliminary, they are quite exciting. There is an unexpectedly large number of families with multiple incidence of autism that have been identified to date. These families could represent a subtype of autism that deserves further clinical and biomedical research.

Practical Importance of Family-Genetic Research

While research in this area is of undoubted theoretical significance, it must be said that the research is at too early a stage of development to have much practical significance. However, genetic research in other developmentally disabled populations has proved to have high practical significance. For example, genetic counseling with certain families can offer exact estimates of the likelihood of having children with certain types of problems. High-risk families can be counseled on the likelihood of having a child with certain particular types of problems, such as Down's syndrome or PKU. In the "softer" psychiatric areas, such as genetics of affective disorders in schizophrenia in which there are undoubted genetic components, genetic counseling has yet to find its proper role. However, the findings to date from the multiple-index families do suggest genetic factors operating in one subgroup or possibly more than one subgroup of autistic individuals. They also suggest that the genetic diathesis is for more than just autism alone but rather for a broader spectrum of cognitive and linguistic disabilities. Further research may lead to information that will have practical significance in terms of genetic counseling.

THE IMPACT OF THE AUTISTIC CHILD ON THE FAMILY

Recently, in a review of research related to autism, McAdoo and DeMyer (1978) stated that they believed that the most productive approach to research in the area of family factors in autism would be to focus on the autistic individual as a source of chronic stress on the family. Despite the fact that there is a fairly large body of literature dealing with the situations of families of handicapped children in general, systematic research on the effects of autism on the family is still just beginning (Bristol, Chapter 17, this volume).

DeMyer (1979) has written an interesting compendium of her clinical experiences in which she details the major events occurring in the lives of autistic children and describes the reactions of the families to each of these events. DeMyer found that families are intensely affected by the multiple failures of their autistic children, and that these failures affect each parent as an individual, the marital relationship, the parent–child relationship, and the other children in the family. DeMyer found that mothers were most severely affected by the autistic child's problems, with approximately one-third of the mothers having major depressive symptoms. Problems associated with the rearing of the autistic child weakened the affectional bond between parents in more than half of the families DeMyer saw, and prominent thoughts about divorce were expressed by more than one-quarter of the parents. Other children in the family were also affected by the autistic child, and approximately one-third of the siblings expressed feelings of neglect because so much time was given to the autistic child. DeMyer found that the family difficulties did not diminish as the autistic child grew older; rather, the parents of autistic adolescents reported numerous problems dealing with psychosexual development, puberty, the reactions of others to the adolescent, and the locating of appropriate educational facilities and professional services. The parents also frequently expressed fears that they were going to be perpetual caretakers, as well as worries about whether they had adequate finances and psychological resources to resist institutionalization of the child.

Holroyd, Brown, Wikler, and Simmons (1975) attempted to isolate some of the factors influencing levels of stress in families of autistic children. They evaluated 29 families, rating each family with a ''stress level'' score derived from a 285-item questionnaire and a personal interview. Comparisons of families with and without institutionalized autistic children revealed no significant differences in stress levels. Among the families with noninstitutionalized autistic children, however, there was a correlation between stress levels and the age of the autistic child, with more stress being present in families with older autistic children.

Bristol (1979, and Chapter 17) examined factors affecting stress in mothers of autistic children. Forty mothers of 4- to 19-year-old autistic children were interviewed in their homes using Holroyd's questionnaire on resources and stress, Bronfenbrenner's sources-for-help checklist, and a schedule of recent experiences. Bristol, like Holroyd, found that older autistic children were associated with higher levels of stress in mothers, and that this association held even when outside events, life changes, maternal age, and degree of child's dependency were controlled for.

Marcus (1977) reported that clinical experience with parents of autistic children indicated that parents were markedly affected by the children's disabilities, with constant fear, worry, anxiety, and apprehension being typical. The main areas where parents expressed serious concern were the children's linguistic handicaps, the children's behavioral abnormalities, and the problems of relating to others, particularly professionals. The parents typically responded with bafflement, confusion, and fear to the children's anomalous perceptual and auditory handicaps. The autistic children's lack of human relatedness presented great difficulties to the parents in loving and relating to a child who essentially gave them nothing in return. Interestingly, Marcus found that more parents considered professionals to be more harmful than helpful, and that they resented the relentless questions they found themselves being asked. All of the parents Marcus saw expressed fears that their situation would get worse as their autistic child grew older, bigger, and more difficult to manage. Marcus concluded that the parents of autistic children are confused, distressed, and worried, and that there is an urgent need for research examining factors that might contribute to more effective coping: internal supports, access to social activities, attitudes of acceptance, and development of appropriate expectations.

O'Moore (1978), in an Irish study, interviewed the mothers of 25 autistic children, aged 3 through 14 and living at home, with the goal of elucidating problem areas. Topics systematically covered in the interview included daily activities with the autistic child (feeding, dressing, toileting, play, discipline), special family events (shopping, trips, holidays), and aspects of overall family life (behavior of siblings, health of family members, social contacts). In contrast to some previous reports, O'Moore found that the majority of the siblings of autistic children appeared to be well adjusted, although it was pointed out that the siblings were not externally evaluated. As has been found in other studies, O'Moore found that the majority of the mothers suffered from depression, for which few sought medical help. As DeMyer also detailed, there were numerous difficulties imposed by the characteristics of the autistic child upon daily management and other aspects of family behavior.

Culbertson (1977) interviewed 10 families of autistic individuals aged 8 to 25 years regarding the helpfulness of professionals to the family. Culbertson found that the diagnostic history of most autistic children was a tedious and depressing one, with between 6 and 15 professional contacts being made before a final diagnosis was reached. Consultations included psyhologists, neurologists, psychiatrists, orthopedists, speech and language specialists, pediatricians, social workers, mental health clinics, and institutions. The establishment of treatment plans for the autistic children was similarly disappointing: Seventy percent of the parents reported that at the time the child received a definite diagnosis of autism, the professional recommendation was for the parents to engage in therapy. Many parents reported being in therapy for up to 7 years, during which time no other treatment was recommended by professionals, and parental attempts to discuss specific treatment for the children were ignored. The parents in Culbertson's study rated the most effective professional actions as defining the child rather than the parent as the problem, providing educational and behavioral programming, and giving a definitive diagnosis of the child's condition. The parents cited various ineffective professional actions, including inattentive listening, parent-as-problem model of treatment, nondirective therapeutic approach, recommendations to institutionalize the child, and withholding of information.

Leighton (1969) reported on impressions from "the other side" of the professional table. She noted that working with parents of autistic children is an especially difficult task because of the multiple problems that must be addressed. These include issues of parental expectations for the child, parental guilt and/or allocation of blame, appropriate placement for the child, practical help for the family, and reducing emotional pressures placed on the family. Leighton concluded that the two most difficult problems for parents of autistic children are the wide intellectual gap that exists between the child and the parents, and the vulnerability of the parents to the lack of empathy and approval from community members.

Several studies of siblings of autistic children are in progress, and one is reported in Chapter 14 by Sullivan. Sullivan (1979) compiled a collection of reports by five siblings of autistic children and found that all the siblings learned early in their lives about stress and pressure and that they tended to mature early, often taking on the role of the elder sibling, even if their chronological age was younger than the autistic child's. Two different responses to this pressure were found in the siblings: Some siblings identified with parental attitudes of sacrifice for the autistic child (these siblings often became members of helping professions as adults); other siblings preferred a life-style of self-expression, often ignoring the autistic child and the rest of the family at the expense of personal guilt and family resentment.

Berger (1980) examined self-concepts of siblings of autistic children. Twenty siblings of autistic children scored significantly higher on the Piers-Harris Scale than did the general population. Interview data also supported the hypothesis that these children had positive self-concepts. Berger concluded that professionals should consider including siblings in therapy programs with families in order to emphasize the strengths of the family instead of focusing solely on the family's weaknesses.

Practical Significance of Research on the Impact of the Autistic Child on the Family

Some issues that might be looked at more closely in this area include the effects of various types of intervention, the effects of various types of respite care, and the effects of good schooling, not only on the behavior of the autistic individual but also on changes in family functioning (such as depression in either parent, marital discord, family discord of other types, parent–sibling interaction, behavior and academic performance of siblings).

This is a relatively untapped area, but the research that does exist in this area suggests it is likely to be a fruitful one, both from the standpoint of helping the family and from the standpoint of looking again for other areas of multimodal therapeutic intervention. It is likely that every autistic individual will need to be involved in a multimodality therapy program. Elements of these programs have generally been described individually, but the additive effects of various types of intervention on the autistic individual and on family functioning have rarely been studied. The benefits to the autistic individual that accrue from improvement in functioning in various family subsystems likewise is relatively neglected.

THE ROLE OF THE FAMILY ON THE DEVELOPMENT OF THE AUTISTIC CHILD

Research on Family Factors that Influence Language Development

There have been essentially no studies of family factors that may be associated with the language development of autistic children. However, the literature on family factors associated with language development in nonautistic children warrants some mention here.

Children with certain demographic backgrounds (females, firstborns, children from small families, and children from upper and upper-middle social classes) have superior language development (Gerber and Hertel, 1969; Lehman, 1971; Ramey, 1978; Rubin, Hultsch, and Peters, 1971; Scott and Siefert, 1975). These data suggest that these children receive more language stimulation in their environments, better nutrition, and greater selection for higher education and language facility (Bee, Van Egeren, Streissguth, Nyman, and Leckie, 1969; Bernstein, 1961; Friedlander, 1970; Halverson and Waldrop, 1970; Lieven, 1978; Peters, 1980; Rubin *et al.*, 1971). Several studies of children acquiring language have been done using detailed naturalistic observations over long periods of time, and these studies have also shown that the children with the largest amount of language stimulation have the most rapid linguistic progress.

Nelson (1973) did a longitudinal study of middle-class children and found that the children with the greatest language development had been exposed to the largest number of adults, had received the largest number of weekly outings, and had watched the least amount of television. No association was found between the syntactic form of the mother's speech and the children's rate of language development, however.

Cross (1978), Newport, Gleitman, and Gleitman (1977), and Salzinger, Patenaude, and Lichtenstein (1975) found that the children with the greatest language growth tended to be those who received an extensive amount of feedback, reinforcement, and expansions of their own utterances from their mothers. Like Nelson, Newport *et al.* and Cross found no associations between children's language development and syntactic complexity of mothers' speech.

In one of the more complex studies on child language acquisition, Wells (1980) followed a large number of children over a 2-year period using multiple samples of speech interactions in the home. Wells found that the children whose language acquisition showed the most rapid progress were those who received the greatest amount of adult speech, who had the highest frequency of adult expansions, and who heard the most adult references to joint activities. Wells concluded that "there are qualitative aspects of adult speech to children which are facilitative of the child's language development" and which are independent of social class or family position.

In addition to the observational evidence of the significance of linguistic input for the child's acquisition of language, there is experimental evidence of the value of certain environmental factors. Cazden (1965, 1966) experimentally investigated the effectiveness of modeling (systematic use of well-formed utterance of a particular structure) and expansion (repetition of the child's utterances with systematic additions in terms of structure) versus time spent with the child in a free-play situation. She found that the children in the "modeling" group learned the structure best, and that the children in the "expansion" group learned better than the children in the "free-play" group. Odom, Liebert, and Hill (1968) experimented on modeling a grammatical structure embedded in both grammatical and ungrammatical sentences. They found that children's use of the structure was increased by both the grammatical and the ungrammatical modeling. Feldman and Rodgon (Note 1) compared "contingent" expansions, expansions of all utterances, and modeling on the acquisition of a syntactic structure in young children. They found both types of expansions to be superior to modeling, and "contingent" expansions to be the most successful method of increasing syntactic usage. Malouf and Dodd (1972) compared imitation, expansions, and modeling in children's acquisition of a word-order rule. They found that imitation and expansion were more effective than modeling, but that modeling was more effective than no technique. Whitehurst, Novak, and Lorin (1972) manipulated the amount of conversation and amount of imitative prompts used by the parents. They found that the acquisition of new words by the child could be controlled by raising the amount of conversation and the imitative prompts provided by the parents. Nelson (1973) compared use of expansions and modeling to no intervention with three groups of 3-year-olds matched for mean sentence length. They found that after biweekly sessions for 11 weeks, the "expansion" group had advanced language development on a number of measures. The modeling group had not advanced significantly over the controls. Scherer and Olsway (Note 2) examined the role of mothers' expansions on children's production of certain semantic relations. They found that mother's expansions facilitated children's development of semantic structures.

Research on Family Factors Associated with Improvement in Autism

The only research that we are familiar with that has addressed the issue of the role of family factors in the outcome of autism is by Dubpernell (1979). In this study, 58 autistic children ranging in age from 5 through 19 years were divided into two groups. Parents of children in the experimental group were asked to provide three social experiences per week above what they usually provided for the child, and parents of children in the control group were given no particular instructions. The assessment methodology included parental interview, Vineland Social Maturity Scale, Adaptive Behavior Scale, a checklist of social experiences, and questionnaire information on personal data, all administered before and after the 12-week experimental period. Dubpernell found significant differences in the behaviors and social adjustment of children in the experimental group and concluded that familial social experiences play an important part in the development of social maturity in autistic children.

Role of Family as Therapeutic Agents for the Autistic Child

One area where there has been research involving autistic children is the area of therapy involving family members as therapists. A variety of different types of therapy involving the family have been examined, including behavior modification involving the parents or siblings as therapists, language therapy using the parents as therapists, family or group therapy, and psychotherapy of the parents. This is an area of work that is only recently gaining attention, and much of the published literature consists of single-case reports (Boudry and Pfaehler, 1976; Coppage and Veal, 1979; Fodor, 1973; Goldstein and Lanyon, 1971; Johnson, Whitman, and Borloon, 1978; McDade, 1981; Moore and Bailey, 1973; Schell and Adams, 1968; Singh, 1978; White, Hornsby, and Gordon, 1972; Wildman and Simon, 1978), which have invariably described some degree of success for each of the different types of therapy involving the family. The majority of the literature has been concerned less with evaluating success than with establishing feasibility, and reporting any changes occurring subsequent to treatment as "treatment success."

Kozloff (1969, and Chapter 10) described an early method of parents doing therapy aimed at changing both the social behaviors and the communication behaviors of their autistic children. Four families were observed initially, during the parent-treatment phase, and at follow-up from 1 to 10 months after the treatment phase. Kozloff reported that the treatment had been successful, and that parents had reported changes after treatment in the speech, cooperation levels, and socialization activities of the children.

Kane, Kane, Amorosa, and Kumpmann (1976) reported on a feasibility study in which parents of autistic, mentally retarded, and organically disturbed children acted as therapists in teaching language and self-help skills to the children. Parents were trained in charting children's behaviors, as well as in acting as therapists. All parents were successful in charting behaviors and in carrying out the therapy program, even though considerable time commitments were required.

Casey (1978) reported on the success of mothers of autistic children teaching manual communication to the children. Data were recorded for four children daily both in the therapy situation and in the regular school setting. It was found that the manual program facilitated generalization of communicative behavior to the child's total environment, and that the acquisition of manual communication techniques was associated with a decrease in inappropriate social behaviors.

Koegel, Glahn, and Nieminen (1978; see also Chapter 11, this volume) used an experimental format to assess the generalized effects of several different training programs involving parents. In the first experiment, it was found that a brief demonstration of how to teach the autistic child new behaviors was sufficient to teach parents how to teach children those behaviors. However, generalization to new child-target behaviors did not take place. In the second experiment, sections of videotapes showing highly specific training procedures were shown. It was found that viewing the entire package of tapes was necessary before the adults were able to improve the autistic children's behaviors. The authors concluded that very thorough training of parents was necessary before parents were able to function as effective therapists for autistic children.

Lovaas (1978) specified a very detailed training method and videotaped feedback of parental therapeutic attempts. While Lovaas stated that his program was highly successful in the treatment of autistic children, no actual data were provided. Lovaas's program demands a major commitment from parents in terms of time and attention to the program, and we feel that it is unlikely that this approach will appeal to the "average" parent who may not be able to devote the amount of time demanded.

Simpson, Swenson, and Thompson (1980) examined the effectiveness of a parent-applied procedure for reducing self-stimulatory responses in school-age autistic children. While the home intervention procedure was effective in the home, the children's performance in the classroom did not seem to be changed by the home intervention procedure. The authors concluded that generalization effects of treatment across settings must be specifically programmed to be at all effective.

Harris, Wolchik, and Weitz (1981) investigated the effectiveness of parents teaching speech behaviors to their 11 autistic children. At posttreatment, significant gains were found in the speech behaviors of the children. However, at 1-year follow-up, although the children had maintained their gains, there was no evidence of any further improvement. The authors concluded that continued formal teaching is necessary.

Two large-scale programs have evaluated the effectiveness of parents as therapists, or "home-based therapy" with autistic children. One is the work of the Rutter group in England (Hemsley, Howlin, Berger, Hersov, Holbrook, Rutter, and Yule, 1978; Howlin, 1981; Rutter, 1980) and the other is the work of Schopler and his colleagues in North Carolina in the TEACCH program (see Chapter 4 by Schopler, Mesibov, Shigley, and Bashford; Schopler, 1978; Schopler, Mesibov, and Baker, 1982; Schopler, Mesibov, DeVellis, and Short, 1981). These programs differ in a number of ways, with the British one being a more narrow and more research-based approach that focuses on language development in autistic children of grossly normal performance intelligence. The TEACCH program accepts all autistic children and attempts to treat whatever behavioral problems are considered most serious by the parents. The British program uses more stringent research methodology, with behavioral changes being measured in the home, control groups of both untreated autistic children and outpatient-treated autistic children matched for variables shown to be related to outcome being used for comparisons, and the efficacy of treatment being evaluated in terms of relatively long follow-up. Both the British program and the TEACCH program have reported considerable success with a number of children and families, and, equally important, both programs are beginning to isolate some of the factors that are most highly associated with success in the parental therapy programs.

The British study reports significant changes within the first 6 months of home-based treatment for children, with treatment being more successful in dealing with social, emotional, and behavioral problems than in dealing with language development *per se*. When language improvement is achieved, it tends to be in the area of social use of language, not in the area of grammatical development. While a great deal of individual variation has been found in the improvements made across children, the British study shows that significant changes occur for almost all children. The children who seem to be the most likely to benefit from home-based treatment are those who are verbal but have very limited language initially.

The TEACCH program has been favorably received by both the parents and the professionals involved in the program. Questionnaires returned by 348 families who participated in the program had an average "helpfulness rating" of 4.6 (on a scale of 1–5). Areas where the parents rated the program as most effective included managing the children's behaviors, understanding the children, teaching the children, feeling competent as parents, and enjoying the children. Analyses of the returned questionnaires suggest that different subgroups of families responded better to different aspects of the program, with, for example, lower SES families showing the greatest improvements in social and self-help skills of the children. Blind ratings of both the children's behavior and the parental teaching styles before and after participation in the TEACCH program showed significant improvements after as little as 2 months of treatment. In addition, the long-term effectiveness of the program is attested to by the unusually low institutionalization rates of children who have participated in the program.

Practical Significance of Research on the Family's Role in the Development of the Autistic Child

Parents of autistic children should be encouraged to expose their children to the maximum amount of effective communication and interaction. Even with mute or nonverbal autistic children, some communication is possible and should be attempted. Parents should try to gain their nonverbal child's attention and to provide clear, simple linguistic input. With children who have some language, parents should try to engage the child in conversation by asking questions or giving commands. When children do verbalize, they should be given the parent's complete attention. Positive reinforcement, either verbal or using whatever type of other reinforcement is meaningful to the child, should be given.

Although the literature on normal children is as yet unclear about which type of systematic exposure is best—modeling, imitating, prompting, or expanding— we suspect that whatever technique is finally shown to be the most effective one with normal children may not necessarily be the most effective one with autistic children. Therefore, we cannot recommend a particular method of providing structured linguistic input to autistic children, particularly longitudinally.

At the present time, there is really a dearth of research on family factors and the outcome of autism. While several studies have been done examining various family factors in relation to the outcome of "childhood psychoses" or "childhood schizophrenia," the diagnostic criteria used do not clearly define autistic children. The one study done specifically on autistic children does suggest some association between family outings and good prognosis, but the interrelationship between these variables is unclear. At the present time, we feel it is premature to draw any conclusions in this area. We can only advocate further research that uses clearly defined diagnostic criteria and a prospective format, and that at-

tempts to control for factors such as severity of disorder and other initial dif-
ferances in children that may be associated with outcome.

The parental decision on whether to become a therapist for his autistic child
is a difficult one. The parent of a handicapped child faces enormous burdens, and
a commitment of more time and energy may be asking more than many parents
can give. Teaching any child is a difficult task even for professional educators
(Dunlap, Koegel, and Egel, 1979), and the unique handicaps of the autistic child
(disruptive behaviors, self-stimulation, lack of motivation, and stimulus overselectivity) make him especially difficult to teach. Any parent considering a
home-based treatment program should be cautioned that this is no easy task.

Nonetheless, the research has now shown that, in many instances, a home-
based treatment program is a highly feasible approach and may even be more
effective than outpatient treatment. The research is now showing which children
seem most likely to benefit from home-based treatment and which treatment
approaches are most successful. We believe that in the next few years there will
be even more concrete data on this treatment modality and that this is generally a
very promising approach. We feel that any parents who express an interest in
attempting this type of work after being forewarned of the commitment of time
and energy necessary should be encouraged to take part in such a program.

SUMMARY AND CONCLUSIONS

This chapter has reviewed research issues in families of individuals with
autism. It can be seen that of the major areas covered, most of the research has
been done on the family as an environmental etiologic agent, with less than
fruitful results. Research on possible family-genetic factors, research on the
impact of the autistic individual on the family, and research on the role of family
factors on the outcome of autistic individuals has been much less in volume but
possibly more fruitful in outcome.

We feel that the literature to date does not provide any convincing evidence
that the family is an environmental etiological agent in the development of
infantile autism. The studies proposing that the family is an environmental
etiological agent, either through ''severe early stress'' or through ''deviant parent personality,'' suffer from some serious methodological flaws. While we do
not feel that ''deviant family interaction patterns'' have been shown to play an
etiological role in autism either, we do feel that the research has not ruled out the
possibility of some type of communication deficit existing in parents of autistic
children that might signal a potential genetic (rather than environmental)
etiologic factor.

The literature on the family genetic factors in the development of infantile autism is in too early a stage of development to be very conclusive or to have much practical value in terms of genetic counseling or identification of high-risk families. Nonetheless, the preliminary data do suggest that genetic factors may operate in at least one or possibly more than one subgroup of autistic individuals.

What research has been done in the area of the impact of the autistic child upon the family clearly shows that the parents and families of autistic individuals are under severe stress for long periods of time. Serious discord, depression, and financial distress seem to be major problems that continue for many years, with the families of more severely handicapped children and older children being more seriously affected than the families of younger children. It is not now clear what the best methods are for helping these "families in distress," and research is desperately needed in this area.

The research on language development in normal children has shown consistently that exposure to linguistic interactions is associated with progress in language development. While this type of research has not been systematically done with autistic children, we feel that the data with normal children are promising enough to warrant efforts to provide additional language stimulation with autistic children. The literature on language teaching, which shows that grammatical development can be facilitated by means of systematic presentations to the child in terms of modeling, imitating, prompting, or expanding, also has implications for autistic children and warrants the efforts of families in systematically exposing their autistic children to basic language structures. Unfortunately, the lack of additional research on family factors that may influence the outcome for autistic children prevents even guesses as to further approaches that the family can make that may be useful.

One area with promising results is the area of the "family as therapists" for the autistic child. While the data are by no means conclusive, there is some evidence that home-based therapy programs are effective in helping autistic children and are very effective in relieving family stresses and concerns. We hope that in the next few years there will be even more data on *which children and families* are most likely to benefit from *which* programs and in *which areas* the largest gains can be made.

The lack of firm conclusions to be drawn from the research on the family and autism is disappointing. In several areas of family research, little more is known than that further research is needed.

REFERENCE NOTES

1. Feldman, C. F., and Rodgon, M. *The effects of various types of adult responses in the syntactic acquisition of 2- to 3-year-olds.* Unpublished manuscript, University of Chicago, 1970.
2. Scherer, N. J., and Olsway, L. B. *Role of mother's expansions in facilitating language learning.*

Paper presented at the American Speech and Hearing Association Conference, Los Angeles, November 1981.

REFERENCES

Alanen, Y. Some thoughts on schizophrenia and ego development in the light of family investigations. *Archives of General Psychiatry,* 1960, *3,* 650–656.

Allen, J., DeMyer, M. K., Norton, J. A., Pontius, W. O., and Yang, E. Intellectuality in parents of psychotic, subnormal, and normal children. *Journal of Autism and Childhood Schizophrenia,* 1971, *1,* 311–326.

August, G. J., Stewart, M. A., and Tsai, L. The incidence of cognitive disabilities in the siblings of autistic children. *British Journal of Psychiatry,* 1981, *138,* 416–422.

Bee, H. L., Van Egeren, C. F., Streissguth, P., Nyman, B. A., and Leckie, M. S. Social class differences in maternal teaching strategies and speech patterns. *Developmental Psychology,* 1969, *1*(6), 726–734.

Berger, E. W. *A study of self-concepts of siblings of autistic children.* Unpublished doctoral dissertation, University of Cincinnati, 1980.

Bernstein, B. Social class and linguistic development: A theory of social learning. In A. H. Halsey and C. A. Anderson (Eds.), *Education, economy and society.* Glencoe, Ill.: Free Press, 1961. Pp. 288–314.

Block, J. Parents of schizophrenic, neurotic, asthmatic and congenitally ill children. *Archives of General Psychiatry,* 1969, *20,* 659–674.

Boudry, C. L., and Pfaehler, P. Double focus treatment of a psychotic young girl and her parents. *Revue de Neuropsychiatrie Infantile et d'Hygiene Mentale de l'Enfance,* 1976, *24*(1–2), 25–33.

Bowen, M., Bysinger, R., and Basamania, B. The role of the father in families with a schizophrenic patient. *American Journal of Psychiatry,* 1959, *115,* 1017–1020.

Bristol, M. M. *Maternal coping with autistic children: The effect of child characteristics and interpersonal support.* Unpublished doctoral dissertation, University of North Carolina at Chapel Hill, 1979.

Bronfenbrenner, U. Doing your own thing—our undoing. Child Psychiatry and Human Development, 1977, *8,* 3–10.

Cantwell, D. P., Baker, L., and Rutter, M. Families of autistic and dysphasic children. II. Mothers' speech to the children. *Journal of Autism and Childhood Schizophrenia,* 1977, *7,* 313–327.

Cantwell, D. P., Baker, L., and Rutter, M. Family factors. In M. Rutter and E. Schopler (Eds.), *Autism: A reappraisal of concepts and treatment.* New York: Plenum, 1978.

Cantwell, D. P., Baker, L., and Rutter, M. Families of autistic and dysphasic children. I. Family life and interaction patterns. *Archives of General Psychiatry,* 1979, *36,* 682–687.

Casey, L. O. Development of communicative behavior in autistic children: A parent program using manual signs. *Journal of Autism and Childhood Schizophrenia,* 1978, *8,* 45–59.

Cazden, C. *Environmental assistance to the child's acquisition of grammar.* Unpublished doctoral dissertation, Harvard University, 1965.

Cazden, B. Subcultural differences in child language: An interdisciplinary review. *Merrill-Palmer Quarterly,* 1966, *12,* 185–218.

Coppage, K. W., and Veal, M. C. Establishing functional language in an autistic child: A cooperative approach. *Journal of Communication Disorders,* 1979, *12,* 447–460.

Cox, A., Rutter, M., Neuman, S., and Bartak, L. A comparative study of infantile autism and specific developmental receptive language disorder. II. Parental characteristics. *British Journal of Psychiatry,* 1975, *126,* 146–159.

Creak, M., and Ini, S. Families of psychotic children. *Journal of Child Psychology and Psychiatry and Allied Disciplines,* 1960, *1,* 156–175.

Cross, T. G. Mothers' speech and its association with rate of linguistic development in young children. In C. Snow and N. Waterson (Eds.), *The development of communication.* New York: Wiley, 1978.

Culbertson, F. M. The search for help of parents of autistic children or beware of professional "group think." *Journal of Clinical Child Psychology,* 1977, *6,* 63–65.

DeMyer, M. K. *Parents and children in autism.* New York: Wiley, 1979.

DeMyer, M. K., Alpern, G. D., Barton, S., DeMyer, W. E., Churchill, D. W., Hingtgen, J. N., Bryson, C. Q., Pontius, W., and Kimberlin, C. Imitation in autistic, early schizophrenic, and nonpsychotic subnormal children. *Journal of Autism and Childhood Schizophrenia,* 1972, *2,* 264–287.

DeMyer, M. K., Hingtgen, J. N., and Jackson, R. K. Infantile autism reviewed: A decade of research. *Schizophrenia Bulletin,* 1981, *7*(3), 388–451.

DeMyer, M. K., Pontius, W., Norton, J. A., Barton, S., Allen, J., and Steele, R. Parental practices and innate activity in normal, autistic, and brain-damaged infants. *Journal of Autism and Childhood Schizophrenia,* 1972, *2,* 49–66.

Dubpernell, A. L. *The effect of familial social experiences on the social maturity of the autistic child.* Unpublished doctoral dissertation, Wayne State University, 1979.

Dunlap, G., Koegel, R. L., and Egel, A. L. Autistic children in school. *Exceptional Children,* 1979, *45,* 552–558.

Eisenberg, L., and Kanner, L. Early infantile autism. *American Journal of Orthopsychiatry,* 1956, *26,* 556–566.

Fodor, I. E. The parent as a therapist. *Mental Hygiene,* 1973, *57*(2), 16–19.

Folstein, S., and Rutter, M. A twin study of individuals with infantile autism. In M. Rutter and E. Schopler (Eds.), *Autism: A reappraisal of concepts and treatment.* New York: Plenum, 1978.

Fraknoi, J., and Ruttenberg, B. A. Formulation of the dynamic economic factors underlying infantile autism. *Journal of the American Academy of Child Psychiatry,* 1971, *10,* 713–738.

Frank, S. M., Allen, D. A., Stein, L., and Myers, B. Linguistic performance in vulnerable and autistic children and their mothers. *American Journal of Psychiatry,* 1976, *133,* 909–915.

Friedlander, B. A. Receptive language development in infancy: Issues and problems. *Merrill-Palmer Quarterly,* 1970, *16,* 7–51.

Gerber, S. E., and Hertel, C. G. Language deficiency of disadvantaged children. *Journal of Speech and Hearing Research,* 1969, *12,* 270–280.

Goldfarb, W., Goldfarb, N., and Scholl, M. The speech of mothers of schizophrenic children. *American Journal of Psychiatry,* 1966, *122,* 1220–1227.

Goldfarb, W., Levy, D., and Meyers, D. The verbal encounter between the schizophrenic child and his mother. In G. Goldman and D. Shapiro (Eds.), *Developments in psychoanalysis.* New York: Hofner, 1966.

Goldstein, S. B., and Lanyon, R. I. Parent-clinicians in the language training of an autistic child. *Journal of Speech and Hearing Disorders,* 1971, *36*(4), 552–560.

Halverson, C. F., and Waldrop, M. F. Maternal behavior towards own and other preschool children: The problem of "ownness." *Child Development,* 1970, *41,* 839.

Hanson, D. R., and Gottesman, I. I. The genetics, if any, of infantile autism, and childhood schizophrenia. *Journal of Autism and Childhood Schizophrenia,* 1976, *6,* 209–234.

Harris, S. L., Wolchik, S. A., and Weitz, S. The acquisition of language skills by autistic children: Can parents do the job? *Journal of Autism and Developmental Disorders,* 1981, *11,* 373–384.

Hemsley, R., Howlin, P., Berger, M., Hersov, L., Holbrook, D., Rutter, M., and Yule, W. Treating autistic children in a family context. In M. Rutter and E. Schopler (Eds.), *Autism: A reappraisal of concepts and treatment.* New York: Plenum, 1978.

Hinde, R. A. The family influences. In M. Rutter (Ed.), *Scientific foundations of developmental psychiatry*. Baltimore: University Park Press, 1981.

Holroyd, J., Brown, N., Wikler, L., and Simmons, J. Q. Stress in families of institutionalized autistic children. *Journal of Community Psychology*, 1975, *3*(1), 26–31.

Honjo, S., and Wakabayashi, S. A clinical study of infantile autism in twins. *Japanese Journal of Child and Adolescent Psychiatry*, 1981, *22*(1), 91–102.

Howlin, P. A. The effectiveness of operant language training with autistic children. *Journal of Autism and Developmental Disorders*, 1981, *11*, 89–105.

Johnson, M. R., Whitman, T. L., and Borloon, N. B. A home-based program for a preschool behaviorally disturbed child with parents as therapists. *Journal of Behavior Therapy and Experimental Psychiatry*, 1978, *9*(1), 65–70.

Kane, G., Kane, J. F., Amorosa, H., and Kumpmann, S. Parents as participants in the behavior therapy of their mentally retarded children. *Perspectives Psychiatriques*, 1976, No. 58, 293–303.

Kanner, L. Autistic disturbances of affective contact. *Nervous Child*, 1943, *2*, 217–250.

Kaufman, B. N. *A miracle to believe in: They loved a child back to life*. New York: Doubleday, 1981.

Kaufman, I., Frank, T., Heims, L., Herrick, J., and Willer, V. Four types of defense in mothers and fathers of schizophrenic children. *American Journal of Orthopsychiatry*, 1959, *29*, 460–472.

Klebanoff, L. B. Parental attitudes of mothers of schizophrenic, brain-injured and retarded and normal children. *American Journal of Orthopsychiatry*, 1959, *29*, 445–454.

Koegel, R. L., Glahn, T. J., and Nieminen, G. S. Generalization of parent-training results. *Journal of Applied Behavior Analysis*, 1978, *11*(1), 95–109.

Kolvin, L., Ounsted, C., Richardson, L. M., and Garside, R. F. Studies in the childhood psychoses. III. The family and social background in childhood psychoses. *British Journal of Psychiatry*, 1971, *118*, 396–402.

Kozloff, M. A. *Social and behavioral change in families of autistic children*. Unpublished doctoral dissertation, Washington University, 1969.

Lehman, G. Family composition and its influence on the language development of the 18–34 month-old child in the American lower and middle class family. *Journal of Behavioral Science*, 1971, *1*(3), 125–130.

Leighton, D. J. Casework with the parents of autistic children. *British Journal of Psychiatric Social Work*, 1969, *10*(1), 17–21.

Lennox, C., Callias, M., and Rutter, M. Cognitive characteristics of parents of autistic children. *Journal of Autism and Childhood Schizophrenia*, 1977, *7*, 243–261.

Lieven, E. M. Conversations between mothers and young children: Individual differences and their possible implications for the study of language learning. In C. Snow and N. Waterson (Eds.), *The development of communication*. New York: Wiley, 1978.

Lovaas, O. I. Parents as therapists. In M. Rutter and E. Schopler (Eds.), *Autism: A reappraisal of concepts and treatment*. New York: Plenum, 1978.

Malouf, R. E., and Dodd, D. H. Role of exposure, imitation and expansion in the acquisition of an artificial grammatical rule. *Developmental Psychology*, 1972, *7*(2), 195–203.

Marcus, L. M. Patterns of coping in families of psychotic children. *American Journal of Orthopsychiatry*, 1977, *47*(3), 388–399.

Massie, H. N. The early natural history of childhood psychosis. *Journal of the American Academy of Child Psychiatry*, 1975, *14*, 683–707.

McAdoo, W. G., and DeMyer, M. K. Personality characteristics of parents. In M. Rutter and E. Schopler (Eds.), *Autism: A reappraisal of concepts and treatment*. New York: Plenum, 1978.

McDade, H. L. A parent–child interactional model for assessing and remediating language disabilities. *British Journal of Disorders of Communication*, 1981, *16*, 175–183.

Moore, B., and Bailey, J. S. Social punishment in the modification of a preschool child's autistic-like behavior with a mother as therapist. *Journal of Applied Behavior Analysis,* 1973, *6*(3), 497–507.

Nelson, K. Structure and strategy in learning to talk. *Monographs of the Society for Research in Child Development,* 1973, *37*(Serial No. 149).

Netley, C., Lockyer, L., and Greenbaum, G. Parental characteristics in relation to diagnosis and neurological status in childhood psychosis. *British Journal of Psychiatry,* 1975, *127,* 440–444.

Newport, E. L., Gletiman, H., and Gleitman, L. Mother, I'd rather do it myself: Some effects and noneffects of maternal speech style. In C. E. Snow and C. A. Ferguson (Eds.), *Talking to children: Language input and acquisition.* Cambridge: Cambridge University Press, 1977.

Odom, R. D., Liebert, R. M., and Hill, J. H. The effects of modeling cues, rewards, and attentional set on the prediction of grammatical and ungrammatical syntactic constructions. *Journal of Experimental Psychology,* 1968, *6,* 131–140.

Ogdon, D. P., Bass, C. L., Thomas, E. R., and Loroi, W. Parents of autistic children. *American Journal of Orthopsychiatry,* 1968, *38,* 653–658.

O'Moore, M. Living with autism. *Irish Journal of Psychology,* 1978, *4,* 33–52.

Peters, A. M. The units of language acquisition. *Working Papers in Linguistics,* 12, University of Hawaii, Linguistics Department, 1980.

Ramey, C. T. Observations of mother–infant interactions and implications for development. In F. D. Minifie and L. L. Lloyd (Eds.), *Communicative and cognitive abilities: Early behavioral assessment.* Baltimore: University Park Press, 1978.

Rice, C., Kebecs, J. C., and Yahalom, J. Differences in communicative impact between mothers of psychotic and nonpsychotic children. *American Journal of Orthopsychiatry,* 1966, *36,* 529–543.

Ritvo, E. R., and Ritvo, E. C. Genetic and immuno-hematologic factors in autism. In C. Perris, G. Struwe, and B. Jansson (Eds.), *Biological psychiatry 1981* (Proceedings of the IIIrd World Congress of Biological Psychiatry, Stockholm, June 28–July 3, 1981). Amsterdam: Elsevier/North Holland Biomedical Press, 1981.

Rubin, K. H., Hultsch, D. F., and Peters, D. L. Nonsocial speech in 4-year-old children as a function of birth order and interpersonal situation. *Merrill-Palmer Quarterly,* 1971, *17,* 41–50.

Rutter, M. Infantile autism and other child psychoses. In M. Rutter and L. Hersov (Eds.), *Child psychiatry: Modern approaches.* London: Blackwell Scientific Publications, 1977.

Rutter, M. Language training with autistic children: How does it work and what does it achieve? In L. Hersov, M. Berger, and A. R. Nicol (Eds.), *Language and language disorders in childhood.* New York: Pergamon Press, 1980.

Rutter, M., Bartak, L., and Newman, S. Autism—A central disorder of cognition and language? In M. Rutter (Ed.), *Infantile autism: Concepts, characteristics, and treatment.* Edinburgh: Whitefriars Press, 1971.

Salzinger, S., Patenaude, J. W., and Lichtenstein, H. A descriptive study of the effects of selected variables on the communicative speech of preschool children. In A. Aaronson and R. Rieber (Eds.), *Developmental psycholinguistics and communication disorders. Annals of the New York Academy of Sciences,* 1975, *263,* 99–106.

Schell, R. E., and Adams, W. P. Training parents of a young child with profound behavior deficits to be teacher-therapists. *Journal of Special Education,* 1968, *2*(4), 439–454.

Schopler, E. Changing parental involvement in behavioral treatment. In M. Rutter and E. Schopler (Eds.), *Autism: A reappraisal of concepts and treatment.* New York: Plenum, 1978.

Schopler, E., Mesibov, G., and Baker, A. Evaluation of treatment for autistic children and their parents. *Journal of the American Academy of Child Psychiatry,* 1982, *21,* 262–267.

Schopler, E., Mesibov, G. B., DeVellis, R. F., and Short, A. Treatment outcome for autistic children and families. In P. Mittler (Ed.), *Frontiers of knowledge in mental retardation: Social, educational, and behavioral aspects.* Baltimore: University Park Press, 1981.

Scott, R., and Siefert, K. Family size and learning readiness profiles of socioeconomically disadvantaged preschool whites. *Journal of Psychology,* 1975, *89*(1), 307.

Simpson, R. L., Swenson, C. R., and Thompson, T. N. Academic performance in the classroom as a function of a parent applied home management program to severely emotionally disturbed children. *Behavior Disorders,* 1980, *6*(1), 4–11.

Singh, N. N. Reprogramming the social environment of an autistic child. *New Zealand Medical Journal,* 1978, *87*(606), 135–138.

Sullivan, R. C. Siblings of autistic children. *Journal of Autism and Developmental Disorders,* 1979, *9,* 287–298.

Tinberger, E. A., and Tinberger, N. Early childhood autism: An etiological approach. *Journal of Comparative Ethology, Supplement,* 1972, *10,* 1–53.

Wells, G. Adjustments in adult–child conversation: Some effects of interaction. In H. Giles, W. P. Robinson, and P. M. Smith (Eds.), *Language.* Oxford: Pergamon Press, 1980.

White, J. H., Hornsby, L. G., and Gordon, R. Treating infantile autism with parent therapists. *International Journal of Child Psychotherapy,* 1972, *1*(3), 84–95.

Whitehurst, G. J., Novak, G., and Lorin, G. A. Delayed speech studied in the home. *Developmental Psychology,* 1972, *7*(2), 169–177.

Wild, C. M., Shapiro, L. N., and Abelin, T. Communication patterns and role structure in families of male schizophrenics: A study using automated techniques. *Archives of General Psychiatry,* 1977, *34*(1), 58–70.

Wildman, R. W., and Simon, S. J. An indirect method for increasing the rate of social interaction in an autistic child. *Journal of Clinical Psychology,* 1978, *34*(1), 144–149.

Williams, S., and Harper, J. A study of etiological factors at critical periods of development in autistic children. *Australian and New Zealand Journal of Psychiatry,* 1973, *7*(3), 163–168.

Wolff, W. M., and Morris, L. A. Intellectual and personality characteristics of parents of autistic children. *Journal of Abnormal Psychology,* 1971, *77*(2), 155–161.

Zevin, B. Family communication with schizophrenic and nonschizophrenic siblings. *Proceedings of the 81st Annual Convention of the American Psychological Association, Montreal,* 1973, *8,* 471–472.

4

Helping Autistic Children through Their Parents
The TEACCH Model

ERIC SCHOPLER, GARY B. MESIBOV, R. HAL
SHIGLEY, and ANNE BASHFORD

If you sought help for an autistic child during the 1960s, you would soon discover that the professional mental health arena was programmed to respond in ways now considered obsolete and reviewed in Chapter 1. Psychoanalytic theory was the orienting perspective in this country. Accordingly, autism was widely regarded as a form of social withdrawal from pathological parenting. As a result of such psychogenic formulation, autistic children were often treated with inappropriate psychotherapy, excluded from special education in public schools, and committed for institutional placement to protect them from the presumed cause of their disorder—their own parents.

If, on the other hand, during the same period a professional who did not subscribe to psychogenic theory examined autistic children and their families (Rimland, 1964), a significantly different understanding of autism could emerge. One such effort was the North Carolina program for the Treatment and Education of Autistic and related Communication handicapped CHildren (Division TEACCH), which began as a research project in 1966. This research program was based on the founders' (Schopler and Reichler, 1971) extensive clinical experience with such severely disturbed children and their families.

ERIC SCHOPLER and GARY B. MESIBOV • Division TEACCH, University of North Carolina, Chapel Hill, North Carolina 27514. R. HAL SHIGLEY • Eastern TEACCH Center, Greenville, North Carolina 27834. ANNE BASHFORD • Southeastern TEACCH Center, Wilmington, North Carolina 28401. This project is supported in part by grants from the National Institute of Mental Health (NIMH RO1-MH15539) and the Office of Education (OEG 0-8-070827-2633 [032]).

This experience led them to believe that these children suffered from some form of brain abnormality rather than a parentally induced behavior disorder. They also became convinced that the best potential for the child's improvement would be found through parental efforts, interests, and skills, efforts that should be enhanced and made more effective through parent–professional collaboration. That the developmental progress of young chldren is linked to parents is not a new formulation, though it was rarely applied to severely disturbed children. The idea that parents of autistic and similar children could collaborate as cotherapists for the child's benefit had not been considered, and was all the more intriguing for going against accepted mental health practice and knowledge. The psychogenic theory explicitly blamed parents for the child's autism (Bettelheim, 1967). Even many behaviorists were convinced that parental failure to provide an appropriate reinforcement history caused the autism syndrome (Ferster, 1961). Nevertheless, clinical support for cotherapy increased with each family seen in the TEACCH program. At the same time, it also provided an increasingly intriguing basis for empirical research. The convergence of this clinical experience with empirical research evolved into our statewide program, Division TEACCH (Reichler and Schopler, 1976). We had been sufficiently convinced by the effectiveness of our parent involvement emphasis that it was made part of the TEACCH model at three different levels. In this chapter we will trace the involvement of parents at the level of research and conceptualization, at the level of program organization, and at the level of clinical procedures. The parent–professional relationships that have evolved from this involvement are then defined.

RESEARCH AND CONCEPTS

The guiding philosophy of our program grew from a primary commitment to improve our ability to help and to understand these children and their families. Since the criteria for determining the most appropriate treatment are not necessarily the same as those for conducting systematic research, clinical insights sometimes precede research findings. However, we have always tried to maintain a close tie between clinical practice and research, an effort that is often more convincing to professional colleagues than so-called basic research. Empirical verification of clinical insights has included the following studies.

Schopler and Loftin (1969) investigated the widely held belief that parents of autistic and schizophrenic children suffered from thought disorders. They found that when parents were tested in the context of psychogenically oriented psychotherapy for their autistic child, they obtained higher thought-impairment scores than did parents of mentally retarded or normal children. On the other hand, when such parents were tested in the context of their successful child-rearing experiences with their nonpsychotic normal children, they did not differ

significantly in their thought-impairment scores from parents of mentally retarded or normal children. These findings clearly suggested that there was no
evidence for a formal thought disorder in parents of autistic children. Therefore,
it must also follow that parents had a more realistic understanding of their autistic
children's problems than most professionals gave them credit for.

In a subsequent study Schopler and Reichler (1972) examined the ability of
parents to perceive their autistic children realistically. They asked parents to
estimate their autistic child's level of mental functioning, language development,
and social development before any testing took place. When parents' estimates
were then compared with subsequent formal test results, a significant correlation
was found. As a group, the parents were able to assess their children's current
development levels quite accurately.

Such evidence further supported Schopler's (1971) formulation that parents
were more the victims than the creators of their children's autism, and that there
were sound empirical bases for pursuing better ways of understanding and treating autistic children by pursuing a parental perspective. Moreover, professional
misunderstanding of parents had been sufficiently pervasive in the past that to
make any impact it appeared necessary to provide services for these children that
are comprehensive—including their lives at home, at school, and in the community—and that are targeted at a broad age-span. Our development of comprehensive services from a parental perspective could best be accomplished with an
eclectic approach—the recognition that many professional disciplines were concerned with these children and were now finding procedures and treatment techniques. Many of these seemed extremely effective with some children, but not
with others. It became clear that at this time only individualized assessment and
treatment could offer optimal adaptation for child and family. Along with an
emphasis on individualized and eclectic treatment, the following concepts provide major guidance in the philosophy of the TEACCH model.

Generalist Model

Traditionally within the mental health professions, service delivery systems
emphasize specialization. Psychologists conduct psychological evaluations,
speech therapists provide speech therapy, occupational therapists provide sensory-motor integration therapy, physicians offer medical evaluations, psychiatrists
perform psychiatric evaluations, and so on. This is an understandable phenomenon considering the long and intense training that is required by professionals in various disciplines. Because graduate training is heavily specialized,
these kinds of treatment services are a logical and predictable outcome. Unfortunately, such a system poses a number of problems for a family seeking help with
their handicapped child.

One commonly hears parents state that they have received contradictory opinions and advice about both the diagnosis and appropriate forms of treatment for their handicapped child. In both the literature and the clinical community, professionals are matched against one another, and often the child and the family are the losers. Rather than the needs of a child being met in a consistent and systematic way through a variety of specialized disciplines, fragmentation of a child's evaluation and treatment are often the result.

In order to avoid some of these difficulties, the TEACCH program utilizes a generalist model, focusing primary attention on the needs of the child and families rather than on the needs of the various professional disciplines. Clinic staff are designated as psychoeducational therapists and serve on diagnostic teams providing whatever treatment or services are needed by the child and his or her family. These therapists have educational backgrounds in diverse fields, including special education, early childhood education, psychology, counseling, social work, speech and language, and related fields. Moreover, we expect our special education teachers to be knowledgeable in a broad range of topics, including behavior modification, language development, social development, family interactions, and traditional special education issues. A frequently voiced argument against the generalist model is that there is too much knowledge to reasonably expect any therapist or teacher to become proficient in each area. However, we have found the converse to be more compelling. Teachers and therapists, like parents, have to deal with all aspects of the child's life, regardless of their degree of expertise. Specialists can be found for consultation when needed. But only generalists and parents are willing to relate to and communicate in behalf of the entire child.

Evaluation–Treatment Continuity

Another important principle in the TEACCH program is that evaluation and treatment components are closely related to each other and are part of the same process. Diagnostic questions are given priority according to their relevance to the child's needs and parents' concern, rather than because of specialized professional interests. Likewise, diagnostic procedures and results are not kept secret from parents. Parents often observe psychological testing, and children's records are not routinely classified confidential from their parents. Honest and open discussion on the relationship between assessment and treatment not only is in the child's best interest, it also improves the parent–professional relationship. When a family comes for an evaluation and discusses many of their intimate feelings, triumphs, and tragedies, a certain bond forms between them and the evaluation staff. It is neither reasonable nor cost-effective to send them to another agency once a diagnostic evaluation is completed. Moreover, the whole purpose of conducting an evaluation is to provide insights into the unique strengths, needs, and difficulties of an autistic child and his /or her family. The main purpose in discovering these is to be able to provide appropriate, individualized services. Therefore, it is essential to any comprehensive treatment effort that evaluation and treatment be kept in close relationship with each other.

Developmental Perspective

The concept of development is emphasized for several reasons. First, it serves as a reminder that children, normal or otherwise, grow and change with age. Although few people would disagree with this statement, far too many are not aware how specific behaviors, such as a child's comprehension or ability to reason, are shaped by his /or her developmental level. Even fewer people know how an autistic child's symptoms and behavior problems are affected by development. Far too often both professionals and parents evolve complex motivational explanations for problems rooted in developmental delays. Second, a developmental framework provides a means to describe and understand the characteristically uneven learning patterns manifested by autistic children. In the same child various functions often operate on different developmental levels. Therefore, the most relevant teaching techniques can often be best approximated from the appropriate techniques for a particular developmental level. For example, if a 5-year-old boy has the motor coordination of a normal 5-year-old but has the language comprehension of a 2-year-old, this boy can best be taught to ride a tricycle by using simple speech appropriate to his language level. Although autistic children are not like normal younger children, their problems can often be understood in terms of the similarities and common needs of chronologically younger ones. Moreover, that connective bridge becomes increasingly important as autistic children remain in the community and public schools with normal children.

Interaction Concept

This concept represents three important principles for the TEACCH model. First, it serves as a reminder that professional–family relations are defined not only by the expertise communicated from the professional to the parent but also by the parent's resources, aspirations, and questions directed at the professional. When both sides to that relationship are understood, the potential for mutually satisfactory results is enhanced. Second, and equally important, is the recognition that handicapped children and even infants have an impact on their parents every bit as real as the effect parents have on their children. Third, the interaction concept is probably most important for the TEACCH model in evaluating the outcome of educational and other intervention efforts. That is, the outcome is the product of two kinds of change. Either the child acquires better skills or reduces dysfunctional behavior, on the one hand, or the environment (home, school, community) develops greater acceptance of the child's deficits, on the other hand. Either of these interactions will produce improved adaptation for the child. Both parents and professionals must recognize that with a chronic disability like autism, both kinds of change must be pursued.

ORGANIZATIONAL STRUCTURE

As we recognized the necessity for developing comprehensive services for autistic children and adults (Reichler and Schopler, 1976), it became evident that improved adaptation for the developmentally handicapped child must occur in the three major areas of his life: home and family life, school and special education, and the community and its shared responsibility. It was clear that parent involvement would have to play an important role in each of those three levels.

Home and Family Adjustment

The main location for improving home adjustment with individual children and their families is the TEACCH Center. North Carolina has been divided into five areas, each served by a regional TEACCH Center. All five centers are located near campuses of the University of North Carolina, thus enhancing the potential for student involvement through training and research. Center staff (therapists) collaborate with parents in diagnostic assessment, the development of behavior management techniques, and special education procedures.

The diagnostic process at each center occurs mainly in a one-way observation room. This will be described in greater detail later. After completing the evaluation, the therapist demonstrates certain special education procedures and behavioral techniques while the parents observe. These are written out in a home teaching program, implemented by parents and/or siblings at home. In subsequent sessions parents demonstrate their use of the home program while the therapist observes. Parents frequently introduce new procedures from their own observations and experience aimed at finding the optimum individualized teaching program for each child. An indexed collection of these teaching activities has recently been published as part of the TEACCH assessment series (Schopler, Lansing, and Waters, 1983).

School and Special Education

During the research phase of the TEACCH program, while the parents-as-cotherapists model was being developed, it became unavoidably clear that the child's special education was a central concern for each and every family. As their part of the cotherapy team, the professional staff found it necessary to develop a good working relationship with every teacher who had one of our children in his or her classroom. Two developments during this period deserve special note. One was that the staff was surprised by how frequently teachers were willing to take special pains with autistic children, even though (maybe because) they had no previous training or experience with such children. When consultation and information was offered, most teachers were eager to collaborate. The second observation was that as mothers became more effective in using and developing home teaching programs, they became interested in pursuing a special education career. Four out of 10 mothers from the original cotherapy research sample became special education teachers (Schopler and Reichler, 1971). We established public school classrooms for autistic children in North Carolina, 5 years before it became a federal requirement, after answering two questions: (1) Was it feasible to teach autistic children in the public schools? (2) What was the political motivation for including such children? After all, most of the mental health rhetoric suggested negative answers to both of these questions. However, we had learned otherwise from two sources. During the research phase we saw that a surprising number of teachers were willing to include such difficult children in their classrooms and provide for them individually when appropriate support was supplied. From the parents we learned the importance of having their handicapped child included in public schools, not just because they recognized the importance of education but also because they knew that the society shared child-rearing efforts through the schools with parents of other children. Exclusion of autistic children from public education was to subject these families to one of the severest forms of social isolation possible in the United States during the 1970s.

After the state extended the cotherapy project to a statewide basis through special legislation in 1972, special education classrooms became a structural part of the TEACCH program. Their number and administrative organization have changed with time. The original legislation included funding for 9 TEACCH classrooms located in public schools. This was part of the research, testing to see if autistic children could be taught in public schools. When the results were positive these were soon increased by 31 more, but funded by the local educational authorities. With the acceptance of these classrooms as part of the state special education program, funding for all TEACCH classrooms was covered by the North Carolina Department of Public Instruction and local education authorities. Regardless of these changes, however, the involvement of parents in their children's education was always maintained as central to the child's educational program. The reasons for this program emphasis was neither obscure nor mysterious. One of the central educational problems for autistic and similar children is their inability to generalize learned experience from one situation to another. Their tendency to repetition is usually anchored in attachment to some concrete feature of the situation. For example, such a child can learn that his teacher is wearing a red sweater. But when his sister wears a red scarf, the color identification becomes a new problem. Clearly, the parents are central agents in generalizing their child's learning from school to home and community.

The degree and kind of parent involvement with TEACCH classrooms varies both among families and among school systems for many reasons. Families with greater financial resources and fewer children often have more classroom involvement time than more pressured families. The age of the child is another important factor, with young children often evoking more consistent parent involvement than adolescents. Four different levels of parent involvement are used in TEACCH classrooms.

At the most intense level, a mother will function as an assistant teacher and work in the classroom on a regular basis, usually with children other than her own. The second level of intensity involves parents working in the classroom at irregular intervals and at special events like birthday parties or field trips. For example, one of our teachers injured her back and was out of class for a week, and one of the mothers immediately offered to substitute. Another of our teachers, making a home visit, found the mother nervously trying to tint her hair for the first time. Having had experience with this procedure, the teacher helped her do a fine job. Parents and teachers are supportive with each other in attitude, words, and actions. They compliment each other on success achieved with the child and are supportive when progress is slow and negligible. The details of their mutual support is defined by the situation and the individuals involved. At this level parents may also collaborate with the teacher by engaging in certain teaching activities.

The third level involves weekly meetings with the teacher and occasional visits to the classroom when the teacher wants to demonstrate a newly discovered, effective teaching intervention. Conversely, as parents are involved in the classroom, teachers are encouraged to make home visits to improve their understanding of the child and also to build their collaborative relationship with parents. The fourth and least intensive level of parent–teacher collaboration is a monthly conference between parent and teacher. This is considered a minimum requirement because even when parents lack transportation to the school, they can at least make a monthly phone call to the teacher.

Parent involvement with the classroom has varied over time. Before the passage of PL 94-142, parents and teachers were frequently eager for collaboration. After 1977, when handicapped children's right to education became legal, fewer parents wanted to be in the classrooms. Both they and the teachers now saw their child's education as a legal right rather than as the result of a collaborative effort. This response did not come as a surprise. For the teacher, having a parent in the classroom often meant extra work in organizing another adult into the daily schedule. For the parent, it meant giving up time from other activities and family needs. However, in nearly every case where intense parent–teacher collaboration was seen as a special opportunity, the result was a well-integrated educational program, providing a deeply satisfying experience for those involved. More detailed information on the school program is available in Schopler and Bristol (1980) and Schopler and Olley (1982).

Advocacy and Community Relations

If our concern with the autistic child's adjustment within his family led immediately to working with the school system, then our work with the school led directly to community relations. It was clear that special services were needed beyond what the schools could supply.

In order to facilitate the autistic child's access to community facilities that are taken for granted by nonhandicapped people, several kinds of parent–professional groups were developed to advocate such access. Each of our TEACCH classrooms has a parent group attached to it. They meet around special activities, needs such as transportation, and special education procedures or behavior modification techniques. Conflicts and differences between teachers and parents are often mitigated by the presence of therapists in school-related parent groups. Each of the five regional TEACCH centers also has a parent group affiliation. These groups meet for special seminars, lectures, and social occasions. The center staff usually organizes the program and make babysitting or child care provisions for parents who have to bring their children.

Each of the parent groups attached to classrooms and centers are also part of the North Carolina Society for Autistic Adults and Children (NCSAAC), a chapter of the National Society for Children and Adults with Autism (NSAC), discussed in Chapter 6 by Warren. NCSAAC's executive board meets every other month, and the meeting place rotates to different regions in the state. TEACCH staff participate in these meetings, which are usually aimed at developing needed services and at informing the community about the needs and problems of autism. Program development and programmatic changes in the TEACCH program have had their beginnings in these parent group meetings. This has included the development of summer camp programs, adding two regional TEACCH centers to the original three, and adding both research and services for adolescents and adults with autism.

The need for adolescent and adult services became especially clear during the past few years, and our staff took an active role in planning and developing such services. First came a group home for autistic adolescents, soon followed by three more. TEACCH established the position of coordinator for adolescent and adult services, and he became active in developing a fuller spectrum of services (Mesibov, Schopler, and Sloan, 1983). These included respite care programs, vocational training, social skill training groups, vocational job advocacy, and better integration of autistic clients with sheltered workshops and group homes already established for other developmental disabilities.

Another aspect of parental involvement relates to TEACCH's training efforts. Each year new teachers, group home staff, and therapists are trained during our annual in-service training program. This is an intensive 2-week training effort that covers the main topics new staff should know about when working with autistic clients. Central to this training experience is the direct participation of trainees with some of our autistic children and their parents. Beginning with our first in-service training in 1972, parents have been willing to bring in their children and answer questions discussed many times before. Classrooms are set up for the purpose of training new staff, and parent panels are used to teach the valid distinctions between parent and professional perspectives as well as their commonalities. Parental participation in our training program has always been enthusiastic. They are quick to recognize that any inconvenience to them for having their children used as training "subjects" is well repaid by having appropriately trained professionals available in the future.

We have discussed some of the administrative structures designed for the purpose of fostering and promoting parent–professional collaboration in the area of family adjustment, special education, and advocacy in the community. In the next section we will discuss some of the clinical procedures and how these foster the parent–professional collaboration pioneered and developed by the TEACCH program.

CLINICAL PROCEDURES

An appropriate and thorough evaluation involves intensive contact with several sources of information, including the child, the family, and the school. The two major purposes for carrying out these diagnostic evaluations are classification and individualized assessment.

Diagnosis and Assessment

Diagnostic classification involves identification of the characteristics children in a diagnostic group have in common with each other. The purpose of this labeling is primarily administrative, to decide whether the referred child may be accepted in a program for autistic children. A diagnostic label is also part of the answer to the parents' question "What's wrong with my child?" For this part of the assessment we use our diagnostic rating scale, the Childhood Autism Rating Scale (CARS) (Schopler, Reichler, DeVellis, and Daly, 1980). Parents rely heavily on professional expertise during the classification phase and assume mainly a traineelike role.

Although parents often attach great significance to the diagnostic label, the best help to improve home adjustment usually comes from improved understanding of the child. This is best accomplished through individualized assessment of the child's unique learning problems and behavioral characteristics. The primary instrument used in our developmental assessment of the child is the Psycho-educational Profile (PEP) (Schopler and Reichler, 1979), which provides the teaching strategies (Schopler, Reichler, and Lansing, 1980) needed for an optimum individualized teaching program (Schopler et al., 1983).

In addition to the assessment based on the testing or direct observation of the child, assessment information from the teacher is important for developing an effective special education program. However, the most frequently overlooked source of information is the child's parents. Too many professionals have a negative attitude about parents who are not managing their difficult child most effectively. They draw the erroneous conclusion that such parents are not a reliable source of information. This is unfortunate since parents have spent the most time with their children. They usually know them best and also have the highest motivation for developing the best possible family adjustment, even when they have difficulties managing the child. Parents usually provide the most useful developmental history information and the clearest picture of current behavior problems. They also have the most extensive information for distinguishing the teaching techniques that worked for them from those that were ineffective. Moreover, effective and relevant help cannot be given without knowing family priorities, concerns, and expectations. For this phase of the relationship it is well for staff to take a trainee role while parents train them on these important issues.

Extended Diagnostic

Once our evaluation has been completed and the results interpreted to the family, we offer parents the opportunity for extended diagnostic sessions where they can extend their skills and understanding of their child. The extended diagnostic usually involves weekly sessions for a period of 6–8 weeks. Once a family enters into this phase, two therapists are assigned to them, one assuming the role of the "child therapist" while the other is designated the "parent consultant."

The child therapist is responsible for working with the child and learning how to work with him/or her more effectively. Utilizing test results, direct work with the child, and information from the parents, the child therapist proposes cognitive and behavioral goals, which are outlined and implemented in home teaching programs. These programs specify activities and techniques that involve the parents in teaching and managing their children in structured work sessions. The child therapist discusses the suggested goals with the family to make sure they are acceptable and meaningful. The child therapist then proceeds to teach the parents how to carry out these teaching programs. The parents learn from the written instructions in the program as well as from observations of the child therapist working with their child. The parents also demonstrate their efforts with their child in the clinic during these extended diagnostic sessions and receive direct feedback from the child therapist. Through ongoing dialogue between the parents and the therapist, the parents participate in the development of new responses that bring about desirable changes in the child's learning and behavior patterns. Therefore, treatment gains are not exclusively credited to the child therapist's efforts and skills but are the result of a parent–professional collaborative effort.

The parent consultant is the therapist who continues to gather information from the parents and who works to improve their understanding of their child's disability. The parent consultant has a listening, supporting, understanding role with the family. The consultant helps the parents organize their priorities for their home setting. Current problems and past experiences are reviewed with the parents to extract useful information for effecting change. The parent consultant sits with the parents while they observe the child therapist working with their child. The consultant calls the parents' attention to relevant issues, management and teaching techniques, and changes in strategy during the session. It is the parent consultant who usually has the major responsibility for enlisting the parents in the cotherapist process. The parent consultant also helps the parents realize that they are the major resources for bringing about enduring change.

The extended diagnostic provides a structure for getting to know a family and learning from them. The child therapist and the parent consultant may also draw from other information sources such as teachers or relatives who have had meaningful contact with the child. The extended diagnostic is a time for gathering any information that contributes to a better understanding of a child and his/or her family.

During the time-limited extended diagnostic, efforts are directed toward the accomplishment of specific teaching and behavioral goals. Using assessment data and other information that has been accumulated during the diagnostic evaluation, the therapists select goals that are developmentally appropriate as well as relevant to the child's functioning in the family. Another criterion in choosing goals is a high probability for attainment within the contract period.

The first visit during the extended diagnostic phase might typically involve the parents meeting with the parent consultant while the child's therapist interacts with the child in another room. During this and subsequent sessions, the child therapist conceptualizes ideas for an initial home teaching program, a written version of the proposed goals, and specific activities and techniques, which are then discussed with the parents. This sequence is usually completed by the second or third clinic meeting. Then the child therapist demonstrates the program while the parents and the parent consultant observe through a one-way mirror.

During the next few weeks, the parents carry out the program at home. Usually the program requires 30 to 60 minutes each day, depending upon the child's developmental level and attention span and the specific family situation. Ideally, both parents are involved, but more often it has been the mother who has done the home program sessions.

Parents are encouraged to demonstrate their home programs during a clinic session as soon as possible. These demonstrations provide opportunities to reinforce parental competency. Initiative and generalization of concepts and skills are recognized. When there are problems, the parents examine them together with the parent consultant and the child therapist so that everyone participates in the learning process.

At the end of the extended diagnostic period, the director of the clinic meets with the parents and therapists to review problems and progress from each person's perspective. A decision is reached on future plans. These may involve an additional extended diagnostic period, another agency, or special classroom placement without clinic contact.

We have reviewed how parent–professional collaboration is structured and fostered in our organizational and clinical procedures in order to improve adaptation at home, in school, and with the community. In order to provide this kind of comprehensive service mandated for the TEACCH program, a number of different treatment goals must be pursued. In developing the TEACCH model we have found it useful to evolve four different kinds of parent–professional relationships. These will be summarized next.

PARENT–PROFESSIONAL RELATIONSHIPS IN THE TEACCH MODEL

Prior to the development of the TEACCH model for parent–professional relationships we had seen the dominance of two other models. At the risk of oversimplifying these two we will designate one the medical and the other the behavioral model. The former refers to the relationship in which the physician is the expert on the diagnosis and treatment of a disease and the patient or the parent is primarily a passive participant of treatment. On the other hand, in the behavioral model, although the behaviorist must still be expert on the most recent scientific technology for behavior modification, the emphasis is on training the parent in behavioral techniques, which gives the parent an active role as a trainee.

In the TEACCH program we have found that neither of these two parent–professional models is adequate to the task of delivering cost-effective and comprehensive services for autistic and developmentally disabled clients. Instead, we have found from the cotherapy model that there are four quite distinct forms of parent-professional relationships. When the cotherapy relationship is characterized by mutual respect between professionals and parents, they are each able to shift to the appropriate form as needed.

1. *Parent as trainee* and professional as trainer is the model developed quite effectively by bevariorists. It is based on the recognition that the professional has seen many similar children and that he or she also knows the most recent developments in new treatments, including special education, behavioral procedures, and drug intervention. The professional also knows how to make the correct diagnostic classification. The parent needs this information in order to understand the child's disorder and what can be done about it. This forms an important element in the parent–professional relationship during the phase of the diagnostic session involving classification. It is also the dominant emphasis in the therapist's demonstration during the extended diagnostic session.

2. *Parent as trainer* and professional as trainee is a much less familiar relationship component. It is based on our recognition that parents are in most cases the foremost experts on their own handicapped child's behavior. They have lived with the child longer than anyone else and have spent more time teaching early social behaviors such as communication skills, toileting, eating, dressing, and washing. Parents also tend to have higher motivation for living harmoniously with their child than anyone else, especially in the younger age range. However, this form of relationship can be used only when professionals are convinced that they can have reasonable trust in most parents' accounts of their children's development or problem, and if they are convinced that the child's improved adaptation is a mutual task they share with parents. This form of relationship is used when parents provide assessment information to staff, when parents demonstrate to staff effective interventions they developed in their home teaching sessions or classroom participation, and also when they train new staff or legislators.

3. *Emotional support,* the third form of relationship, signifies the mutual emotional support given by professionals to parents and vice versa. The parents' need for emotional support becomes clear when our staff understands that these parents have the same stresses endured by everyone else, but with the addition that they also have a handicapped child, a child who does not learn at the same rate as other children. This results in frustration and disappointments to which

the family must adjust and make special provisions. Once our staff develops even an approximate understanding of parenting a handicapped child, they can provide the needed emotional support, even when there are disagreements between them and parents about behavioral interpretations and techniques. Conversely, the parents must understand the extra effort required by professionals to work with clients slow to respond and less able to provide the positive feedback needed by professionals. Parents must understand the professionals' desires to be effective teachers, therapists, or houseparents for autistic clients. We have found that when neither parents nor professionals are misinformed about each other's needs, they spontaneously tend to offer mutual emotional support quite easily, and need very little training to practice it.

4. *Community advocacy* is a form of the parent–professional relationship in which the objective is to develop community understanding and acceptance of their children's special problems and to develop needed and cost-effective services. A common front is developed from the other three aspects of the relationship, and individual differences are at a minimum in this role. When parents and professionals form a meaningful collaborative relationship they are also politically most effective. It is somewhat more difficult to characterize the difference between parents and professionals in this community advocacy role than in the three previously described forms of parent–professional interaction. This is because community advocacy takes so many shapes, and a parent's contribution is as versatile as his or her career, be it writer, lawyer, administrator, or physician. Therefore, the division of labor between professionals and parents is not readily predetermined, though usually parents, more than professionals, represent a political constituency, while professionals are seen as those who meet that constituency's needs. Once they are in agreement about their collaboration, their respective contributions are readily negotiated.

Earlier we described how the TEACCH organization structure supports, and facilitates collaboration between, professional staff and parents. The four relationships cited above do not correspond neatly to different program facets. Instead, they have evolved from the specific content of the cotherapy relationship. For example, during the extended diagnostic period, described earlier, the parent is most frequently in the trainee role and the therapist in the role of the trainer. However, both the parent and the therapist may shift from trainee to trainer several times in the same conversation. We have resisted pressures to develop a "parent training package" because these roles evolve best out of task-oriented conversations in which the staff are committed to provide the best problem-oriented help they are capable of offering and the parents are committed to seeking the best answers they can find for maintaining their family with a handicapped child. We have found that the parent–professional relationship develops best out of appropriate administrative and clinical structures rather than from scientific parent-training techniques.

CONCLUSION

Eighteen years ago our research project demonstrated that parents of autistic children could be effective cotherapists and developmental agents for their own children. Since then the evolution of the TEACCH program has been an ongoing demonstration of the service, training, and research progress that can be developed out of a parent–professional cotherapy relationship. In this chapter we have attempted to summarize the working concepts and the research that grew out of this parent–professional collaboration. We reviewed the organizational structures conducive to this collaboration and the types of clinical procedures and relationships that enable the collaborative effort to be translated into effective service. We do not yet have enough of the needed service in place, nor have we solved all the problems represented by these developmentally handicapped children and adults. But we have learned that parents and professionals can collaborate in a task-oriented effort to alleviate this devastating handicap, and when parents and professionals treat one another with respect and affection, the specific skills and perspectives of each can be used to maximize the development of autistic children. In North Carolina, the parent–professional relationships are strong and growing, which makes us optimistic about the future for our autistic residents.

REFERENCES

Bettelheim, B. *The empty fortress—Infantile autism and the birth of the self*. New York: Free Press, 1967.

Ferster, C. B. Positive reinforcement and behavioral deficits of autistic children. *Child Development*, 1961, *32*, 437–456.

Mesibov, G. B., Schopler, E., and Sloan, J. L. Service development for adolescents and adults in North Carolina's TEACCH Program. In E. Schopler and G. B. Mesibov (Eds.), *Autism in adolescents and adults*. New York: Plenum, 1983.

Reichler, R. J., and Schopler, E. Developmental therapy: A program model for providing individualized services in the community. In E. Schopler and R. J. Reichler (Eds.), *Psychopathology and child development*. New York: Plenum, 1976.

Rimland, B. *Infantile autism*. New York: Appleton-Century-Crofts, 1964.

Schopler, E. Parents of psychotic children as scapegoats. *Journal of Contemporary Psychotherapy*, 1971, *4*, 17–22.

Schopler, E., and Bristol, M. M. *Autistic children in public school*. Reston, Va.: ERIC Clearinghouse for C.E.C., 1980.

Schopler, E., Lansing, M. D., and Waters. L. *Individualized assessment and treatment for autistic and developmentally disabled children. Vol. III. Teaching activities for autistic children*. Baltimore: University Park Press, 1983.

Schopler, E., and Loftin, J. M. Thought disorders in parents of psychotic children: A function of test anxiety. *Archives of General Psychiatry*, 1969, *20*(2), 174–181.

Schopler, E., and Olley, J. G. Comprehensive educational services for autistic children: The

TEACCH model. In C. R. Reynolds and T. R. Gutkin (Eds.), *The handbook of school psychology*. New York: 1982.

Schopler, E., and Reichler, R. J. Parents as cotherapists in the treatment of psychotic children. *Journal of Autism and Childhood Schizophrenia,* 1971, *1,* 87–102.

Schopler, E., and Reichler, R. J. How well do parents understand their own psychotic child? *Journal of Autism and Childhood Schizophrenia,* 1972, *2,* 387–400.

Schopler, E., and Reichler, R. J. *Individualized assessment and treatment for autistic and developmentally disabled children. Vol. I: Psychoeducational profile.* Baltimore: University Park Press, 1979.

Schopler, E., Reichler, R. J., DeVellis, R. F., and Daly, K. Toward objective classification of childhood autism: Childhood Autism Rating Scale (CARS). *Journal of Autism and Developmental Disorders,* 1980, *10,* 91–103.

Schopler, E., Reichler, R. J., and Lansing, M. D. *Individualized assessment and treatment for autistic and developmentally disabled children. Vol. II: Teaching strategies for parents and professionals.* Baltimore: University Park Press, 1980.

III

Parents as Advocates

5

Developmental Changes in Families with Autistic Children
A Parent's Perspective

MARY S. AKERLEY

> Happy families are all alike; every unhappy family is unhappy in its own way.
> Tolstoi, *Anna Karenina*

Trite as that beginning may be, I chose it because it has an emphasis we need. Note that it does not say, "Every family with an autistic child is unhappy in its own way," just "every unhappy family." In thinking about this topic—developmental changes in families with an autistic child—I kept running into dead ends: Of every example of change that our son Ed wrought in our lives, I could say, "It would have happened anyway—or something very like it." So what we are going to be looking at here doesn't have as much to do with autism as it does with stress and different ways of reacting to it.

I am the mother of four children, the youngest of whom has autism. He is now what is termed "high-functioning" and "near-normal," but he started out life as a potential backward resident. He was utterly passive, irrationally fearful, and almost totally devoid of any behavior. He didn't crawl, play with toys (even inappropriately), or babble any pretalk syllables. He did rock back and forth on all fours, eat, sleep, and scream. We, as individuals and as a family, were often angry or sad because of him, but I don't believe we were ever an unhappy family.

Many of the changes he forced upon us were helpful in our personal growth and in our development as a family. And when he made progress, he brought us indescribable joy. Perhaps Tolstoi was wrong about happy families; surely that joy is unique? But even as I write that sentence, I see the error. The joy we

---

MARY S. AKERLEY • 10609 Glenwild Road, Silver Spring, Maryland 20901.

experienced the first time Ed answered a question is qualitatively the same as the joy we felt when our "normal" son Bill finally got an A in math—only the degree is different.

The same is true of our sorrows. I believe that families with autistic children are no more or less happy than families in general, and, if they are unhappy, it is not necessarily because of the autism. Autism is a stress, with the same positive and negative potentials as any other stress.

This is really the principle of normalization, taken one step further. Unfortunately, parents are usually so caught up in the difficulties of living with their autistic child (and understandably so) that they come to perceive themselves and the other children as deviant, qualitatively different from the rest of the world. And the professionals with whom they come in contact are usually specialists whose focus is, equally understandably, on the "special" child and his disability. The effect is frequently an exacerbation of the family's difference. This chapter will suggest ways in which the family's potential for normal, healthy development can be enhanced in spite of the presence of an unremitting stress.

OVERALL CONSIDERATIONS

There are three factors that need to be considered regardless of what developmental level the family has reached. Please note: There are no "answers" or even suggestions in this section of the chapter, only things to think about when one is deciding how to help.

The first is the position of the autistic child in the family. First children are always an experiment; when the first child has a developmental disability, the parent may easily conclude that the experiment has failed. Youngest children are often "babied"; when the baby actually does function like a much younger child, the tendency to overprotect, to hold back, is both justified and exacerbated. It may become very hard to separate necessary protection from that which is purely anxiety-based.

Middle children, according to the conventional wisdom, are the most well adjusted. There is no reason to assume that this would not be the most favorable position for an autistic child as well, but it may add to the stress felt by his younger sibs. They will never experience "normal" family life and, because of the unusual amount of attention required by the autistic child, they may not get even the normal attention usually accorded the baby. (If they do, it may mean that the parents have decided to "neglect" the autistic youngster; but that, as we shall see, may be all to the good.)

The second general consideration is the nature of the family itself; some simply have better coping skills, greater tolerance of stress, more resilience than others. Some also have access to more support and help and/or fewer stresses with which to deal. A friend of mine, the mother of eight children (all normal), met another of my friends one evening at a party at our home. Friend number one and her college professor husband were our houseguests for the weekend, so the next morning we had ample opportunity to gossip about the previous night.

Friend number one was sharply critical of friend number two, a fairly well-to-do mother of three very young children, who had apparently made the mistake of discussing how the stresses of motherhood were getting to her. Number one was completely unable to understand or empathize with number two's situation because she seemed to have so much support with relatively little to unnerve her. I was put off by number one's intolerance, but it made me very aware that family demographics don't give a complete picture. Certainly number one's situation was superficially the harder one: more kids (lots more!) and fewer financial resources. But an analysis that stops there fails to take into account the *individual* coping resources of the two very different women involved.

A related concern is the effect of the disabled child on the marriage itself. In the 1970s the Cerebral Palsy Association of Maryland claimed that the divorce rate for couples with a handicapped child was almost double the national average (55% as opposed to 33% overall). Here autism seems to dictate a different result: On the basis of personal observation, I would say the divorce rate among families with an autistic member (at least those I know through NSAC, now the National Society for Children and Adults with Autism) is lower than the national average. In fact, I can think of heroic extremes in the opposite direction. There's an Ohio couple with a severely handicapped adult son. He's *hers,* not theirs; she died recently, but the stepfather is not about to abandon ship. In fact, all along, in spite of his own very serious health problems, he has been a leader in the struggle for human and civil rights for people with autism. I knew them for many years before I found out that the young man was not his biological child.

At the age when they should have been enjoying grandparenthood, a California couple adopted a young child they knew had autism. They, too, have become activists in the field. Someday, some researcher looking for a worthy topic will study the enhancing effects autism has on family strength. He or she will do it, I hope, with the proper respect for and deference to the families it has demolished, but also with the awareness that some of them would have broken anyway, whatever the stress.

I can say from personal experience that autism in the family has made us better parents to all our children, more able to deal with situations that otherwise would have unhinged us. I believe it is a question of perspective: When you, as a parent, are afraid one of your children will never function, the fact that one of your "intact" kids is flunking French *and* math doesn't seem so devastating.

Finally, there is the "autism filter." Perhaps because autism is a low-incidence disorder, the families touched by it sometimes seem to regard themselves as the most put-upon of the suffering. The proper answer to "Why me?"

is "Who else?" We have friends whose children are in jail, wasted on drugs, or lost to them through psychic or physical distance. None of these families have autistic members, but their pain is no less than ours. Autism does not make a family different if sorrow is the differential; we do not love more—or hurt more—because our sorrow springs from a different well. Sometimes we forget that; when we do, we need to be reminded of it—gently.

DEVELOPMENTAL MILESTONES

Up to now, this discussion has been very general because it concerned concepts and considerations that apply over time. But kids, even handicapped kids, and their families develop, and that's what this chapter is really about.

I'm using here the concept of "family" that means heterosexual married couples with children. From that perspective, we can identify four major familial developmental milestones: (1) the birth of a child, especially the first; (2) a child's starting school, particularly significant when that child is first- or last-born; (3) adolescence—of *any* child! and (4) leaving home to begin independent adult life, again most significant when it is the first- or last-born child.

Note that these milestones, while marking the child's life, are equally significant for the family (sometimes more so), and that is the perspective emphasized here. For example, starting school is equally significant for every child in a family, but the day the first child starts school and the day the last child does have a greater impact on the *family* than do the first days of the middle children.

Birth

The first milestone, birth, is regarded as an occasion for congratulations and rejoicing. The stressful aspects are downplayed or ignored, and that is unfortunate because when new parents experience perfectly predictable negative reactions, they then feel guilty and abnormal. Babies are supposed to be all sweetness and light, even when they keep Mommy exhausted and make Daddy jealous. A baby is an intrusion into what was a closed set; the set must expand to accommodate the newcomer, and that requires the kind of change we call growth. Fortunately, the baby grows too: It becomes physically less demanding and develops social behaviors very early, behaviors that reinforce and reward the parents. The parents are thus spurred on to greater efforts, leading to more growth in the child; a positive cycle has been established.

But suppose the baby has autism? Ironically, a lot of what the parents do to show their love and care will be wrong for this baby. For example, hugging and cuddling are considered essential in establishing bonding between parent and child and subsequent healthy emotional development. But for an autistic baby, to whom touch may be neurologically abhorrent, hugging and cuddling may be painful experiences, precipitating, or at least intensifying, the familiar symptom of aversion to being touched. Too, instead of being reinforced by the baby's development, the parents will feel frustrated and even rebuffed by their child's failure to respond or, even worse, by his apparently negative reactions to them. They may try even harder and experience even greater frustrations as a result, or they may eventually give up.

Either way, an antigrowth cycle (for all involved) has been started. If this is a first child, the implications for subsequent children cannot be ignored. One mother of an autistic firstborn put it this way: "It affected all our subsequent parenting. We had to learn the ropes with a defective educational toy." We do learn parenting from our children, and deviant children generate deviancy in their pupils.

Similarly abnormal reactions occur between the new infant and any siblings, but with a different emphasis. The other children will become frustrated and give up sooner with the baby, so that by the time the autistic child is a toddler, he will be excluded from their play as a matter of course. This elective separateness is going to generate further parental concern and reactive behavior. Depending on their own states of mind, the parents will either excuse it or try to change it, worrying that their other children are becoming either selfish or cruel.

The foregoing analysis has been predicted on a very unlikely assumption: identical, or at least harmonious, responses from both parents. Parents' expectation for and attitudes toward their children differ and so, therefore, do their crisis-coping mechanisms. Those are two negatives that do *not*, when combined, yield a positive. Rather, they are another source of frustration and, sooner or later, friction.

Nor is it just the birth itself that precipitates problems. Each developmental milestone in the toddler and preschool years brings new pain and new separateness from the normal world. Everyone is familiar with the somewhat humorous anxieties of the first-time parents if their baby doesn't sit up or talk or feed himself when the baby books or the grandparents or the neighbors say he should. We've all heard the joke about the child who had reached age 5 without ever saying a word. His frantic parents had tried everything without success. Then, one evening at dinner, he said, "This steak is tough!" His excited parents could hardly believe their ears: "You spoke! You can talk! Why haven't you ever said anything until now?" "Because," their son replied, "I didn't have any complaints until now."

That stupid joke has probably been inflicted on every parent of an autistic child sometime during the child's early years. It is meant to be reassuring, offered as such when the parent shares with some friend or family member his or her fears about the child's not talking. But imagine the concern a first-time mother feels when her child doesn't even come close to meeting *any* of the developmental milestones on the pediatrician's chart. She doesn't want jokes, she wants at least one small success to reassure her—and to give her something to brag about at the next neighborhood coffee klatch. She is beginning to feel very isolated from her peers: Her child isn't doing any of the things their children are; their children aren't still screaming all night (if indeed they ever were) or rocking back and forth or presenting any of the other problems her child is. It is beginning to occur to her that something may be wrong with her baby.

There may be no more crucial point in the family development than this one. It is at the point where help is sought that they have taken their first giant step forward: They have admitted that something is wrong. Up to now they have been struggling through the preliminary stages of grief, especially denial. In many ways this first step is similar to the one taken by an alcoholic when she attends her first AA meeting. In admission of the problem lie the seeds of acceptance. In acceptance lie the seeds of growth.

But suppose that, when the alcoholic makes that first brave statement, "My name is Mary Smith and I am an alcoholic," her listeners, other alcoholics to whom she has turned for help, say "Oh, no you're not. You're really just overly concerned. There's nothing wrong with you. Lots of people drink more than you do." The chance for growth will be effectively extinguished. That reaction seems so improbable, yet it happens routinely to parents of developmentally disabled children. The pediatrician, wishing to reassure them, tells them that they are just overanxious parents and that their child is "just a little slow." By now, enlightened professionals have acknowledged the devastating effect this can have on the child's habilitation; I have yet to see or hear much on what it does to the parents.

I cannot stress too heavily how important it is for the professional to acknowledge the problem when the parents seek his help. To do less is to stifle their growth. Even if the pediatrician or teacher or social worker really believes that the kid *is* fine (but "just a little slow"), what real harm will be done by accepting the parents' assessment? At most, they will spend some time and money that they didn't really have to. Their concern is real and, one way or another, it must be attended to.

If the child does have a developmental disability, holistic professional help is needed. Besides appropriate intervention for the child, the parents need services that will make them feel less abnormal and that will reduce the almost inevitable focus on the handicap. They need a source of competent sitters so that they can go out just like their peers—routinely. This becomes even more important as the child grows older, if he still cannot be left alone. Parents of normal teenagers or of adult children do not need sitters; they are free to go out whenever they please. This means that parents of older handicapped children need regular reliable care not just for relief but for normalcy as well.

They will very likely need some short-term reality-based therapy, so they won't feel they have to apologize for their child's existence or make excuses to strangers for his behavior whenever he makes a public appearance.

They need help in managing time for their other children. It is here that parents and professionals, in their zeal to help the child and their enthusiasm for the task, may fall into the trap of "too much." The professional, convinced that there is no habilitation without data, may ask the parent to chart every finger-flick in a 24-hour period. The parent, convinced that somewhere there is a cure, religiously complies. The result is that normal son cannot be driven to his trumpet lesson and normal daughter gets bounced from Brownies because her mother can't take her required turn as assistant troop leader. The parents will be afraid that if they miss a single digital disturbance, the cure will not take—a risk they are not willing to assume. The professional very likely does not realize how literally her directions will be taken, nor does she usually take into account the parenting needs of the normal children. Actually, the parents may need to be told outright that it's perfectly OK to "neglect" their handicapped child from time to time in order to be good parents to their other children (or just to be good to themselves!).

This "neglect" will sometimes produce an unexpected benefit: The autistic child may be forced to develop in order to survive. When Ed was about 3, I was forced to use a local nursery two mornings a week for his care. Although this did not upset him, it was clear that he didn't like it. But after about 2 months there he began to use words to communicate, and eventually the place became such a treat for him that I used it more often. My husband and I are convinced that he realized that he *had* to speak there if he was going to get whatever he wanted or needed (i.e., in order to "survive"). Over the years since, we have observed similar leaps ahead during times when other obligations forced us to cut down on the amount of attention we gave him.

If there are no other children, the parents should be encouraged to have another child. The chances of its being autistic are, we all know, very slight, and I believe the advantages of what will in all probability be a normal experience of parenthood far outweigh any risk. The parents who seem to have the hardest time coping are those whose disabled child is their only child. One such mother, now divorced, told me just recently that she wished she'd had another child. Her son, who has schizophrenia, is almost 20. We agreed that parents who have no normal children are deprived of a very reinforcing element in their lives, one that could make a significant difference in their handicapped child's life as well as in their own. This goes back to what was said earlier about learning parenting from our children; if we get a chance to learn some normal parenting skills, everyone will benefit.

Then too, siblings are great role models and playmates for a handicapped child, who otherwise might not have either. They also act as a brake on the parents' very natural tendency to immerse themselves in the disability. And they have needs flowing from the presence of the disabled child in their lives. They need a chance to talk about their feelings and fears, and they need a role to play in their sibling's life. They can be taught how to play with their handiapped brother or sister, and they need to be reassured that it's all right to get angry at him or be resentful of the amount of attention she gets. (A note of caution here: Participation in a program for siblings may be perceived as just one more sign of the family's abnormality. If so, the idea should be dropped immediately; it can always be offered again at a later time if that seems appropriate.)

Starting School

The second major milestone for kids and parents is starting school. Overall, this development is usually a stress-reliever, particularly for the parent doing the bulk of the child care. It is a little time off each day. However, the new anxieties of "outsiders" evaluating one's child and the child's own vulnerability to outside influences do arise. Put more simply: Any parent will assure you that no child learns cuss words until he goes to school.

These stresses are almost nonexistent if the child is autistic because by now, one hopes, the child has been evaluated several times and the parents have become comfortable with professional reports. As for influences reaching our autistic kids, we are always delighted if *anything* gets through to them! If the parents are lucky enough to have a choice of schools, the decisions they face are not much different from those facing any parent: Each option will have its pluses and minuses to be weighed. Since most of our kids start out in self-contained special programs, the really big decision gets postponed until the child has been in school for a while. That is, of course, the decision about whether to mainstream and, if so, when.

This seems the perfect place to digress a bit and talk about two related problems that occur in normal parenting but that are exacerbated when the child has a disability, particularly one that impairs his judgmental abilities. The first is the "when to protect and when to push" dilemma; as you can see, that has a direct bearing on mainstreaming.

The professionals involved with the family can be of tremendous assistance here, especially if they keep in mind that they're dealing with a problem that every human parent faces. (Animal parents seem to do much better here; mother robins know instinctively when to push the baby birds out of the nest.) By this time in the child's life, virtually everything he does or doesn't do is assessed through what I call the "autism filter," so I suggest that before any decisions are made, that filter be discarded.

For example, Sonny wants to ride his bike to school, but Mom and Dad aren't sure he's ready. Of course, the threshold question is: "Can he ride a bike?'' We needn't even ask if he knows the way; if he's been there once, and if he's autistic, he does. The *crucial* question is: ''If he didn't have a handicap, what would the answer be?'' That is usually the right answer here as well. Parents may have a very hard time accepting this, especially if this is an only or firstborn child. They don't know what is normal for any given age. Professionals can tell them and can reassure them about the rightness of ''letting go'' (or the wisdom of holding on for now, although I think that's much less likely to be a problem). The professional can ask, in a noncritical manner, just what it is that the parents are afraid might happen; when they answer that they're afraid their child might have an accident, the professional should point out that the concern is certainly legitimate, but it's one every parent has about bike-riding.

I don't mean to oversimplify; I think the ''push or protect'' dilemma is one of the toughest we parents face. We face it with all our children, but our autistic children do develop more slowly and do need more protection; however, they also need more pushing. The best thing professionals can do here, besides helping the parents reach a decision, is to point out that it is not so terrible to make a wrong decision. All parents make mistakes with all their kids. Mistakes are nothing to feel guilty about; they are a normal part of the developmental process.

The other digression is closely related; it has to do with helping parents develop realistic goals for their children. That, of course, can cut either way. At one extreme are the parents who are utterly convinced that their child is and always will be totally helpless; at the other are the parents who are sure that, with the right help, the kid will get into Harvard. Although expectations can never be static (I am acquainted with one young man who was mute and putting his head through walls when he was 15 and who now, at 19, is talking a little and holding down a part-time job!), one can help families avoid egregious errors in planning for their child's present and future services. If, at 15, an autistic student is still not reading, it's clearly time to shift gears and set aside academic goals for a more practical program of life skills and vocational training. The parental disappointment that is bound to accompany such a revision is normal, not just in this context but in the overall framework of family life. One of our children decided not to go to college. She has the academic potential but not the interest. Of course, we are disappointed; we think she's making a mistake. *We* would be making an even bigger one, though, if we insisted that she live up to our expectations and tried to coerce her into going.

That disparity between what we want for our children and what our children want for themselves is at the root of our grief. Once we recognize this, it is easier to set sensible goals and to be of real help to our children. When Ed was very young, he was invited to a neighborhood birthday party. Of course, I declined for him; neither he nor the party would have benefited from his presence. But I was not so cool and rational when the day itself arrived. The party, complete with balloons in the trees and a pony ride, was only two houses away—clearly visible and audible from our patio, where Ed was autistically driving his matchbox cars in circles. I looked at him, I looked at the party, and I wept. He seemed to me to be hopelessly outside life. But then I realized the real reason for my tears. Ed wasn't unhappy about missing a party; he was having a perfectly fine afternoon. I was unhappy because he wasn't! In other words, his expectations for himself differed from mine for him. He didn't want for himself what I wanted—not for him as an individual, but for him as a normal, 3-year-old boy. I think I smartened up a lot that afternoon. I realized I would have to adopt as goals for him what would make him happy and fulfilled as he was, not as I wished him to be. (This is not to suggest in any way that no attempt should be made to mitigate the effects of his autism; rather, it is an acknowledgment of his difference, rather like the awareness that has freed black people from their former feeling that they had to straighten their hair.)

I suspect that professionals fall into the same trap, but perhaps to a lesser extent. Let me give you one more illustration that will, I promise, take us back to mainstreaming. After several years in special private programs, Ed moved on to public school. He was placed in a self-contained learning disabilities classroom in a regular neighborhood school. In his third year there (6th grade), he got a brand-new teacher, just out of college and with all the enthusiasm and idealism one would expect. We met with her perodically during the year; nothing that took place in any of those meetings prepared me for the I.E.P. meeting in the spring. I thought he should stay behind and have one more year in elementary school; the teacher and the principal were ready to move him on to junior high. As we discussed the pros and cons of each position, I became more bewildered by the teacher's reluctance to have Ed in her class again. Finally it came out: She thought she had failed him as a teacher; she didn't feel she had done a good, or even adequate, job with him because he wasn't vastly improved. All of us seem to need reminders from time to time that there is no cure for autism.

As to mainstreaming, the question should be when to do it, not whether to (except possibly in the most severe cases). Difficulties arise, not because the child isn't ready but because the school isn't. Here is a fertile field for professional talents. We need inservices for public school teachers; without exception, everyone Ed has had (including the specially trained L.D. teachers) has known absolutely nothing about autism.

Even more important is the development of effective techniques to prepare the regular education students for their new classmates. The most painful and difficult aspect of Ed's transition to public school was the teasing he endured, especially in junior high. I refuse to believe that it cannot be eliminated, or at least greatly reduced. Mainstreaming itself will help: As handicapped youngsters become commonplace in neighborhood schools, they will stand out less and suffer less because of their difference. But the kids who are there now need help now.

I have two specific projects that I'd like to see tried, projects that apply to all disabilities, not just autism. The first, for very young children, would be a Great Books program that included such works as *Dumbo, The Ugly Duckling,* maybe even *Cinderella,* and others that stress the positive aspects of difference, so we could get right to how it feels to be teased. The other idea is more suitable for older students, middle grades on up. Disabled students could themselves be offered the opportunity to make presentations about their disabilities. The setting could be anything from "show and tell" in the classroom to an all-school assembly, complete with a professional speaker as well. The effect would be twofold: The students (and teachers!) would learn something about the various disabilities they're encountering, and the former "goat" would become an expert, a hero in the eyes of his peers.

Adolescence

We have now arrived at the third milestone: adolescence. This is an ulcer-producer for all parents of all kids. Ironically, autism is a sort of saving grace here: Autistic teens don't get stoned, don't get drunk, don't get pregnant (or get someone else pregnant), don't get busted, don't skip school, don't "hang around," don't cruise, don't party—in short, they don't have much fun. Here their abnormality begins to shine forth like some awful beacon, illuminating the future. The older they get, the more different they appear. We have now hit my stage of parenting, and what I want for my son may shock some of you who read this, or at least make you uncomfortable, but I hope you will give it some serious thought nonetheless.

Ed is 17; he would like to have what is called in today's jargon a "meaningful relationship." He would also like very much to have some normal friendships. Eventually, he would like to get married.

Good educational programs have worked academic and behavioral miracles. Now that same creative energy must be turned to solving the next-stage problems. There is a widespread belief that adolescents with autism aren't interested in sexual relationships. Don't you believe it. I've talked to several (my own included) who want to marry or just have a girl- or boyfriend. This is the price, if we can call it that, of getting them moving. The Chinese are said to believe that if you save someone's life, you are responsible for that person forevermore. Our autistic children's lives have been saved; now those lives must be made worthwhile. It is vital that programs to teach normal social interactions be developed—and I mean "normal" as the rest of the world sees it. This is the area for many of us parents where "normal" gets turned 180 degrees. The very things we fear our normal kids will do (at least too soon) we hope our autistic kids will do eventually.

We cannot take false comfort by what has been done in the area of sex education for the mentally handicapped to date. We are now able to teach people with cognitive impairments clinically correct concepts, but not what to do with them. Masturbation is not the solution, at least now when it's suggested as a substitute for the real thing. We—parents and professionals—need to think about how to recognize sexual preference and develop it, how to help an autistic adult develop personal values without simply adopting ours, and, finally, how to impart the skills (social and sexual) that will let him implement those values.

Let me give you some examples. Ed wants to spend free time with his peers but he doesn't know how to get the process started. He recently asked if he could invite some school "friends" (really just people that say "hi" to him in the hall) over to play games (e.g., Monopoly). He's relying on techniques that are no longer age-appropriate. At the same time he's not really ready to participate in the kinds of situations teenagers do, because he still doesn't have spontaneous social skills. He is also very vulnerable to suggestions from peers—he was "set up" more than once in junior high, so of course we worry about what might happen if he did go somewhere with a group.

The boy–girl relationships pose more subtle but equally difficult problems because they are so value-laden. I still believe that premarital chastity is a desirable objective, but I also know that view is, to put it mildly, somewhat outdated. With my three so-called normals this has not created any difficulty. They can accept or reject my values, and we can discuss our differences—and often do. Ed on the other hand, takes everything I say very literally. I suppose I should be grateful, but I do see that as a barrier to his own growth and to normal peer functioning. Perhaps a homosexual relationship would be very satisfying to him; how can that option be presented without either encouraging or discouraging it inappropriately?

Or take the easier case: How does one teach a 17-year-old with autism how to ask a girl for a date? There's so much that precedes the asking, subtle clues that the overture would not be welcome, clues that are totally lost on Ed. He thinks if a girl is friendly, she's interested. So far he's limited his interests to regular education students; that's another hazard of mainstreaming. Quite frankly, I think he'd do better with "one of his own kind" (now I really sound like a throwback), but they don't seem to look as good to him. Or their parents don't allow them to go out with boys.

As our kids continue to improve, more will marry or at least have sexual relationships. We do need to develop *good* sex education for them, including some instruction as to technique. Ed and I have had several good old "birds and bees" sessions, and I can see the inadequacy of that for him. He needs information conveyed by what I'd call a knowledgeable peer. Now there's a program for you: Friend to Friend with a new twist. At a minimum, adolescents can be taught how to handle beer, how to dance, how to interact once a social situation has been set up for them.

Leaving Home

Finally, there's the last milestone of parenthood: leaving home. This is where parental fears and hopes seem greatest—and most conflicting. We want it so badly and we fear disaster so much. The last thing I want is a "Best Boy" (a commercially produced film, based on real life, about a 40-year-old mentally retarded man who still lives with his mother, and his brother's efforts to normalize his life), and I feel fairly certain that Ed will be self-supporting and able to live independently. But I do wonder if he'll be happy. And I worry that some of the more complex areas of day-to-day living (health insurance, for example) may be beyond his competence.

The solution is a good trustee or guardianship program, with the level of intervention and assistance tailored to the individual needs of the enrollees. Parents should be able to enroll a son or daughter for services while the parents are still alive, by paying a monthly or annual fee. If they are satisfied with the program, they could then assure lifetime assistance for their dependent child by leaving money to a trust fund in their will; the amount could be based on the dependent's level of need and the family's resources.

Even with such a system (and appropriate community residential facilities) in place, professionals will still have to deal with parental reluctance to let go. When all else fails to persuade them that the time has come, the greatest professional kindness may be the apparent cruelty of reminding them of their mortality. Their child will in all likelihood outlive them. His or her adjustment to independent adult life is bound to be much easier and happier if it is not irrevocably associated with the loss of his parents. The child's grief at and acceptance of his parents' deaths will be hard enough without adding to it his uprooting from home.

Above all, we must do everything we can as professional or personal friends of the family to prevent parental dependence on the other children to care for their autistic sibling. No child should grow up with that cloud over his head; the effects (and I have seen them) are terrifying. I know a young woman who suffers from the worst case of false cheerfulness that I have ever encountered. Her attitude perfectly reflects her mother's when her mother tells people, in Joanie's presence, that "Joanie loves Peter. We never have to worry about an institution because Joanie is going to take care of Peter when we're gone. Joanie wants to—don't you, sweetie?" One gets a clear sense that Joanie has never been asked directly, in private, what her feelings are. Peter, as you may have surmised, is Joanie's brother and is very severely handicapped by autism.

Brothers and sisters, left to their own filial devices, generally care for and about one another as adults. During John Hinckley's trial for the attempted assassination of President Reagan, his brother and sister both testified that they had discussed with each other their concerns about John and how they might help him—this with no apparent parental prodding. Conversely, forcing a child to care for a sibling can create resentment sufficient to bring about the exact opposite of the desired effect. Finally, one might inquire of the parents who are determined to bequeath this responsibility to a normal child or children: "How do you think you'd have managed if, in addition to Peter, you had a hand-me-down handicapped dependent from *your* parents?"

CONCLUSION

When a family recognizes a child's disability, its members want two things: (1) the child cured—that cannot happen, and someone must tell them so early on; (2) to be made whole again, to be like every other family—we can show them that they are.

6

The Role of the National Society in Working with Families

FRANK WARREN

> We persist because we love our children, they need us desperately and few others are willing to take up the fight. We persist because we fear what the future holds and time is short and barriers are great.
>
> We join together because we are few . . . our energy will someday wane, our supporters are limited, and we must make headway now, while we can.
>
> We strive . . . because we know that the very lives of our children depend on it, and we must make change, for their sake, or they will die unseen, their beauty unappreciated, locked up, unloved and alone. (Warren, 1978, p. 242)

THE NATIONAL SOCIETY AS A FAMILY

The National Society for Children and Adults with Autism (NSAC)* can be understood as a family, with all the shades of meaning, all the positive and negative connotations, all the happiness, elation, boredom, work, responsibility, determination, anger, frustration, and peace that "family" implies.

NSAC (pronounced "en-sac") is the only "family" that 340,000 children and adults with autism have in common. We are they and they are us. We are their parents and their siblings and their teachers, they are our children and our brothers and our sisters and our students. Their blood is in our veins and our lives are joined. Their failures are felt in our dreams, and their successes in our aspirations. We are they and they are us.

*This chapter is written from the author's perspective as both a parent of a grown son with autism and a long-time member of NSAC. It is not presented as an official statement of the society.

FRANK WARREN • Community Services for Autistic Adults and Children, 751 Twinbrook Parkway, Rockville, Maryland 20851.

In 1982 a father in a sparsely populated northwestern state, facing a tragedy of misunderstanding that threatened to strip him of his job, his place in the community, a home for his wife and children, said: "I know one thing. I can turn to NSAC and know I will be understood. I can talk about my son with autism and know that what I say will be heard."

This father, a member of the society, held a position of some stature in a small town. Because his son has autism, and because he undertook a treatment program that was foreign to the community's level of knowledge, his job was put in jeopardy, his motives were mistaken, he was accused of child abuse, and a hate campaign was launched against him.

With a call to NSAC, he received support, peer counseling, and the backing of an array of professionals in the field. He was no longer alone, misunderstood, surrounded by uninformed people passing judgment on him. NSAC members telephoned his employers, contacted the press, talked with professionals in his community, spoke with and encouraged his wife, backed him in his decision to hold his ground, and offered him the advice of legal counsel if needed.

This family learned quickly that the NSAC family cares for and supports its own. The assistance came from the state chapter, the national office, members of the national board, members of the Professional Advisory Board. It was given quickly, unhesitatingly, and effectively.

Using the family analogy, one can think of the National Society in a number of ways.

It can be thought of as a fraternal group. NSAC is a single-member organization, all the members are equal, and each shares the common purpose—dedication to the education and welfare of children and adults with autism. Each member, then becomes as a brother or sister to each other member, linked, if not by blood, by common purpose.

The society may also be considered as an extended family. NSAC has, in 1983, 167 chapters and state societies across the country. The purposes of the chapters are the same as the purposes of NSAC as a whole.

1. To promote the general welfare of autistic children and adults at home, in the community, in institutions, and in public, private, and religious schools.
2. To further the advancement of all ameliorative and preventive study, research, therapy, care, and cure of autistic children and adults.
3. To develop a better understanding of the problems of children and adults with autism.
4. To promote the education, training, and recreation of autistic persons and to foster the development of integrated care in their behalf.
5. To promote the establishment of adequate diagnostic, therapeutic, educational, and recreational facilities for persons with autism.

6. To further the training and education of parents and professional personnel for training, educating, and caring for people with autism.
7. To encourage the formation of parent groups, to advise and aid parents in the solution of their problems with autistic offspring, and to coordinate the efforts and activities of these groups.
8. To serve as a clearinghouse for gathering and disseminating information regarding autism.
9. To solicit and receive funds for the accomplishment of the above purposes (NSAC, 1981a).

The function of a local chapter is to bring together those who care about autistic children and adults, so that they may address the purposes of NSAC in the area where they live. I have seen parents weep with relief at their first chapter meeting, when, for the first time in their lives, they met others with the same problems, the same frustrations, the same pleasures. One thing that often confuses untrained professionals is the humor that parents of autistic children find in their children. The humor, from a parent's point of view, is understandable. The options, when considered, often demand it!

NSAC local chapters are charged with advocating for change, with creating understanding of autism in their communities, and with helping families with autistic children meet the day-to-day challenges that they all face.

Continuing the "family" analogy, the governing body of NSAC, its board of directors, is elected by the general membership and is charged with setting policy for the organization and assuring that NSAC staff and chapters pursue society goals. The board can be viewed as the parallel of a family council—not a paternalistic body but a democratic council, drawing its authority from the general membership that elects the board at meetings held each year.

NSAC persists for the love of the children and adults with autism, who must have their "family" to survive.

The following relates the history of NSAC, describes its functions and that of the NSAC Information and Referral Service (NSAC-IRS), looks at how siblings are beginning to fit into the society, and discusses advocacy as viewed and practiced by the society and its members. The chapter concludes with a look at the challenges NSAC faces in the future.

A HISTORICAL SUMMARY

"We persist because we fear what the future holds and time is short and barriers are great."

The National Society for Autistic Children was founded because parents of children with autism knew that many things closely affecting their lives were terribly wrong, they recognized that change had to be made, and they believed that by joining together they could work more effectively to bring about the needed changes.

First, the parents who founded NSAC knew that their children needed help, that no one understood what was wrong with them, and that leadership in all the helping professions were blaming the parents for their children's disability— scapegoating them, to use the view that Dr. Eric Schopler advanced in the early 1970s (Schopler, 1971). Naturally the parents were angry. Naturally the fledgling society was a highly charged and scrappy organization.

Dr. Bernard Rimland, a psychologist and the parent of an autistic son, Mark, published *Infantile Autism* in 1964. This book challenged the prevailing thought regarding autism and advanced the theory that autism is an organic disability, not a severe emotional disturbance caused by poor parenting.

The effect of this work on parents who read it, or who heard about it through the media, was electrifying. Rimland's book had been reviewed at length over a 2-week period in a nationally syndicated health column, and hundreds of parents had written to him. Behavior modification with autistic children, as used by Dr. Ivar Lovaas, was the subject of a feature in *Life* magazine in early 1965. Lovaas shared the letters he received with Rimland, and together they became a resource for launching NSAC. Ruth Sullivan, later to become the first elected president of NSAC, saw a television program about an autistic boy and recognized characteristics of her son, Joseph. She called the writer, Robert Crean, of New York, and he put her in touch with Rimland.

What was to become the organizational meeting of NSAC was organized by Rimland and Sullivan. The meeting was held in the home of Herbert and Rosalyn Kahn of Teaneck, New Jersey on November 14, 1965 (Warren, Note 1).

Rimland was acting chairperson. Dr. Mary Goodwin of Cooperstown, New York, who had done work with autistic children using a device called a "talking typewriter," was guest speaker. Rimland gave parents lists of things to do with their children. Some 60 persons, most from New York and New Jersey, but some from Boston, were present.

"We fell on each other," recalls Sullivan. "It was heady. For the first time we had hope." Most of the parents had never met one another—or any other parent of an autistic child. "It was the most electrifying meeting I have ever been to in my life" (Sullivan, Note 2).

The meeting began at 8:00 P.M. and lasted until midnight. When it was over, NSAC was a reality. The name was selected from the British society of the same name, which had begun 2 years earlier. Later, the society's symbol, a child's face with jigsaw puzzle pieces superimposed upon it, was adopted. This, too, was modeled after the British logo but is a bit different. A design using the autistic son of Duke and Helen Rosenberg of Texas as the model was approved by NSAC (NSAC, 1968).

To some, the logo projects a constant state of confusion over the nature of the disability ("autism is puzzling" was once a slogan) and thus tends to prevent the clear expression of knowledge about autism that does exist.

During the four hour meeting in Teaneck, the group (1) decided to be a national organization, (2) selected a name, (3) adopted purposes that were later incorporated in the society's charter, (4) decided to publish a newsletter for members, and (5) decided to appoint a Professional Advisory Board.

Moosa Grant of suburban Washington was first president of NSAC; Dr. Campbell Goodwin was first chair of the Professional Advisory Board, and within the first few months chapters of NSAC were organized in Cooperstown, Albany, Poughkeepsie, New York City (in that order), and later in California, Virginia, Georgia, North Carolina, Missouri, and Texas. NSAC currently has chapters in nearly every state of the union.

The NSAC *Newsletter,* now called the *Advocate,* published every 2 months, was, for many years, the only source of general information about autism available to families with autistic children. It reached out to isolated families and let them know that they were not alone. It was considered a model newsletter for parents of handicapped children (Neimark, Note 3).

MAJOR EVENTS IN THE HISTORY OF NSAC

- *1965:* NSAC was founded in Teaneck, New Jersey, and was chartered as a nonprofit organization under the laws of the District of Columbia.
- *1966:* NSAC was represented on the Advisory Committee to the Joint Commission on the Mental Health of Children.
- *1968:* The first general election of officers and board members was held.
- *1969:* NSAC held its first national conference in Washington, D.C. The society's bookstore was started.
- *1970:* The NSAC Information and Referral Service (NSAC-IRS) was established. The *Journal of Autism and Childhood Schizophrenia* (now the *Journal of Autism and Developmental Disorders*) was founded.
- *1971:* NSAC began an annual survey of facilities serving children and adults with autism. The society's North Carolina Chapter was instrumental in the founding of the first statewide program for autistic children, Division TEACCH, offering education to autistic children in public schools.
- *1972:* Annual observance of National Autistic Children's Week was begun.
- *1973:* NSAC was represented on the National Advisory Council for Developmental Disabilities.

- *1974:* The research project that resulted in publication of *The Autistic Syndromes,* by Mary Coleman, M.D., was facilitated by the society at its annual meeting and conference in Washington.
- *1975:* Autism was included by specific mention, in the definition of developmental disabilities; persons with autism were thus entitled to benefits under the Developmental Disabilities Act. Public Law 94-142, requiring a "free, appropriate, public education" for all handicapped children, including those with autism, was enacted. The society adopted a functional definition of autism developed by Eric Schopler, Ph.D., as second chairman of the Professional Advisory Board.
- *1976:* The North Carolina chapter of NSAC established the first community-based residence for severely handicapped youth with autism, the Triad Home in Greensboro, North Carolina. NSAC also began its ongoing autopsy project for the study of brain tissue.
- *1977:* NSAC's board of directors adopted the Definition of the Syndrome of Autism developed by Edward R. Ritvo, M.D., and B. J. Freeman, Ph.D., modified and approved by the NSAC Professional Advisory Board.
- *1978:* NSAC's national office moved from Albany, New York, to Washington, D.C.
- *1979:* The society consolidated its Information and Referral Service,

Table I. Historical Data about NSAC

Year	National office location	President	Individual dues	N of chapters	Conference site
1966	Washington, DC	M. Grant (DC)	$5		NA
1967	Washington, DC	M. Grant (DC)	$5		NA
1968	Albany, NY	R. Sullivan (NY)	$5		NA
1969	"	R. Sullivan (NY)	$5		Washington, DC
1970	"	C. Griffith (GA)	$5	63	San Francisco
1971	"	C. Griffith (GA)	$5	70	Nashville
1972	"	R. Miller (CA)	$5	67	Flint, MI
1973	"	L. Wheeler (TX)	$10	76	St. Louis
1974	"	M. Akerley (MD)	$10	81	Washington, DC
1975	"	J. Kyne (CA)	$10	84	San Diego
1976	"	H. Lapin (CA)	$10	105	Chicago
1977	"	E. McClelland (MO)	$15	106	Orlando
1978	Washington, DC	E. McClelland (MO)	$15	157	Dallas
1979	Washington, DC	R. Fredricks (CA)	$15	154	San Jose
1980	Washington, DC	D. Nacewicz (MD)	$15	160	Washington, DC
1981	Washington, DC	D. Nacewicz (MD)	$15	157	Boston
1982	Washington, DC	S. Baumann (FL)	$15	167	Omaha

which had operated from Huntington, West Virginia, since 1970, with the new Washington office.

- *1980:* The society cooperated with the U.S. Office of Education in conducting an "Invisible College on Autism," which resulted in publication of *Critical Issues in Educating Handicapped Children and Youth,* currently distributed by NSAC. The NSAC definition of autism is reflected in the *Diagnostic and Statistical Manual* of the American Psychiatric Association (DSM III).
- *1981:* The U.S. Department of Education removed autism from the category of "severe emotional disturbance" in the regulations of Public Law 94-142, The Education of All Handicapped Children Act. The society held its first international conference on autism in Boston.
- *1982:* The U.S. Department of Education funded the NSAC National Personnel Training Project (NSAC-NPT) for 3 years. The society's 5-year project to establish a section on autism in the National Institute of Neurological and Communicative Disorders and Stroke (NINCDS), a part of the National Institutes of Health (NIH), was completed. Martha Bridge Denckla, M.D., was appointed chief of the new section.

Some Historical Data

The growth of NSAC can be charted by the number of chapters in operation at a given time. Early data on chapters are incomplete, since the society did not have a formal chartering system until about 1970. NSAC listed parent groups in Canada until 1973, when the society decided not to charter chapters outside the United States. Table I provides more historical data about NSAC.

NSAC AND HOW IT FUNCTIONS

"We join together because we are few . . . our energy will someday wane, our supporters are limited, and we must make headway now, while we can."

NSAC presents itself as an organization of people who help each other with the problems of autism, not as a bureacracy established to provide services. NSAC is a national self-help group, not an organization of people who support a service delivery system.

NSAC is made up of parents, family members, teachers, researchers, psychologists, psychiatrists, agency representatives—people of all sorts who are interested in autism. In recent years NSAC membership has also included people with autism. While there is currently no comprehensive breakdown of members by category such as "parents" or "teachers," NSAC began, in 1982, keeping computerized records in this manner. It is projected that NSAC membership is 80% parent/family, 15% teacher, and 5% other professional based on several months' membership recruitment and renewal records.

If this proves true, it means that NSAC rolls include 4800 parent/family members, 900 teachers, and 300 other professionals. Thus, the great bulk of NSAC membership is made up of parents and family members.

There are three major ways in which parents and families of people with autism learn about NSAC and what it offers: (1) contact with local chapters, (2) Contact with the NSAC Information and Referral Service, and (3) attendance at the NSAC annual meeting and conference.

Local Chapters

NSAC local chapters, as mentioned, are charged with the responsibility of carrying out the purposes of NSAC in the areas they represent.

A chapter may be chartered by the society with as few as 10 members—but no less. Membership of less than 10 in a local chapter places that chapter in jeopardy of losing its status, and the charter can be removed. Chapter memberships range from 10 to 200 members, with an average of 40 members at present.

As a practical matter, NSAC is more interested in promoting chapter activities—advocacy for individuals with autism and their families, dissemination of information on autism, publication of a chapter newsletter, promotion of appropriate service delivery through monitoring programs and lobbying for funding of good programs—than in keeping watch over local chapter membership (though it does all of these). Chapters that develop annual plans, including systematic efforts to reach and involve parents in their area, have been shown to grow in size and effectiveness.

Service Delivery by Chapters

NSAC chapters, in order to participate in the Combined Federal Campaign (a coordinated solicitation plan for government employees governed by federal regulations), must provide "real and meaningful" services in their locality. For NSAC, this means information and referral, the dissemination of information, a newsletter, parent and family support through regular meetings, organized advocacy work, and the promotion of appropriate public education and human services. Chapters have much latitude in determining their "real and meaningful" services.

An NSAC bylaws amendment, effective July 1, 1977, prohibits NSAC chapters from providing "an on-going direct service program having paid staff," such as a school, group home, or residential facility, unless that chapter sets up a separate corporate entity to operate such a program. Chapters are not prohibited from having paid staff to carry out information and referral, advocacy, and other chapter activity, as described earlier.

Information and Referral Service

Parents and families often come into contact with NSAC through the NSAC Information and Referral Service (NSAC-IRS). The NSAC-IRS was established in 1970 and operated from the Huntington, West Virginia, home of Ruth Sullivan from 1970 until 1973, when it received federal funding and could afford its own office. The NSAC-IRS moved to Washington, and its activities were consolidated with the national office, in 1979.

The NSAC-IRS concept is simple. Any parent—or any person with a question about autism—may contact the IRS. If the answer is available, it is given immediately. If information is not readily available, the query is referred to another source, often a member of the Professional Advisory Board or, depending on the nature of the request, a different agency for action. If IRS staff receive numerous questions on a subject, an information packet is prepared and kept on file.

A network of individuals across the country feeds the IRS information for dissemination, and periodicals are scanned for new data.

Requests made to the NSAC-IRS range from questions about education programs to appeals for help in dealing with a school system or a human service agency. Nearly every imaginable query regarding autism has been, at some time, posed to the NSAC-IRS. Here are some examples.

- An Ithaca, New York, mother appealed to NSAC-IRS to help her get her child admitted to school. He had been excluded for over a year.
- A mother in Florida needed help in getting her son out of jail. He had been picked up by police and charged with a narcotics violation.
- A professional in Japan sought information about programs for autistic children in the United States and about professionals who could be invited to speak in Japan.
- A father in Argentina sought an appropriate program for his son in the Washington area.
- A young woman with autism wanted help in finding a job (NSAC hired her in the national office).
- A California mother sought advice about residential placement.

- A Virginia mother, whose 3-year-old had just been diagnosed, thought she could call NSAC and hear a tape recording on autism. Instead, she found the sympathetic ear of another parent and a support group near her home.
- A family called from a motel in Birmingham, Alabama, seeking an NSAC contact in Huntsville. They received it.

Calls and letters arrive daily and are answered and logged by NSAC staff. By far the most numerous requests are from students who receive prepackaged information, including lists of books to look up in libraries or to order from the NSAC bookstore.

NSAC Annual Meeting and Conference

The late Dr. Carl Fenichel, director of the League School in Brooklyn, attended the first annual meeting and conference of NSAC in Washington, D.C. He said: "As a veteran of almost two decades of meetings all over this country . . . I found this one to be by far the most productive, exciting and memorable one I have ever attended. I was deeply moved and impressed by the people as well as the program. The dedication, enthusiasm, total involvement and interaction of the parents and professionals was a rare and heartening experience that I would love to see replicated elsewhere. . . ."

The 1969 NSAC conference was different from most meetings on handicapped children at that time. It was not organized or attended by professionals alone. It was a serious scientific meeting put together by a coalition of parents and professionals interacting on an equal footing, with the parents acting as coordinators and the professionals as resources.

NSAC conferences from that time onward have attempted to maintain that theme. Conferences have been held in every part of the country, from San Francisco to Boston, from Nashville to Omaha, from Orlando to San Jose, from Flint, Michigan, to Dallas. In every case, NSAC parents have organized, orchestrated, and carried out the conferences.

In the mid-1970s NSAC began to promote regional conferences for people who lived too far from annual conference sites. Regional conferences are held under the auspices of NSAC, and local chapters bid to host them. Three or four regional conferences are held each year, with attendance ranging from 150 to 800 persons.

Parents attend the annual and regional conferences to learn more about autism, and new developments in the field, and for the opportunity to meet and speak with people who are engaged in exciting new work—either in the form of research findings or in services and education for persons with autism. Many families bring their children—both autistic and nonautistic. The society provides child care services at the annual meetings—and most regional meetings—for handicapped and nonhandicapped children. The cost is kept at a minimum, as a matter of policy. In addition, many members attend the annual meeting especially for the annual membership meeting of NSAC, at which time elections are held and important issues resolved.

The society attempts to hold its conferences in locations that will attract the most interested persons, will be as inexpensive as possible, for parents, and will provide an opportunity for parents to enjoy new experiences—since many parents have little opportunity to "get away" during the year.

A bound book of *Proceedings* is produced each year from papers presented at the annual meeting and conference. These have been published each year since 1969. The 1981 International Conference on Autism in Boston resulted in a 350-page volume including over 100 presentations. Major presentations were reproduced at some length, while concurrent presentations were summarized. The *Proceedings* included names, professional credits, and list areas of interest of scores of investigators and service providers, both those who presented and those who were considered for inclusion, as a resource for parents and professionals.

Practically every major event in the field of autism, or services to persons with autism, has been heralded by a presentation at the annual meeting and conference of NSAC. The first meeting in 1969 featured Dr. Leo Kanner, who described autism in 1943 and who is recognized as the person who first brought this disability to public attention.

Parents who had read Dr. Kanner's work were swept with a sense of relief and a renewed feeling of self-worth when they heard him say to the general session of that 1969 meeting: "Because I reported some characteristics of some parents . . . I have been misquoted. . . . Those of you who have come to me know . . . I never said 'parents did it.' I hereby acquit you people as parents."

And they fairly leapt to their feet with applause when he referred to Bettelheim's *The Empty Fortress* as "the empty book."

The concept of parents as cotherapists with their children (Schopler and Reichler, 1971), the group home movement (Lovaas, 1977; Sloan and Dossett, 1977), deinstitutionalization and the concept of normalization (Dussault, 1980; Gold, 1979; Krug, 1980; NSAC, 1981b; Solnit, 1977), the criterion of ultimate functioning (Donnellan and Brown, Note 4), advocacy for public education of autistic children (Gilhool, 1974; Schopler, 1980), assessment for the purpose of meeting direct needs (Reichler, 1980; Donnellan and Brown, Note 4), megavitamin therapy (Rimland, 1979), the role of protection and advocacy systems and how to use them—all have found a forum for discussion and dissemination at annual NSAC meetings.

NSAC and Siblings

NSAC, as a formal organization, has not paid a great deal of attention to the brothers and sisters of autistic children over the years, though several efforts have been made to provide an organized way for them to meet each other, learn, and advocate.

In the early 1970s a youth society was formed and functioned for a few years. In 1981 a Siblings Committee was established, beginning its work with money collected by passing the hat at the 1981 awards banquet in Boston. The chair of that committee was Laura Prieser of Maryland, who, with members of her committee set up a network of siblings across the country. The committee has produced a booklet of writing by brothers and sisters of autistic children and adults, and other material for distribution to siblings. The booklet is available through the NSAC national office.

At the 1983 NSAC Executive Committee meeting, a formal study of siblings was authorized to be conducted in cooperation with investigators at Johns Hopkins University and the Siblings Committee.

Parents of children with autism have been urged in the past to institutionalize their handicapped offspring because professionals felt that "normal" children were placed in a position of neglect, since so much of the parents' attention was demanded by the handicapped child. Few studies, however, have been done to determine what, if any, effect an autistic child has on his or her brothers and sisters.

NSAC parents, as a rule, reject the "neglect" notion and adopt the attitude that their autistic child's brothers and sisters experience valuable growth as a result of living with their autistic sibling.

NSAC provides siblings with the opportunity for peer support, wider involvement in advocacy efforts for persons with autism, and a chance to learn about new developments through NSAC chapters, conferences, the Information and Referral Service, and the Siblings Committee. In 1981 NSAC employed a sibling, Ken Laureys, as assistant to the Government Affairs Office. At this writing, Laureys is also staff to the Siblings Committee.

ADVOCACY

"We strive . . . because we know that the very lives of our children depend on it, and we must make change, for their sake, or they will die unseen, their beauty unappreciated, locked up, unloved and alone."

Advocacy, taken to its Latin roots, means simply "to speak for." In legal terms, advocacy is what an attorney is paid to do for his or her client, the implication being that the client needs the superior knowledge or ability of the lawyer to gain some particular goal.

While the attorney client relationship is important for the understanding of advocacy, it carries with it a "we–they" connotation. NSAC is, as the name implies, a society of people who dedicate themselves to certain purposes, and who, together, advocate for people with autism. NSAC is not a separate group apart from parents, which advocates for them and their children. The society works for change that will allow persons with autism to realize their own goals, as best they can be understood, and NSAC historically has asserted that parents of autistic offspring are the persons with the highest degree of investment in the lives of persons with autism, understand their own children better than anyone, and are, therefore, most able to understand the personal goals of their offspring and to translate that understanding into policies guiding the operations of the society. That is partially the reason NSAC has never has more than two non-parents at a time as members of its governing board.

The NSAC–parent relationship does not parallel the attorney–client relationship. It is not a "we/they" relationship, it is "us." While the formal operations of the organization requires that certain functions be specialized, and that form be followed, the relationship between NSAC and the person with autism is more like that of parent–child.

The Advocacy Bureaucracy

When the child advocacy movement began in the 1960s, NSAC did not jump on the bandwagon for two reasons: (1) The child advocacy movement appeared to be promulgated by mental health professionals who seemed to concentrate on problems in the parent–child relationship; and (2) NSAC parents, because of the early notion that "refrigerator mothers" and "concentration camp families" caused autism, naturally resisted all professionals who seemed to devalue the parent's positive role in the lives of their children.

An NSAC spokesman, in a formal statement to the Joint Commission on the Mental Health of Children in 1968 (Warren, Note 1), took sharp issue with the concept of child advocacy, stating: "If I have a toothache, I don't need someone to tell me I need a dentist—I just need a dentist!" In other words, don't give us professional advocates, just give us good programs—we'll advocate for ourselves.

The commission did not acknowledge the NSAC statement and did not mention it in its final report (Sullivan, Note 2). This report led to the formalization of child advocacy efforts within government structure. In later years NSAC received funding from agencies growing out of the commission study in order to publish a handbook on facilities serving persons with autism.

In spite of disagreements with the formulators of the child advocacy movement, NSAC has, at all levels, functioned as a strong advocate for handicapped children and adults. For example:

1. NSAC participates as a member of the Consortium Concerned with Developmental Disabilities (CCDD), made up of major national organizations such as United Cerebral Palsy Associations (UCPA), Association for Retarded Citizens (ARC), Epilepsy Foundation of America (EFA), and has played an active role in the passage and protection of PL 94-142, the Education for All Handicapped Children Act; the Developmental Disabilities Act; and a variety of housing, Social Security, vocational rehabilitation, transportation, education, and budgetary issues before Congress each session since 1973.

2. NSAC advocates caused autism to be recognized as a developmental disability in the federal definition adopted in 1975. Later, as part of the effort to broaden the definition to include other disabled children and adults, NSAC stood with the noncategorical definition that was adopted by a slim margin in 1978 (Akerley, 1979).

3. NSAC members have played and continue to play an active role on boards of directors of state developmental disabilities councils, protection and advocacy systems, and other advocacy agencies. In Washington state the founder and first president of the Washington chapter heads the state's advocacy agency, Troubleshooters, Inc. Emma McClelland, past NSAC president from St. Louis, was elected secretary of the National Association of Developmental Disabilities Councils in 1982. No data are available on the number of NSAC members holding leadership positions in advocacy agencies, but the perception of the national office is that it is significant.

4. The NSAC Information and Referral Service staff provides advice and counseling by phone to parents seeking advocacy strategies

Advocacy as a Matter of Policy

Advocacy became the official policy of the society in 1977, though it had been practiced from the beginning. In 1977 the membership approved a bylaws change acknowledging that "a major purpose of each chapter and state society is to advocate on behalf of autistic persons," and directed that chapters no longer operate direct service programs, but advocate for their development (NSAC, 1981a).

It was not until 1980 that the society decided under what policy programs should be developed. At the board of directors' meeting in 1980 a resolution was offered and passed that set off 12 months of heated debate and resulted in the society's Community Policy Resolution, which was finally approved in July 1981. The resolution is reproduced on p. 114.

THE WORK AHEAD

NSAC's challenges in the years ahead were presented in a succinct manner by Richard S. Nacewicz, NSAC president from 1980 through 1982. He said:

> The decade of the 1980s presents many barriers to the achievement of a free, public education for all of our children, vocational training for our youth, homes and jobs for our young men and women. And the causes and remediation of autism remain an elusive goal for the research we support and the investigators we encourage.
>
> The following examples show, in brief, the challenge of our work ahead:
> * Custodial institutions still wait for the majority of adults with autism when their parents die—though technology to serve them better exists. Community support systems are fragmented, disorganized or non-existent.
> * Families still pay, in time, money, frustration and legal battles; for the education which is provided free to others; and to which our children are entitled under law.
> * Approximately 30 community living arrangements, such as group homes and supervised apartments, serve a tiny fraction of the 200,000 adults in need.
> * Reserach grants to investigators in our field are few and far between. Autism, unlike cancer, heart disease and scores of other disabling conditions, is accorded a fragment of the funds, both government and otherwise, that serious research must have.
> * And families still suffer needlessly from a lack of professional assistance and understanding—a situation that can only be resolved through education.
>
> It is the work of the National Society to solve these problems and overcome these barriers. It is our single-minded purpose to cause change that will benefit this most needy population. And we will pursue this purpose with all the resources . . . we can muster. (Nacewicz, 1980)

Suz Baumann, elected to her first term as NSAC president in 1982, addressed parents of autistic persons in a paper delivered in Alexandria, Virginia, in April of 1983:

> NSAC says to parents: Listen. You are not alone. There are thousands of us like you, who face the same problems, who love our children the same as you love yours; who understand what you face, who share your hopes, your dreams, your anger and your sorrow; who will stand with you and will support you, and together we shall bring change for you and your children—for all of us and our autistic offspring, both children and adults. We have accomplished much through the intensity of parental interest, and the dedication of those professionals who understand the disability. We will continue this intense work, as long as one autistic child goes without schooling, and as long as one adult with this disability is alone, isolated from help and appropriate care, in desperation and despair. NSAC shall not give up. NSAC shall persist. (Baumann, Note 5)

COMMUNITY POLICY RESOLUTION

In order to develop, learn, grow and live as fully as possible, persons with autism and other handicapping conditions require access to services which allow for comprehensive, systematic, and chronological age appropriate interactions with persons without identified handicaps. Such interactions can best occur in domestic living, educational, vocational, recreational and leisure environments.

Specifically, handicapped individuals should: 1) participate in family-like or other normal, community-based domestic living environments; 2) receive educational services in chronological, age appropriate, regular educational environments; 3) receive training in and access to a wide variety of vocational environments and opportunities regardless of functioning level; and 4) participate in a wide range of normal recreational and leisure environments and activities that involve persons without identified handicaps.

NSAC believes that the above conditions can best be met by providing quality community-based services. Therefore, be it resolved that NSAC will work toward the rapid but responsible termination of living environments that separate, regiment and isolate people from the individual attention and sustained normal community interactions necessary for maximum growth, development and the enjoyment of life.

Adopted July, 1980
NSAC Board of Directors

Addendum July, 1981
This resolution:
• Emphatically affirms the intention of this nation, its people and their government to assure the human, civil and constitutional rights of *all* of its citizens, including those with autism and other handicapping conditions. This policy on human dignity is a reaffirmation of these civil, human and constitutional rights.
• Recognizes the wide range of needs of people with autism and recognizes the corresponding range of options required to match those needs.
• Encourages quality services which offer the lifestyle choices enjoyed by all other local community members. This is the meaning and the intent of community-based services. These services shall be developed appropriate to the needs of each individual person with autism.
• Recognizes their need for individualized programs, to be carried out in the least restrictive setting, optimally in a regular domestic living, educational, vocational, recreational and leisure environment.
• Community-based technology exists now, offering quality individualized services appropriate for people with autism in less restrictive settings, and such services must be expanded. Thus, where equal or better, community-based services shall be the programs of choice. The responsible termination of unnecessarily restrictive alternatives requires the availability of these more appropriate options in the community.

From the *Advocate*, Vol. 13, No. 4, page 7, July, 1981.

REFERENCE NOTES

1. Warren, F. *NSAC, the mouse that roared.* Unpublished manuscript, 1977.
2. Sullivan, R. Personal communication, summer 1977.
3. Neimark, S. Personal communication, summer 1977.
4. Donnellan, A., and Brown, L. *Development of educational curricula which meet the criterion of ultimate functioning.* Paper presented at the International Conference on Autism, Boston, 1981.
5. Baumann, S. *Purpose and function of NSAC, the National Society for Children and Adults with Autism.* Unpublished manuscript, April 1983.

REFERENCES

Akerley, M. NSAC, its future within the system. *Proceedings of the National Society for Autistic Children,* 1979, 98–110.

Dussault, W. L. E. Implementing PL 94-142 and Section 504 of the Rehabilitation Act of 1973 to acquire services. *Proceedings of the National Society for Autistic Children,* 1980, 23–46.

Gilhool, T. Autistic children, their right to free public education. *Proceedings of the National Society for Autistic Children,* 1974, 124–132.

Gold, M. Preparing for a meaningful adult life. *Proceedings of the National Society for Autistic Children,* 1979, 35–42.

Krug, D. Severely autistic adolescents in a normal high school setting. *Proceedings of the National Society for Autistic Children,* 1980, 63–80.

Lovaas, O. I. Teaching homes, an alternative to institutionalization. *Proceedings of the National Society for Autistic Children,* 1977, 29–30.

Nacewicz, R. S. Message from the president. *Annual report of the National Society for Children and Adults with Autism,* 1980, 2.

NSAC. *Minutes of the NSAC Board of Directors,* September 13, 1968.

NSAC. *By-laws of the National Society for Autistic Children, Inc., operating as NSAC, the National Society for Children and Adults with Autism,* 1981. (a)

NSAC. Community policy resolution. *Advocate,* 1981, *13*(4), 7. (b)

Reichler, R. J. Diagnosis and its implications. *Proceedings of the National Society for Autistic Children,* 1980, 95–110.

Rimland, B. *Infantile autism.* Englewood Cliffs, N.J.: Prentice-Hall, 1964.

Rimland, B. Update of research on the use of B-15. *Proceedings of the National Society for Autistic Children,* 1979, 111–133.

Schopler, E. Parents of psychotic children as scapegoats. *Journal of Contemporary Psychotherapy,* 1971, *4*(1), 17–22.

Schopler, E. Implementing the mandate for appropriate education of autistic children. *Proceedings of the National Society for Autistic Children,* 1980, 115–132.

Schopler, E., and Reichler, R. J. Parents as cotherapists in the treatment of psychotic children. *Journal of Autism and Childhood Schizophrenia,* 1971, *1*, 87–102.

Sloan, J. L., and Dossett, B. Recent program developments and efforts to establish community-based group homes. *Proceedings of the National Society for Autistic Children,* 1977, 87–120.

Solnit, A. J. Changes in the meaning of handicapped children's rights in a changing world. *Proceedings of the National Society for Autistic Children,* 1977, 74–86.

Warren, F. The child as victim. *Journal of Autism and Childhood Schizophrenia,* 1978, 10, 240–242.

7

The Professional's Role as Advocate

SIEGFRIED M. PUESCHEL and JAMES C. BERNIER

INTRODUCTION

We live in a culture that places great value on individual achievement and ingenuity. Throughout our lives we are educated to develop our potential without emotional or professional support. Indeed, to experience a need for such support often provokes a vague sense of guilt or shame, even if our need is legitimate or beyond our control. Nothing illustrates this emphasis on self-reliance more dramatically than having a disabled child.

Whatever the disability, this one fact changes a family's life and somehow places it outside the network of normal expectations. The very nature of being disabled implies that one is incapable of participating in the mainstream. There are countless testimonies of individuals who are physically disabled, but keenly perceptive, that indicate they feel a pervasive devaluation of them as persons because of their difference and increased needs (Zola, 1982). Many persons with serious mental handicaps are not able to experience this devaluation, but their families are highly aware of the prejudice. Being a parent in such a situation may be extremely difficult, not only because of the multitude of emotional and psychological issues to deal with but because at times one must make demands on a system that is not designed to meet the child's special needs. The child's problem is, after all, the parent's problem, and placing new demands on the system makes the process of advocacy a daily reality.

As professionals in an agency designed to serve developmentally disabled children, we have become increasingly aware of our need to provide parents with appropriate advocacy assistance in many situations. Parents may experience deep

SIEGFRIED M. PUESCHEL and JAMES C. BERNIER • Child Development Center, Rhode Island Hospital, Providence, Rhode Island 02902.

satisfaction with services provided in the community, yet be critically aware of their dependence on the providers for guidance. Moreover, they must look to professionals to help them attain the services they need and to plead their cause. At such times professionals who are knowledgeable of local resources and responsibilities will be of great importance. Also, parents will look toward such persons as experts to assist them in developing and gaining access to new programs, in designing new approaches, and in cultivating public awareness. All of these are aspects of advocacy.

The Professional's Role

Although it is true that advocacy is an important service that must be provided, it is also true that for most professionals it is not a central element in their daily work. Because of heavy work load and limited time, it is often difficult for them to intervene in many of the areas in which the families might need help. One can offer guidance but most of the actual contact, exertion, and effort that advocacy requires must be made by the parents. Though it may be necessary for a professional to intervene personally, most often a family with the proper guidance can be as effective, and perhaps more effective, in obtaining necessary changes, at least for the more common situations. By training the parents in proper methods, the professional can in a practical and more consistent fashion participate in the advocacy process in a variety of ways. This training is what we perceive as the professional's central role in advocating for a disabled individual.

A MULTILEVEL APPROACH TO ADVOCACY

Autism is an ongoing problem, and conflicts are bound to arise over such issues as proper modes of management and the responsibilities for service provision. Therefore, advocacy and advocacy training are, of necessity, an integral part of longitudinal management. This is a multilevel process, one that penetrates the various strata of the autistic child's life. The person who views advocacy as a narrow function, which deals only with "an unwieldy public machine" or in developing "public awareness," misses the more important underpinnings of parental education, counseling, and support. In a sense, all dealings with families of autistic children should proceed in a manner that strengthens service delivery, whether it is speaking with a family on behalf of the child or addressing the public sector to provide what is necessary.

It is important to remember that the most successful advocacy takes place in the milieu of a parent–professional partnership. Maximum outcome depends on a partnership that seeks to obtain what is best for the child and his family.

We will outline the elements of a successful parent–professional interface during the initial stages of diagnosis and in this way hope to address the core of the advocacy process, while at the same time respecting the infinite variation in circumstance and context. In addition, we will discuss the advocacy process in several aspects of the child's life. Particular attention will be paid to securing medical and educational services. Also, the role of the advocate in determining the appropiateness of an educational program will be considered. Since eligibility for various assistance often depends on technical information, we will dwell on the necessity of investigating specific agency policy requirements in order to secure services. Finally, some suggestions will be offered in providing counseling for future needs. All this can be done only in general terms, for as Buscaglia (1975) points out, ''Since each agency may vary in its function, procedures, and eligibility requirements from regional to county to state to federal programs, it is difficult to be specific regarding service information.''

Advocacy during the Initial Phase

Perhaps at no other time in a family's development is the need for professional multilevel intervention so important as during the initial phase of discovery, diagnosis, and entry into the service system. This stage also illustrates how education and counseling are an ongoing part of the advocacy process.

This early experience can be profoundly disorienting as parents struggle to deal with their own emotions and insecurities, while seeking to come to terms with the very practical issues of management, which sets the tone for future action. In most cases, the family is not familiar with autism, nor are they familiar with issues relating to special education and specialized services. It is quite easy for the professional to forget that this may be totally new to the parents and that they are in a state of bewilderment and confusion. Until this time they may have known that something was wrong but were not really prepared to understand or accept the depth of their child's problem. Perhaps the parents had hoped that whatever was wrong would eventually be outgrown or that it represented a transient phase in the development of an otherwise healthy youngster. In most cases, parents are able to see only in retrospect that the child's development was deviant at an earlier point than when they initially experienced concern.

Sartre (1956) said: ''Before a child is born, even before he is conceived, his parents have decided who he will be.'' Whether we accept this statement or not, it does point to a fundamental fact in parenthood. Each of us has a set of expectations for our children, some of them conscious and others hidden. Under normal circumstances, these expectations are refined, abandoned, or modified in a gradual manner. Though this is not necessarily a painless process, it is a common experience for parents in our culture.

Discovering that your child is autistic or has some kind of developmental disability is another matter. However the parents choose to adapt, the central fact is that their expectations for their child need to be radically altered. Though they may not express it, one may expect that the parents will experience an intense loss, the loss of the "normal child" they anticipated raising. Further, because their own emotional life is so woven into their children's, one can expect that they will experience at least a temporary loss of self-esteem, which may be expressed in an undermined sense of self-confidence, confusion, fear, and other manifestations. In some, a sense of hopelessness and despair may prevail during the initial phase of adjustment.

Informing Interviews

Parents tend to remember well the time when they were given "the bad news." Highly critical or casual comments made at this time may have an indelible impact. Anyone familiar with the field of developmental disabilities rapidly accumulates a repertoire of tales concerning mishandled informing interviews. In the wake of such an experience, the parents' ability to come to terms with the child and his handicap is seriously affected.

Even if handled expertly and compassionately, this first encounter is a difficult task. It sets the tone for how the family will view the child and his prospects, and how the "newly disabled family" will present itself to the community. It is in this sense that we say that the professional advocates for the child and his family by preparing the family so that the family itself can better pursue the child's needs.

During this initial stage, it is important to present the relevant information in simple, though accurate, terms. Any attempt to "spare the parents' feelings" by presenting a less than realistic representation of the facts ultimately serves to subvert creditability. In addition, it can be a disservice to the child by increasing the likelihood of inappropriate intervention on his behalf.

By dealing with the issues in a sensitive though direct manner, the professional serves as a model for necessary parental behaviors. Handled well, this phase enables the parent and the professional to form a partnership that will be a foundation for future mutual efforts. This relationship is critical if they are to work together effectively in their approach to the child. In most cases, parents are looking for honest answers and opinions, though they may be quite difficult to give as well as to receive. However grim the findings, most parents do have the internal resources to survive if they are presented in a sensitive, empathic manner.

We have found that though they may be initially distressed, the families return to where they have heard an honest response, even if an answer was uncertain. Such treatment conveys a basic trust in them as parents and as decision-makers. The association that develops from such interaction enables the parents to effectively advocate for the child as well as to know when they can most benefit from professional intervention because they have been able to explore the parameters of their own individual competencies. Then, knowing that they bear the brunt of responsibilities in procuring services, the family can turn to the professional in confidence for support and aid in navigating the sea of opinions, layers of bureaucracy, and divisions of responsibility that they are inevitably going to face.

During this initial encounter, it is important that the professional gives hope in a situation that appears hopeless. He is in a unique position to help the parents to a positive beginning, and in doing so he should attempt to mobilize existing parental strengths. If the professional's positive attitude and sincere involvement in the care for this child prevails, the parents will sense that he is interested in their child as a human being.

Parents often assimilate only part of the information provided to them during the initial counseling session. It is therefore paramount that follow-up sessions be scheduled to communicate more details to them when they can cope better and can ask more realistic questions. They will be concerned about many aspects of the future of their autistic child. While the professionals cannot predict the future, they can inform parents of the significant changes in society's attitudes that have taken place over the past years. While a few decades ago most children with autism were institutionalized, today society recognizes the need for appropriate services for handicapped children in the community. In addition, progress in the biomedical and behavioral sciences made during the past 20 years, renewed research efforts, attempts to improve educational opportunities, and a somewhat better informed society will provide encouragement and a more positive outlook into the future. These changes will affect the parents' attitudes and coping abilities.

The initial phase should also be a time to prepare parents for possible differences of opinion in evaluators. For example, some facilities apply the label of autism only when strict Kannerian criteria are met, while others are more current in their usage. Treatment philosophies may differ too. Though most facilities now use behavioral principles, their emphasis on reinforcement of punishment as a means of shaping or extinguishing behavior may vary. Therefore, some advance preparation will be helpful in getting the parents past this confusing period. In our own setting, this responsibility is assumed by a patient coordinator. In other situations, individual evaluators may have to shoulder this responsibility when they judge it appropriate.

Securing Medical Services

When discussing with the parents the medical findings of their child, it is important that the professional not only enumerates the pathological findings but also emphasizes that this is first and foremost a child in need of nurturance and care. Usually, the child with autism does not have any significant abnormal physical features and his respiratory, cardiac, gastrointestinal, genitourinary, and musculoskeletal systems are usually unaffected. On occasion, ophthalmologic and auditory dysfunctions may require consultations with specialists. At times, when an autistic child is suspected to have a seizure disorder, neurological evaluation, electroencephalographic studies, and other laboratory procedures might be indicated. Appropriate treatment and follow-up should be forthcoming if the child has been identified to have a definite seizure disorder. Hence, it is the professional's role to advocate for appropriate care and management.

Moreover, the autistic child, as any other child, will need routine health maintenance by a pediatrician who is willing and able to provide care for a developmentally disabled child. The child will need regular checkups, immunizations, and other preventive health measures as well as treatment when ill. Another necessary service is regular dental examinations by a dentist capable of handling children with autism.

Some parents may be dissatisfied with the results of an evaluation and may look for a ''cure'' for their child. While understanding for such action can be offered, ''shopping around'' in search for the ''cure'' should be discouraged. However, there is no reason why parents should not obtain a second opinion by a qualified provider. When a true trust relationship between parents and professionals exists, parents are then less likely to engage in unnecessary and costly false-hopes-evoking endeavors. We have found that parents gravitate toward programs that project the most confidence and not necessarily one that matches the needs of the individual child.

Securing Educational Services

Once it has been determined that a child is autistic and the parents have been informed, the next important matter is obtaining appropriate educational and other services. With the advent of early intervention programs and of Public Law 94-142 as well as other legislation dealing with education for the handicapped, educational placement is often less difficult than in the past. Nevertheless, for a family in crisis and unaccustomed to looking for special services, placement is a difficult task.

Advocating for Early Placement

When the child is below 3 years of age, we recommend that he be enrolled in an early intervention program, since the reports from the literature on early intervention indicate that the child's behavior and rate of learning can be modified by early competent management and training (Simeonsson, Cooper, and Scheiner, 1982). Specifically, early intervention will attempt to enhance an autistic infant's sensory-motor and social development. It is agreed today that it is the quality rather than the sum of total stimulation that shapes the mental and behavioral development of the young autistic child. It is therefore the structure and the content of a stimulation program that should be emphasized rather than the indiscriminate use of nonspecific stimuli. Frequently, for autistic children, a combination of strong visual, auditory, and tactile stimulation has to be used to elicit adequate responses. The most important aspect of any early intervention program is to respond positively to those reactions that show that the autistic infant has engaged in some activity resulting in a new learning experience. Even unimpressive and slow progress may ultimately add up to a point where it will make a difference in the capacity to cope better with a number of tasks that most children with autism are able to learn. Thus, it is of importance that the professional recommends enrollment in an early intervention program. In addition, the parents may foster their child's development at home by applying the same techniques of stimulation that the professionals use.

Just as early intervention programs enhance the development of the child with autism, nursery school is a most appropriate adjunct to a family's daily efforts to care for their autistic child. Both the autistic child and his family often need the extra reinforcement that can come from nursery school. Here, social interaction, discipline, working on self-help skills, improving gross and fine motor coordination, and learning to live with all types of behavior are essential components. Furthermore, learning to play is one of the most valuable skills a child can acquire in nursery school, as play is a natural means of growth and learning. Again, sensory stimulation is of most significance in that the child will learn to feel, touch, taste, smell, listen, and see. The acquisition of self-help skills including toilet training, dressing, feeding, and personal hygienic measures is emphasized. Nursery school can open a new world for the autistic child and his family. For parents, it is important to see their child functioning out of the home. The few hours taken up by the child's attendance at the nursery school allows the mother time to perform other tasks or to pursue her own interests. Therefore, advocating for appropriate nursery school experience is the professional's obligation.

Concerning the school years, parents and teachers frequently ask, "Is the child ready to enter school?" Perhaps the real question should be "Is the school ready for the child?" Since many of the developmental functions one would expect of the normal child are not usually observed in the child with autism when he enters school, the educational program will have to be adapted to his ability and special needs. Therefore, we do have to ask, "Does his school provide all the elements necessary to educate a youngster with autism? Is the teacher ready to learn about the child's problem in order to help him most effectively?'' And finally, ''Will the educational program assist the student in preparing him for life?'' Hence, the professional should follow the child's progress in school and represent his interests and needs at various stages during the educational process.

Role of Advocate in Determining Appropriateness of Educational Services

In the event that appropriate services are not readily available, the professional's role as advocate includes assisting the parents in obtaining proper educational services and in determining which options best address their specific needs. Parents should be made aware that not all professionals will view their child's needs or diagnosis in precisely the same fashion. Some professionals may indicate to parents the hopelessness in autism. Many such professionals previously recommended institutionalization, and there still are a few who may do so today. They are often uninformed of the unavailability of institutional placement as well as its detrimental effect upon the child. Others may view education of an autistic child as wasted time and effort. Most professionals, however, will be more knowledgeable and will exhibit a more positive attitude. They will advise parents appropriately and will attempt to secure educational services for the child according to his needs.

Financial and programmatic constraints in the local school system as well as a lack of federal funding sources can also lead to inappropriate placement. We are all aware of school systems that test the limits of our patience by placing children inappropriately because there happens to be a convenient space in an existing classroom. For example, a local administration recently wanted to place an autistic child in a classroom for the deaf. The primary rationale, other than the obvious financial considerations, was that the autistic child's problem was primarily a communication deficit! Fortunately, such obvious mismanagement was dealt with rather easily. This incident does illustrate, however, that all parties have vested interests that cannot be ignored. As uncomfortable as it may make us, we must often address the fact that the interests of our colleagues (teachers, physicians, psychologists) will influence what they offer. This can create contingencies in which we must step in and actively support the parents in obtaining the appropriate services, as parents may not be cognizant of these more ''political'' issues.

It is more common, however, to encounter a system that tries to meet the child's needs but has financial constraints that prohibit full compliance. In addition, the child's needs may be perceived differently and for that reason may alter the recommendations in a significant way. For example, a common predicament we have faced is the offer to place autistic children in special education classes programmed to meet the needs of mentally retarded children. Parents understandably can be confused and upset by this, feeling that their child is not receiving a suitable education. However, experience has led us to look at the details of the offer, because essential elements of what we consider to be proper management may be present. If, for instance, a class for the mentally retarded is behaviorally based, is suitably individualized, has an acceptable home training component, and has specialized language and socialization services, it may be adequate for certain children with autism. In fact, such a circumstance can provide the opportunity to redirect the family's attention from the diagnosis to the substance of effective programming. This, in turn, lays a foundation for a well-directed future advocacy effort by the parents because it educates them about what is essential for the child. This is the fundamental function of the professional's advocacy: to train the parents to be their child's advocate by teaching them how to discern what is more suitable in the education of the autistic person. When the parents have a better focus on their child's needs, their advocacy is more credible and more likely to be successful.

An inherent danger in this, of course, is the temptation to concentrate on what is pragmatic or obtainable to the detriment of what is possible or desirable. To a local school system, practicality is a measure of budgetary, personnel, and organizational concerns; to the parents, it is a measure of how well a particular program meets their own and their child's needs. Zola (1982) points out: "Is there a country elsewhere in the world where the statement 'Let's be practical' is the hallmark of so much thinking? As a result there is a push to focus more on the practical possibilities of our limitations, than the unknown potentialities of our strengths." Striking the balance should be our goal.

Proper Agency Definitions in Effective Advocacy

As professionals we are all aware of instances in which a specific diagnostic description is necessary in order to engage a delivery system. An appropriately worded description is a very practical service that can greatly assist a family in obtaining help for their child. For example, using the types of information various bureaucracies need for determining eligibility could mean the difference between acceptance and rejection. Often, the aid offered by agencies is limited by policies that are outdated or phrased in a way that restricts eligibility beyond the intent of the law or regulatory statutes. In such cases, there are often "buzz words" or detailed descriptions of the circumstances of eligibility that, if provided, will result in an adverse decision.

As an example, for several months we had been referring children to the local Social Security Administration to apply for Supplemental Security Income. From what we could determine, the family met the financial criteria and the children met the disability requirements and thus they should have been accepted. Frequently, however, the applicants were found ineligible. We invited some representatives of this program to a conference at our facility and asked them whether new policies had been implemented of which we were unaware. In addition, we needed to assess our understanding of some basic policy issues. What emerged from this meeting illustrates the difficulties we are seeking to illuminate. We learned that the regulations require a score on certain standardized tests as a measure of intelligence. We, however, are primarily concerned with functional assessment and de-emphasize IQ scores. Therefore, we did not provide such scores. As a result, many of our patients had been declared ineligible. Once we were aware of the problem, we could take some corrective measures.

Another issue regarding the same problem was the type of medical information we had been furnishing. It was our custom to send our most recent medical notes on some of our handicapped individuals. At times, statements such as "the patient appears healthy and is making good progress" would be included in the dictation. Those assertions were made in the context of previous evaluations that had extensively delineated the areas of deficiency. Taken out of context, they were seen as indicating little or no involvement. The program in question desired a more elaborate description of our patient, focusing on the disability, while the clinic reports emphasized aspects of growth in areas of competence on which skills could be built. Accordingly, it was necessary to supply the type of information the Social Security office requires in order to advocate effectively for our autistic children.

The specific instances cited above are not isolated cases. We have been baffled by the inconsistency of response on the part of many public agencies (educational, welfare, medical) in this regard. While it is difficult to stay current with policies and legislation in these many fields, an interdisciplinary team facilitates coping with this. For example, a social worker is more likely to be aware of welfare regulations or state funding for items such as residential care. On the other hand, a special education consultant is more familiar with educational policies. It is also advisable to keep in touch with those knowledgeable persons who have coped successfully with the system so that they can be called upon when assistance is needed.

COUNSELING FOR FUTURE NEEDS

Long-term follow-up of each child includes review of the child's interim accomplishments and his difficulties, as well as reevaluation of the child's present functioning with regard to his strengths and weaknesses. On the basis of the data gained from a regular review, a program for medical management and education can be developed. This will often result in changes of advocacy for the child. Parents will have to know of improved services and new developments in the field so that they can be the most effective advocate for their child.

At times the family may be in need of support services. Counseling by social workers, psychologists, or other professionals can help families to cope more effectively. Another service concerns temporary or part-time respite care. Such assistance is designed to relieve family members of the continued burden of providing special care for a child who may be disruptive to "normal" family life. Increasing stress situations thus can be alleviated and parents will be able to pursue leisure activities, take a vacation, or just rest and relax.

Beyond respite care, there are other services that can provide relief to parents at times when they are in need of assistance. Special babysitter services and homemakers are available in many communities to parents with severely handicapped children. Even if parents can leave home and stressful circumstances for only a few hours while a responsible babysitter cares for their autistic child, this will allow the parent to have some "breathing space." While homemaker services may be expensive, they will permit mothers of autistic children to get away from routine home duties, meet friends, and pursue special activities of interest. Such services supporting family integrity will also prevent residential placement of the child with autism.

Another area of advocacy relates to the recommendations of recreational services for the autistic child. Such services can be planned or spontaneous. They can be carried out alone or with others. In summertime, after-school activities or enrollment in a camp may provide recreational outlets for the child. During such leisure-time recreation, parents themselves again will find time to relax.

Adolescence is frequently a challenging time in life for both the young person with autism and his family. While this is often a troublesome period for those of normal intellectual abilities, an autistic adolescent may not possess the capabilities to cope with the demands either of his environment or of his own desire for independence. Many parents are apprehensive about their child being exposed to the risks and responsibilities of growing up and becoming more independent. One factor interfering with the autistic adolescent's independence is parents' and society's tendency to look upon the autistic individual as an "eternal child." Again, the professional involved in follow-up care for the autistic youngster will be guiding the parents and will be an advocate for the adolescent child.

As the person with autism grows older, he will at some time become involved in vocational activities. He will need to be carefully evaluated in a prevocational assessment with respect to his abilities, interests, and social skills. The primary goal of the work experience of an autistic person is not to help him develop specific vocational skills but rather to enable him to attain the good work habits and interpersonal skills necessary to maintain a job, whether it is in a sheltered workshop or in private industry. Cooperation between the public school and the vocational rehabilitation agencies and sheltered workshops is a prerequisite for developing a good vocational program for the individual with autism.

Once the autistic child becomes an adult, different needs may become apparent. As with our other children, there will be a time when he will leave home. Current programming interest has focused primarily on young handicapped children, and there has been little emphasis on the adult with developmental disabilities. There is, however, a growing concern, especially for autistic individuals who live in the community, to provide them with appropriate living arrangements, recreation, and social interactions. In planning community living for the adult with autism, one will have to define the individual needs and then see whether the community is able to meet these needs.

Thus, professionals have an important role as advocates not only in the early phase after the diagnosis has been established but also in longitudinal follow-up when reevaluation requires redefinition of needs. The professional will have to be available throughout the autistic individual's life to represent his emerging interests and needs.

REFERENCES

Buscaglia, L. *The disabled and their parents*. Thorofare, N.J.: Charles B. Slack, 1975.

Sartre, J. P. *Being and nothingness*. New York: Philosophical Library, 1956.

Simeonsson, R. J., Cooper, D. H., and Scheiner, A. P. A review and analysis of the effectiveness of early intervention programs. *Pediatrics*, 1982, *69*(5), 635–641.

Zola, I. K. Denial of emotional needs to people with handicaps. *Archives of Physical Medicine and Rehabilitation*, 1982, *63*, 53–67.

8

Advocacy
Effectively Changing
the System

JAMES E. SURRATT

The need to influence policymakers' decisions on behalf of autistic persons is made more difficult and critical by the low incidence of the condition and by its great severity. Policymakers, whether elected or appointed, local, state, or national, can make life bearable or unbearable for autistic persons and their families. Their failure to provide appropriate help may allow the destruction of families having an autistic person and create even greater obligations for our society. Therefore, effective advocacy techniques are essential to ensure appropriate policy making.

I have served in unusual concomitant roles as the father of an autistic child, superintendent of a school system, teacher of the handicapped, and advocate for handicapped persons. The growth of my son—now 14 years old—has paralleled my career as a school superintendent in North Carolina. I have seen both sides of the issues when advocates have worked to change policy in service areas such as education, and I am convinced that advocates often fail to follow some essential steps that can successfully change the service system.

I have served as president of the North Carolina Society for Autistic Adults and Children (NCSAAC) and as a member of the state board of directors for the Association for Retarded Citizens. At present, I am serving as state chairperson for the Developmental Disabilities Council. Being the parent of an autistic child is a trying role. The school superintendency is one of the most challenging and strenuous roles in which a person can serve. Carrying out these two roles simultaneously has required an efficiency in getting assistance for my son that has led

---

JAMES E. SURRATT • Burlington City Schools, Burlington, North Carolina 27215.

me to some techniques for advocacy. Seeing issues from the roles of both service provider and advocate has helped me to see what successful advocacy entails.

Autistic persons may represent only a small percentage of the populace, but they have far-reaching problems. Those who care for the handicapped are energy-drained by these problems; nevertheless, they must also try to become an effective force to secure help from policymakers at the local, state, and national levels. The basic question is: "How do you shape the commitments of a board, a commission, or a legislature?" One cannot wait until sometime in the future for these policymakers to "come around." Without advocacy, there is no reason for them to change.

Laws and regulations are made by a great many public officials at different levels. At the national level, legislative actions, executive orders, and judicial rulings are all dominant sources of law under which those serving autistic persons must operate. Parallel organs of authority exist at the state and local levels. A governor can set the thermostat for 68 degrees at state institutions by executive order, and unless his actions conflict with actions at a higher level of authority, they will stand. There are also state court decisions and state legislative actions that affect us. Policy or "law" is made by boards of education, superintendents, principals, and teachers. A mayor or chairman of the county commissioners can make policies in emergencies. Even a teacher or a group home parent who decides that children will not chew gum is making "law."

An effective organization of parents and professionals needs to begin at the local level and extend its influence to the state and national levels. With the low incidence of autism and wide geographic differences between persons wanting to affect policy for autistic persons, efficiency in communication is essential. In this chapter, I will summarize the most important principles my experience has taught me for achieving advocacy group effectiveness. They include the following:

1. Recognize that policymakers want to help.
2. Get involved with the selection of policymakers.
3. Work through the legal structure.
4. Know what is wanted.
5. Know what can be done.
6. Document what is needed.
7. Work through channels.
8. Show that what you want is consistent with the philosophy of the policy board.
9. Demonstrate a need for a position.
10. Organize the extended family.
11. Utilize a professional support group.
12. Use existing rights sparingly.

The program for the Treatment and Education of Autistic and related Communication Handicapped Children, Division TEACCH at the University of North

Carolina at Chapel Hill (described in Chapter 4), has demonstrated the feasibility of training parents as cotherapists for their own autistic children. The program was developed on the assumption that the parents understand and care for their children more than anyone else. The TEACCH model has helped parents to become very knowledgeable, not only about their own children but about the entire field of autism as well. Armed with good information, the parents, who are obliged to be their children's best advocates, have become a significant political force in policy formation in North Carolina. The steps to effective advocacy discussed in this chapter are largely an outgrowth of my experience as both a parent and a professional.

RECOGNIZE THAT MOST POLICYMAKERS WANT TO HELP

Often, advocates for exceptional children make mistakes in working with policy-makers that result from their own misconceptions about the motivations of policy-makers. Some argue that public officials seek only political and financial gain. In his study of school boards, however, Marlowe (1979) found that most school board members were responsible persons positively involved with the needs of others. We need to recognize that most policymakers do want to help.

As an advocate and a superintendent, my experience has been that most public officials genuinely feel they can do something beneficial for autistic persons. They are responsive to needs when proper information is available to them. The feeling that officials serve for selfish purposes is counterproductive to good advocacy. Asking, "Why?" rather than saying, "Thank you," when help is offered may also be detrimental to the efforts of others. Recognizing that leaders really want to help may be the single most important factor in the effective representation of autistic persons.

In working to get state support for group homes and for the five regional centers of TEACCH in North Carolina, and in testifying about needs in legislative hearings, I have found that most legislators and other policymakers have a rather limited understanding of autism. They respond favorably, however, if approached in a friendly manner, and they can be helped to see that they have the power to improve the lives of autistic persons. Advocates, by simply attending meetings and hearings and volunteering to serve on study committees, not only impart information but also help policymakers become acquainted with autistic persons and their special needs.

GET INVOLVED IN THE SELECTION OF POLICYMAKERS

An effective way to work with policymakers is to become involved with their election or selection. Being aware of and active in the political process is as important as anything you can do to affect policy for handicapped people. Elected officials must allocate limited public funds to meet societal needs. They are not likely to recognize the needs of autistic persons from personal or staff research, but an effective advocate can help them learn about autism through personal involvement in their campaigns. An effective advocate can also promote the candidacy of parents, professionals, or other persons knowledgeable about autistic persons.

Involvement indicates not only time but often money as well. A contribution of only $10 to $25 may mean a great deal to a candidate running for public office. The sum of money probably will not, in actuality, make a real difference, but it can serve as a form of affirmation and a sign of support. Politicians, for the most part, are genuinely motivated by that kind of affirmation from their constituents, and it is very important (if you think they are the right persons) that you make at least a small donation. Better yet, ask the "right" person to run. Many office-seekers run because someone patted them on the back and said, "You know, I think you would be a super senator!" When the person becomes a candidate, offer your support through both time and money.

WORK THROUGH THE LEGAL STRUCTURE

An obvious way to change policy is to initiate or amend existing legislation. Because changes at the national level are often slow and laborious, advocates for exceptional children will realize results more rapidly when their efforts are focused at the state level. Dorothy Smith (1979) writes that the ordinary citizen can influence state legislators. She points out that when legislators know they can trust you, that you are a person of integrity, and that you are knowledgeable, you can have significant impact on changing an existing program or initiating a new program or policy.

Involvement in the process of making laws should never cease for advocates. The original need for a law changes. Researchers may point out additional needs for autistic persons. Laws may need to be amended to reflect changes. Demographic or technological changes may require new legislation. Even in times of adverse political climate, efforts must be made to protect existing legislation from alteration. The process is continuous and the efforts made by a person or group today establish a course for the future.

In 1972 four or five people in North Carolina were concerned because transportation to Division TEACCH did not exist. (The parents of a child who lived in Greensboro, North Carolina, for instance, would have to transport that child 90 miles each day for treatment.) That small number of concerned people decided that someone ought to help with transportation for such children. Since their problem preceded the enactment of PL 94-142, there was no legal obligation whatsoever for either the state or local school systems to transport TEACCH participants. Although there were less than a half dozen adults involved, they truly believed that they could get legislation passed to provide transportation for those children. They promoted their cause in the state legislature and were successful in getting a bill enacted over the objection, in some cases, of both the educational and the human services bureaucracy. The bill was called Transportation for Autistic and Communication Handicapped Children and Deaf and Blind. Deaf and blind children were added to the bill by state officials to broaden the coverage provided by the legislators. But the important thing is that a small number of people got the bill passed—they did not take anyone to dinner, they did not have a "coffee klatch" in their homes, and they did not pass money to anyone. The legislation was passed because they were trusted by enough lawmakers who understood that they were advocates with integrity and knowledge.

An earlier example of the benefits of lobbying occurred in 1972, when Division TEACCH came into being in North Carolina. Parents of autistic children brought about the statewide program—again, in advance of PL 94-142. A group of parents actually took their children to the General Assembly and onto the floor of the House of Representatives. Legislators had an opportunity to meet the children and to see just how desperate was the need for help. It was a significant event in the lives of the legislators and in the lives of those families in terms of securing services for autistic children. It was not an unpleasant or unsavory demonstration for the parents, but it did require a lot of emotional strength. As a parent of a handicapped child, I know how difficult it is to "use" one's child to get services for autistic children. But fortunately, there are many who have been, and are, willing to do so.

As a result of the actions of those parents in 1972, there are now five regional centers serving autistic persons in North Carolina. Dr. Eric Schopler founded TEACCH in the state, and, as he envisioned, the TEACCH centers work in cooperation with the public school systems. Each school system employs the teachers working in the programs, but TEACCH contracts with the school system for the initial training and continuing staff development services for the teachers. Because most college programs do not include training in teaching autistic children, these TEACCH services are critical. Other legislative victories, accomplished through parents' efforts, include the establishment of a summer camping program for autistic children.

Another avenue to use in working through the legal structure at the state level is to secure the help of influential people. It is vitally important to establish a good relationship with the governor as early as possible because he is important in policymaking in the state. Key governmental officials and business and civic leaders who become committed to the advocacy cause are also important. To educate the public, we must first catch their attention. Popular public figures can acquaint the general population with the needs of autistic persons with a broader coverage than can advocates alone. In North Carolina we have had the help of country music stars such as Conway Twitty, Crash Craddock, and Bill Anderson. Race-car drivers and some of the Harlem Globetrotters have also provided their support.

The advantages of involving other people is twofold: (1) You receive their support and/or money for programs, and (2) you catch the attention of a lot of people who before knew nothing about autism.

Another fact that should not be overlooked is that parents can really accomplish more in the political arena than can professionals, mainly because parents (unlike professionals) are allowed to make mistakes. They are not bound by the same rules and regulations as, for example, a superintendent of schools who wants to keep his job.

KNOW WHAT YOU WANT

The fourth area is knowing what you want from policymakers. Knowing what the problem is will not suffice; you must also have an idea about how to solve the problem. If you seek the help and obtain the attention of a public official—whether he or she is a school board member, a superintendent, the mayor, a legislator, or the governor—but you do not know what you want him or her to do, then chances are their doors will not open to you again. On the other hand, if you know what you want you are likely to elicit a positive response from public officials because they recognize that the parent, as an advocate, has thought through the problem and has some definite direction.

As a superintendent, I have rarely had a person or group call on me to represent a cause who really had a suggested solution to the problem they wanted to discuss. I doubt my experience to be drastically different from that of other public officials. As an advocate, I may seek counseling in many places, but when I call on policymakers, I need a suggested remedy for my concern. If at all possible, I should have a copy of my suggestion in writing to leave at the conclusion of the conference. A written statement not only serves as a reminder to the person called on but also gives me a chance to verify my comments through documentation and provides an opportunity to show how my request may fit into a total plan.

Group homes for autistic persons were established in North Carolina because of the actions of a few parents who knew what they wanted. The parents prepared a list of names of autistic children who were in desperate need of services—children who needed to be in a residential setting. Then they asked for a meeting with a top official in the state in the area of mental retardation. During that meeting, they produced the list of names of autistic children from throughout North Carolina. The parents said, ''It's nice to talk about all the wonderful things we're going to do for autistic children, but would you agree with us to put a degree of accountability in it? The parents of the children on this list have said they need services. Would you meet with us on an annual basis and tell us of the progress made on developing placements for these children? Just these, not all those others. Not those in Florida or California or Illinois. We want to know about these 25 in North Carolina.'' Funds for several group homes for the autistic were allocated soon after the meeting.

The technique these parents used is a powerful one. They gave names and expected some definite accountability for services for specific individuals over a year's time—not generalities and not statistics about autistic children, but needed services for named children. From that one meeting, three new group homes were started. Obviously, there are many ways to work through the legal structure to effect positive policy changes.

KNOW WHAT CAN BE DONE

The fifth factor is a correlate of the fourth—know what *can* be done. Some may argue that those seeking help do not need to know what can be done, that the solutions are the responsibility of public officials. On the contrary, if you want to be successful in getting help for a special child, you *do* need to know monetary capabilities and limitations. Do not ask people for money they do not have or for programs they cannot produce. It does not hurt to let these policymakers know what you want in the future, but in the present, you should ask only for what you believe they can realistically achieve.

Be careful not to lose sight of possibilities. I toured Alcatraz a few years ago. The prison was closed in 1963, at which time the cost per prisoner for 1 year was $30,000. Accounting for inflation, I calculate that the 1963 figure would now exceed $95,000. Such comparisons may be beneficial in determining what can be done by society to serve autistic persons. A public official can understand that the $95,000 could provide residential services for 3 autistic persons or could effectively educate 10 autistic children. A policymaker should easily see that autism is not self-inflicted and that persons having autism deserve as much public funding as does a prisoner. If you conduct appropriate research on costs for programs in your state, you can acquire ample evidence to persuade public officials to set aside comparable funding allocations for the aid of the autistic person.

DOCUMENT WHAT IS NEEDED

I would advise any parent or guardian of an autistic person to keep a written record of every conference, every evaluation, and every conversation with officials concerning that person. Such documentation is the greatest weapon there is to ensure that inconsistencies are not allowed to exist and that the bureaucracy is held accountable for what happens to the individual involved. If residential placement is required, documentation that such placement is beneficial is especially important, since documentation may very well lead to the official position that the person "*must* be served" with residential placement rather than "*may* be served." I am aware of more than one case in which good documentation and the services of an attorney have resulted in residential placement when the service agencies had stated that it could not be provided.

The individualized education programs (IEPs) that are currently required under regulations for education give a great deal of strength to parents and guardians in seeing that appropriate educational programs are in place. Furthermore, they require the education providers to deal with what parents perceive to be their children's educational needs. Since most autistic persons are mentally retarded and have multiple handicaps, the documentation of the labels and stated service needs from school, day care, and vocational rehabilitation officials can serve as a vehicle for accessing those services that are provided for most other handicaps.

Good documentation is essential not only by individuals but also by groups. An advocacy group that documents promises over the years is in an effective position to bring about improvements in service. Such documentation should include a composite of needs as identified by members, in addition to the records of the interaction of the group leadership with public officials.

WORK THROUGH CHANNELS

To accomplish anything effectively, you must learn to work through existing channels. Documentation of the efforts made through the channels is important. Some individuals have lost everything because they did not exhaust all administrative remedies.

First, you need to know what the channels are. If there is a problem with a child, you must begin with the teacher, and then with the principal, followed by the director of special education. If the school system is a large one, there may be a few more channels to go through, but basically these are the steps to take before you approach the superintendent and the board of education. You must work through these channels at the local level first. Failure to do so will only delay a just presentation of your cause. Going through channels is sometimes designated in law (PL 94-142, for example), and a cause may be lost if steps are not pursued in sequence.

There are some other reasons for following appropriate channels. Even the most empathetic professionals may have a bit of emotional reaction if they are left out of a decision-making process when they have expected to be involved. In my experience in working with principals, I have found that a principal becomes upset when someone calls me to complain before he or she calls the principal. That procedure is ineffective. If problems are not resolved at the first level, *then* you proceed to the next level, armed with better answers to questions raised at the first level. In addition, you will have a cool reception from an official at a higher level if lower level administrators have not been involved.

Failure to use the appropriate channels promotes doom from the beginning and allows those with whom you are negotiating to evade the issue and deal with the process followed rather than with the substance of your position. Even if channels are successfully bypassed, those in higher positions will feel some resentment toward you for not following appropriate procedure. This factor is often overlooked in advocacy and is quite costly to those who make the mistake. They have also missed the opportunity to increase their credibility and to add interested people to the cause at each level.

SHOW THAT WHAT YOU WANT IS CONSISTENT WITH THE PHILOSOPHY OF THE POLICY BOARD

Often we overlook a real source of help that already exists. Most policy bodies have a philosophy and stated objectives that are general and broad enough to include the goals you have for autistic persons. Get help for your cause by showing policymakers how they can make an important contribution by improving lives, as their guidelines indicate that they will.

If you really want to accomplish something for autistic children, spend some time trying to determine if the board's goals and philosophy already fit yours. Delicately handled, this process can be very beneficial to an advocacy group. The credibility that can be achieved by a group having done its homework well enough to cite exactly where the goals fit the existing philosophy of the board or commission is a powerful tool. As a superintendent, I have never had anyone advocate for a particular position who had substantiated his or her request on the basis of the philosophy of the board of education I work for. If an autistic child needs vocational training, point to the ubiquitous goal statements in support of vocational education's availability to all students. Such an argument can be quite powerful, and I find that it has helped autistic persons when it has been effectively utilized. The technique is also effective in allowing for the sharing of the praise once an improvement has been made. The policymaker can feel that he or she was responsible for the improvement.

DEMONSTRATE A DEFINITE NEED TO ADOPT YOUR POSITION

The ninth factor in achieving policy changes is convincing policymakers that what you want done is worth doing. The example I cited earlier about the list of 25 names that parents submitted for accountability is appropriate here. The official who made the decisions about residential placement knew most of those children and knew that they were in desperate need of services. The technique was one of the best I have ever used in terms of advocacy. It is hard to argue against a cause that is both right and just.

To be effective in bringing about a change in policy, a group must be able to demonstrate a definite need for its position to be adopted. Convince people that the action you desire is worthwhile. In serving a group with a low-incidence disability like autism, the most essential need is to acquaint people with the problems of the autistic through education and actual contact. As professionals and as policymakers, we find it easy to argue among ourselves. It is difficult, if not impossible, however, to argue against the needs of handicapped individuals when we are confronted with an effective, personal portrayal of their problems.

ORGANIZE THE EXTENDED FAMILY

Because of the low incidence of autism and its devastating effects, it is very important to organize those interested in order to more effectively promote service for autistic persons. Such an organized interest group can become an "overwhelming minority." Autism is about as common as blindness and many times more devastating, but I think that even the most conservative would admit that very little has been spent for those affected—in terms of either aid or prevention.

When a child is born with autism, the parents and siblings need the emotional and political support of grandparents, aunts, uncles, and cousins. An entire family offering support can help the immediate family and also make a great difference in the willingness of policymakers to provide services. Given the low incidence of autism, every supportive voice is important.

For the purpose of seeking support from policymakers, the extended family needs to include supportive service providers. The National Society for Children and Adults with Autism (NSAC) estimates that 340,000 people in the United States are autistic. (Of that number, they estimate one-third to be of school age.) To comprehend the political potential of an autism interest group, let's try to calculate its size. Let's assume that in addition to these 340,000 autistic persons, they could have about 680,000 parents, 1,360,000 grandparents, and at least 340,000 siblings (assuming an average of 1 sibling per autistic person). Furthermore, if only 1 service provider per autistic person were committed to better services, that would add another 340,000 people to the "extended" family. Now let's halve the number of grandparents and reduce the parent number by 25% to account for those who are unable or unwilling to advocate, and we *still* have a group that exceeds 2 million. Two million people are not to be scoffed at politically, especially when they are dealing with a problem that they are familiar with and know to be devastating. So get the interested people you know organized by encouraging them to join NSAC and its local chapters.

I realize the difficulty in thinking that 2 million people would be of one mind. Yet on certain basic issues such as PL 94-142, they would stand together. I have also found that many legislators are themselves related to someone with a major handicap—often autism. Some positive research on the extended families of policymakers can produce excellent results in developing a spirit of cooperation in finding solutions to the problems of autistic persons.

Ironically, the small number of persons touched by autism, though often a great disadvantage, is, in itself, a source of strength. Often, when I have participated in organizations that represent larger numbers of handicapped people, I have found the members' time spent on disagreements within the support group rather than on efforts to obtain assistance for handicapped persons. To illustrate, I recently observed one state organization representing mentally handicapped persons as they spent a great deal of time arguing among themselves over the money set aside by the state to build religious chapels at state institutions. Our parents' group was far removed from the problem under discussion. The small size of the group and the urgency of existing needs helped to prevent that kind of disagreement among group members.

UTILIZE A PROFESSIONAL SUPPORT GROUP

Without a professional support group, you may have some problems dealing with public officials. It is important that you have top legitimate professionals who will support the position you are advocating. Give them recognition for helping you—a small price to pay for the value you receive. Professionals want that kind of affirmation of their value. Utilize that to the advantage of autistic persons. They want credit, and we can see that they get it. The professional opinion adds credibility to a cause. The most effective advocacy for change that I have experienced before a board of education has included expert opinion.

In North Carolina, Dr. Eric Schopler's TEACCH program has always encouraged strong parent involvement in therapy and also in advocacy. Since the inception of Division TEACCH in 1972, many legislative and policy changes have been brought about in the state of North Carolina as a result of a healthy working relationship between parents and professionals. This relationship has been essential in affecting policy in the manner prescribed by the advocacy group.

Through research and study, a strong professional support group lends further credibility to the efforts of the advocacy group. Division TEACCH in North Carolina has served effectively in that effort, as it has provided a statewide network of services to families of autistic and communication-handicapped children. Division TEACCH uses parents as cotherapists, an approach that is particularly effective in helping to build strong parental and professional support groups. The formation of the North Carolina chapter of the National Society for Autistic Children led to the passing of legislation that mandated the TEACCH program. A close relationship between the professional support group and parents in the TEACCH model has been effective, as the professionals have been able to give expert witness, and the parents have been able to use this witness to build support for the program. On numerous occasions involving testimony given before public officials, professionals and parents have formed a persuasive team, with the former citing research and the latter seeking help.

KNOW YOUR RIGHTS AND USE THEM SPARINGLY

A final factor is knowing your rights and making judicious use of them. You have tremendous powers in working with policymakers and administrators to bring about change. You are going to keep living and working with people, however, so you do not want to overkill. Whatever those rights are, make sure you use them only to the extent that you need to in order to produce what is needed for the child. In reality, if you are successful in using the first 11 factors already mentioned, you probably will not need to "use" your rights.

Essentially, you have three major sources of power: PL 92-142, Section 504 of the Vocational Rehabilitation Act, and the state bills that parallel PL 94-142. All are recent laws. They were passed during the 1970s, and we do not yet know their full impact. We do know, however, that they give substantial rights to handicapped persons.

The basic thrust of PL 94-142 is to guarantee a free, appropriate public education for all handicapped children. "Free" means that services are to be provided under public supervision and direction at no cost to parents. The services must meet the standards of state educational agencies and include preschool, elementary, and secondary education, provided in conformity with individualized education programs.

Other services provided through PL 94-142 that few people are aware of include speech pathology, psychological services, occupational training, recreation, physical education, medical and counseling services, transportation, identification and assessment of handicapping conditions for special needs, social work, and parent counseling and training. Under the appropriate circumstances, all of the related services must be provided.

Section 504 of the Vocational Rehabilitation Act provides new rights for residential placement to the autistic person. Once deemed necessary, the placement must be provided at public expense.

Autistic persons have many rights under recent laws. Advocates have an excellent opportunity to bring about improved services by ensuring that the laws are obeyed. However, the changes will be more effective if advocacy groups use legal leverage in concert with the other measures cited for effective advocate strength.

Persons who wish to speak to policymakers on behalf of autistic individuals must realize that they are representing a very small percentage of the total population. We are obligated to be both diligent and persistent if we are to bring about program changes that will benefit the small but very important population of autism.

Our task is to mold or shape the commitments of those in policymaking positions. Otherwise, we will be caught in the syndrome of "too little, too late" for individuals who are in desperate need of services. The 12 factors I have discussed provide a guide for those who want to effect positive policy changes for autistic persons. Even though the numbers are small, those concerned about the welfare and the rights of autistic people can become an overwhelming and influential minority. However, good techniques for advocacy must be used. Failing to use them effectively will only postpone services until they *are* used effectively. On the other hand, a positive and consistent approach will make an enormous difference in the quality of life for autistic persons and their families.

REFERENCES

Marlowe, J. One man's opinion: Why you run for school board office. *American School Board Journal,* 1979, *166* (July), 17–19, 37.
Smith, D. *In our own interest: A handbook for the citizen lobbyist.* Seattle: Madrona, 1979.

IV

Parents as Trainees

9

Parents as Behavior Therapists for Their Autistic Children
Clinical and Empirical Considerations

DAVID J. KOLKO

TRAINING PARENTS AS BEHAVIOR THERAPISTS

Behavior modification procedures used in laboratory and clinical settings have proven useful in managing and treating autistic children (Margolies, 1977). The fact that significant gains were made following limited exposure to a select few behavioral procedures argues convincingly for their potency and applicability in both educational and family settings. In point of fact, behavior modification techniques were incorporated in almost all of the programs designed for autistic children between the years 1971 and 1976 (Sullivan, 1976).

Those treatment gains were lost, however, when the child left these controlled settings. To transfer behavioral improvement across settings and time, the child's home environment had to support the behavior changes. The most widely used solution for programming the child's environment was to train parents to be their child's therapists (Cone and Sloop, 1974; Kozloff, 1973; Schopler and Reichler, 1971).

Dramatic changes made during clinic treatment can be maintained and enhanced by parents in the family system. Follow-up data from a major research

DAVID J. KOLKO • Western Psychiatric Institute and Clinic, School of Medicine, Department of Psychiatry, Division of Child and Adolescent Psychiatry, University of Pittsburgh, Pittsburgh, Pennsylvania 15213. The author expresses his appreciation to Lowell T. Anderson, Ph.D., and Magda Campbell, M.D., for their helpful editorial comments, and to Judith E. Cohen, M. Ed., for her technical assistance.

study show that behavioral improvements were maintained only in those children discharged to parents who had received behavioral training (Lovaas, Koegel, Simmons, and Long, 1973). However, children discharged to institutions or foster homes with untrained parents appeared to have lost much of their nonverbal and verbal improvements.

The fact that children spend most of their time with parents suggests that they are the most likely agents to induce and monitor subsequent behavior change in the home. Moreover, parents exert greatest control over the important environmental events that ultimately shape and influence their child's behavior. Such family-based interventions in the child's natural environment reduce treatment cost and the range of professional services required.

That the training of parents enhances the transfer of treatment gains to novel settings and behaviors was iterated by Freeman and Ritvo (1976) and Hemsley, Howlin, Berger, Hersov, Holbrook, Rutter, and Yule (1978). Hemsley *et al.* (1978) also underscored the potential for broadening both clinically relevant objectives and procedures when parents received professional training. Finally, in many cases, the provision of parent training has established a cooperative working relationship with a treatment specialist and encouraged a strong therapeutic alliance when necessary.

Clearly, a number of benefits accrue to the use of parents as therapists. Perhaps one of the major goals associated with such efforts is to provide parents with the necessary skills to manage, teach, and care for their autistic children at home and in the community (Lovaas, 1978; Schopler, 1978). The utilization of individualized instruction and modeling of different techniques provides the necessary training in effective child management strategies while explicitly pointing out the manner in which they can be most efficiently implemented.

It is expected that when parents become proficient in the utilization of behavioral methods, management at home and in related environments may be greatly facilitated, thereby reducing the characteristic strain often imposed by the necessity to provide constant supervision and care to the autistic child. An assessment of the degree to which this expectation is fulfilled is the primary task of the remainder of this chapter. First, a brief overview of essential therapeutic prerequisites will be discussed.

THERAPEUTIC PREREQUISITES

Enlisting Parental Cooperation

Concurrent with the increasing role played by parents in the treatment process, professionals have placed greater emphasis on establishing a working relationship characterized by reciprocity and concern. Prior to receiving any formalized training, parents have participated in preliminary orientation sessions designed to explicitly document the course of treatment, their role in it, and expectations regarding professional involvement. Some professionals use "work-contracts" (Davids and Berenson, 1977; Israel, 1976; Lovaas, 1978). Parents receive clear guidelines outlining the commitments they are expected to make, attendance requirements, and the consequences for failure to abide by the program's regulations. In addition, parents may be responsible for recording the child's improvements, purchasing programmed instruction materials, and implementing certain procedures at home. Once the entire program is described and understood, the parents may sign legal documents indicating what can be expected from them and program consultants.

Various forms of parent contracts that appear less formal and binding have been employed in additional home-based training programs (Hemsley *et al.*, 1978; Reichler and Schopler, 1976). Reichler and Schopler (1976) provide encouragement of maximal parental involvement in both the home and the school, but they do not require a specified level of intensive participation. Similarly, Hemsley *et al.* (1978) conduct all aspects of treatment in the child's home with the intention that the parents may become more effective as teachers. Thus, there is considerable differential emphasis placed upon the degree of formalized commitment established for parents who seek to participate in a behavioral training program. However, while an optimal level of parental involvement and control has not been suggested, greater attention is being paid to the process by which parents are introduced to and become "engaged" with the therapeutic endeavor (Schopler, 1978). Moreover, the development of support systems has been encouraged to maintain parental commitment (Bristol and Wiegernik, 1979; Harris and Milch, 1981). The range of support-engendering services could include counseling for parents (Schopler, 1976), respite care and access to special education (DeMyer, 1979), or medical services (Bristol and Wiegernik, 1979).

Helping Parents to Think Functionally

As will be reviewed in greater detail in the next section, parent-training efforts have broadened to include instruction in general behavioral or operant psychology principles (Harris and Milch, 1981; Hemsley *et al.*, 1978). Howlin, Marchant, Rutter, Berger, Hersov, and Yule (1973) devote explicit attention to assisting parents to conceptualize their child's behavioral problems in functional terms in order to determine those events that seem to precede and follow each problem. Once these events are known and understood, they may be modified in order to promote more appropriate prosocial behaviors. The parents may evaluate changes in these causal sequences using routine data-collection methods that are amenable to alteration when deemed necessary. Teaching parents to analyze the events that are routinely associated with a given behavior problem not only facilitates the generalized application of a method for assessing problems in the home but also increases the likelihood that effective behavioral solutions will be selected for implementation.

PARENT-TRAINING METHODS

Once parents have consented to participate in treatment, they are exposed to various forms of instruction to facilitate their role as therapists for their children. Among a number of important variables such as the degree of involvement and duration of treatment agreed upon, most programs differ with respect to the specific methods employed to train parents. The studies to be described in this section generally represent three related training methods: comprehensive didactic instruction and practice, modeling, and feedback.

Comprehensive Didactic Instruction and Practice

The most frequently employed form of parental instruction has incorporated training in general behavioral principles, operant psychology, or learning theory in addition to observation and imitation of a professional therapist. Thus, parents receive didactic instruction and systematic practice in behavioral techniques under supervision.

Two early studies described programs that are noteworthy for their inclusion of both aspects of training (Ora and Wiegerink, 1970; Schell and Adams, 1968). In instructing parents to conduct the initial stages of therapy, Schell and Adams (1968) spent 21 sessions teaching record keeping, social learning theory, and operant conditioning techniques to the parents of a 3-year-old boy. The authors provided readings on behavioral and social learning theory, as well as specific techniques and principles of operant conditioning in various textbooks. Subsequent home-based sessions were devoted to answering questions, clarifying procedures, and discussing the treatment program. Gains were made during 3 months of home treatment, which were extended to novel individuals and settings.

In a similarly comprehensive study, Ora and Wiegerink (1970) trained parents in language, motor, and cognitive developmental sequences to facilitate their child's education at home. The parents rapidly learned these sequences and began instructing other parents once their training was completed.

Programmatic extensions based upon the didactic model in terms of subject samples as well as treatment objectives and techniques have also been conducted (Hemsley et al., 1978; Howlin, 1981; Howlin et al., 1973). In these innovative programs, parents viewed one therapist modeling behavioral techniques while another explained their use before learning technical terminology. Improvements were observed in several targeted behaviors as measured using information from individual subjects. Systematic evaluations following treatment also revealed significant changes in treated versus untreated (i.e., control) subjects. The therapeutic diversity of this evaluation is well complemented by its experimental sophistication.

Didactic instruction and practice training methods for parents have also been integrated with training efforts conducted in the child's school. Working with severely handicapped children, O'Dell, Blackwell, Larcen, and Hogan (1977) implemented a comprehensive treatment program comprising a learning and intervention center, a parent-training program, and a training program for teachers in three areas: physical, social, and intellectual. Specific skills were measured and trained according to operationally defined criteria arranged in a five-level developmental sequence. Parents received a 3-week, 90-hour program to learn a broad range of management and problem-solving skills. The program consisted of didactic instruction, coaching, guided observation, and several forms of modeling in actual treatment sessions. The authors reported that 14 of their 58 children had successfully completed the program in that they were soon placed in public schools. This study is one of the few to effectively integrate the implementation of a multicomponent program with a concern for rigorous experimental evaluation. Several methodological strengths characterized this program, including the use of standardized recording definitions, follow-up reports to assess generalization and maintenance, and a competency-based system of training.

Modeling

In one of the earliest behavioral investigations drawing upon professional demonstration (modeling), Wolf, Risley, and Mees (1964) applied positive reward techniques to the behavior problems of a 3½-year-old hospitalized boy. Staff were trained to ignore and punish incompatible behavior. The parents then visited the hospital and observed staff members working with the child. An attendant observed and instructed them in managing the child's behavior. The parents were trained to use punishment techniques on the ward and at home to reduce eating problems, and to use imitation at home to elicit appropriate verbal behavior. Improvements in the child's behavior were observed, which the mother reported had been maintained after discharge. This general strategy of modeling therapeutic techniques during clinic or hospital sessions followed by supervised practice for the involved parent has also been briefly reported by Hewett (1965), Risley (1968), Risley and Wolf (1966), and Wetzel, Baker, Roney, and Martin (1966).

Schopler and Reichler (1971) described one of the earliest demonstration-based treatment programs in which both parents served as primary therapists. The parents observe therapist's demonstrations that are designed to remediate developmental deficits in four major areas. Home programs based upon a home assessment are provided that are occasionally demonstrated by parents to program consultants. The child's behavior changes are documented by parents using a daily log. The authors report anecdotally that parents developed therapeutic skills and that children showed corresponding improvements. Parental involvement in both clinical and research endeavors is highlighted in this particular program. The therapeutic foundation established by Schopler and Reichler (1971), now described as the TEACCH program (see Chapter 4), has evolved into a home- and school-based program of considerable scope and professional involvement (Lansing and Schopler, 1978; Reichler and Schopler, 1976).

Feedback

This particular approach emphasizes live practice in using behavioral techniques with the child followed by feedback regarding their judicious application. Browning and Stover (1971) observed one set of parents working with their child, who had been placed in residential treatment. The parents' skill in rewarding and punishing the child was determined by reviewing videotapes of each therapy session. Staff members not only highlighted correct and incorrect applications but also gave explicit feedback as to the percent of appropriate behavior the child exhibited.

In an innovative application of continuous feedback, Moore and Bailey (1973) experimentally investigated the use of an FM wireless microphone ("bug-in-the-ear") during training sessions with a mother and her 3-year-old girl. The authors cued the mother with simple instructions to apply social praise and punishment to both preacademic behaviors and requests for social interaction. Formal data were collected during sessions in which the therapist and the mother alternated working with the child. It was found that cuing facilitated gains in both targeted areas.

Comparisons of Parent-Training Methods

Only one study was found that was directed toward examining the comparative effectiveness of the aforementioned training methods with the parents of autistic children.

Koegel, Glahn, and Nieminen (1978) were concerned with determining which parent-training methods were associated with more generalized skill deployment subsequent to the training program. Experiment 1 found that didactic training (lectures) and videotape observation were more effective than practice in using specific behavioral techniques alone in facilitating acquisition of a generalized set of skills to teach new target behaviors. Experiment 2 investigated the use of feedback. Three parents viewed two videotapes focusing upon antecedent or consequent control presented in random order to assess the differential effects of such training. The parents showed improvements after viewing the videotapes, and the information contained in each tape was found to be specific to its effects on their performance. The authors noted that didactic training in antecedents and consequences, modeling, and repeated practice are needed to expedite parents' mastery of general behavioral skills.

OVERVIEW OF SPECIFIC BEHAVIOR THERAPY TECHNIQUES

Pinpointing, Observing, and Recording Behavior

The general task of improving the autistic child's disposition is a difficult one and requires clear understanding of the various behaviors in need of modification. To facilitate awareness of the level of different problem behaviors, training has occasionally been provided in specifying problems in terms of specific behaviors and then measuring or recording their frequency of occurrence. Schell and Adams (1968) initiated their treatment program by training parents to keep records of their child's behaviors and their reactions to them for 12 days. Throughout the day, the following information was recorded: the child's behavior, its duration, the setting in which it occurred, and the events that preceded and followed the behavior. Such information eventually became the focus of treatment and ongoing evaluation reviews.

The use of parent-generated records of home progress subsequent to behavioral treatment has been incorporated into the programs described by Harris and Milch (1981), Lansing and Schopler (1978), and Reichler and Schopler (1976). An excellent general description of recording procedures can be found in Baker, Brightman, Heifetz, and Murphy's (1976) *Behavior Problems* training manual.

Attending and Ignoring

The combination of attending to certain behaviors while ignoring other behaviors provides parents with a procedure for increasing the frequency of only those behaviors that are considered desirable or appropriate. The use of attending and ignoring has figured prominently in programs designed to provide rapid control over various problem behaviors, particularly in the absence of explicit punishment procedures. Wetzel *et al.* (1966) trained a mother to withdraw her attention when her 6-year-old boy began to tantrum but to attend whenever he engaged in any appropriate behavior. A similar procedure was employed to modify the child's behavior at home.

Gardner, Pearson, Berkovici, and Bricker (1968) demonstrated that parental attention by the mother was partially responsible for the high frequency of deviant behaviors exhibited by a 6-year-old boy. After being familiarized with certain behavioral principles, the parents were trained to ignore the child's deviant behaviors and to reinstate their attention when an appropriate behavior occurred. Ongoing appropriate behaviors were also rewarded with attention and pleasant physical contact. The procedures were effective in increasing eye contact and verbalizations, and decreasing self-stimulation and screaming.

Wulbert, Barach, Perry, Straughan, Sulzbacher, Turner, and Wiltz (1974) trained the mother of a 5-year-old mute child to reward compliance to commands with social praise and attention, and to ignore noncompliance for approximately 10–20 seconds. Interestingly, the child's entire family began to ignore all instances of self-stimulatory hand-slapping behavior. A comparison with pretreatment levels of compliance indicated considerable improvement following the application of this procedure.

Imitation Training

Imitation training has frequently been employed as a rapid method for facilitating the development of verbal and nonverbal imitation skills in noncommunicative autistic children. Wolf *et al.* (1964) were among the earliest investigators to train the parents of a young autistic boy to use imitation following a hospital treatment program. The parents initially prompted the child to imitate the names of pictures by saying the name of each individually presented picture. The child was eventually trained to say the name in the presence of the picture alone. Once training was extended to the home, the parents observed increases in the use of personal pronouns, requests, and commands, which were evident at follow-up.

A study by Nordquist and Wahler (1973) provides experimental evidence that training resulted in changes in both imitation and compliance, which were evaluated both in the clinic and at home. Interestingly, Nordquist and Wahler (1973) observed that the mother in their study began to use the child's favorite activities, drawing and copying, to reward instances of correct imitation. Tramontana and Stimbert (1970) included the entire family during imitation training, which was found to increase both social behavior and spontaneous verbalization.

Sign Language Training

While these efforts to teach social behavior and communication have relied almost exclusively upon speech and vocal imitation, an interesting recent development involves the instruction of manual signs to facilitate communication. Casey (1978) described a novel training program in which parents taught Signed English to young autistic children in individual laboratory sessions and encouraged them to use signs and verbalizations at home. The children were shown picture cards representing different nouns and actions words, and were rewarded for correct manual signs through social praise. Casey (1978) reported improvements in communication and inappropriate behavior during these sessions that generalized to the classroom. The inclusion of a multiple-baseline design, involving different behaviors and settings, and a 3-month follow-up made use of methodological strengths that allow for empirical documentation of both experimental control and transfer across settings. It must be added, however, that no follow-up for the mother–child interactions was conducted, and that transfer to or follow-up in the home was not assessed. Nevertheless, this study clearly shows that sign language offers an alternative medium for the establishment of rudimentary communication in noncommunicative autistic children.

Token Reward Systems

One of the most frequently employed means for motivating children and facilitating the learning of new behaviors has entailed the delivery of small token rewards contingent upon instances of desirable behavior (Rimm and Masters, 1979). These tokens may then be exchanged for a variety of rewarding objects or activities, such as snacks, toys, movies, or rides. A token reward can be any permanent material, but generally it takes the form of poker chips, points, check marks, stars, or puzzle pieces.

Insofar as token rewards are generally accumulated for a certain period of time before being cashed in, they have only frequently been employed with autistic children. In one of the few applications with autistic children, Zifferblatt, Burton, Horner, and White (1977) implemented a token system for use in the home and at school in which tokens were given for appropriate social and work behaviors. In addition to significant improvements in the children's behavior, it was found that parents could easily and efficiently implement the token economy. In the comprehensive program described by Nordquist and Wahler (1973), the parents altered an imitation program such that the child earned a token, rather than parental attention, for each correct imitative response. The token entitled the child to 15 seconds of television. Interestingly, when television lost its effectiveness, it was replaced with short writing periods, which the child liked.

Time-Out and Mild Physical Punishment

While various forms of punishment have been described in the literature, the most frequently employed means for reducing the frequency of problem behaviors in autistic children involves time-out and mild forms of physical punishment.

A form of punishment through contingent withdrawal of access to rewarding events, time-out has been employed in several parent-training programs. Wolf *et al.* (1964) trained parents to place their child in his room whenever he tantrummed or engaged in self-injurious behavior and to keep the door closed until these behaviors stopped. At that point, the door was opened in order to reward appropriate behavior. The parents' application of the procedure both on the child's hospital ward and at home virtually eliminated the problem behaviors. Moreover, the time-out procedure was applied with comparable success in reducing the frequency of bedtime problems and mealtime disruption.

In a small number of cases requiring rapid control over difficult behaviors, parents have received training in the use of various physical punishment techniques. While physical punishment is generally discouraged, its application has been considered necessary and has been evaluated in a few instances. Risley (1968) observed that time-out as applied by the mother at home was ineffective in reducing the frequency of dangerous climbing in her young daughter. The mother was then trained to deliver a painful shock using a hand hold inductorium paired with a loud "no." Within 4 days, the frequency of inappropriate climbing dropped from 29 per day on the average to 2 per day before being eliminated altogether. Shock also reduced the frequency of fighting with the brother. The mother then replaced shock punishment with spanking and later with a chair time-out procedure in which the child was required to sit in a chair for 10 minutes after each climbing incident.

The application of physical punishment procedures, while frequently effective, has generally followed the ineffective use of alternative, less aversive behavior-management procedures.

Multicomponent Training Programs

Several multicomponent programs have been reported over the past decade that exemplify the complexity of parental involvement and range of techniques employed. In Chapter 11, Schreibman *et al.* outline their program for training the parents of autistic children to serve as general therapists-educators. Five general procedures were found to increase parents' effectiveness when working with their children: (1) identifying the behavior to be modified, (2) presenting proper instructions, (3) prompting correct responses, (4) shaping behavior by rewarding successive approximations to the designated behavioral goal, and (5) providing effective consequences (Schreibman and Koegel, 1981).

A recent parent-training program discussed by Harris and Milch (1981) focused specifically upon training parents to facilitate their children's speech and language at home. The principles of behavior modification and speech training techniques are taught using didactic training and supplemental readings, after which parents learn to increase several speech-related skills, such as eye contact, imitation, and functional speech. There is also opportunity to practice techniques for eliminating various problem behaviors. Parental application of all procedures in structured learning sessions at home is occasionally monitored through direct supervision by program consultants. This program is one of the first to investigate the relationship between parental implementation of behavioral techniques and characteristics of the language environment.

The coordination of a diverse range of educational and therapeutic services in a well-articulated program having school, parent training, and residential components, among others, has been described by Israel (1976). In the school, the child progresses from learning rudimentary preacademic, personal, and social skills in a one-to-one situation to learning academic skills in a group-management situation. Parents are trained in the use of positive reward, ignoring, and time-out techniques to ensure appropriate behavior and later are given recommendations for home instruction. To facilitate community adjustment, the child can participate in residential treatment and a work training program. The absence of data notwithstanding, this program is unique in its attempt to provide the child with a range of integrated services from childhood through the teens and into adulthood.

Of comparable scope and therapeutic involvement is the TEACCH program (see Chapter 4). The program draws upon both parents and teachers in an effort to provide an integrated treatment reigmen consisting of individualized curricula within the context of a special education classroom. A routine diagnostic assessment is conducted to determine the child's developmental level in several areas and to aid in the specification of the home program, a set of instructional tasks used by the mother at home, and the mother and teacher at school. Specific techniques and educational curricula are then jointly determined by the child's mother and teacher, implemented in their respective settings, evaluated, and modified accordingly. The program is sufficiently flexible to permit the deployment of innovative educational strategies on an idiosyncratic basis.

These few studies suggest that the provision of both parent training and specialized schooling results in a variety of social, language, motor, and academic skill improvements. When parents, in addition to teachers, have received training in the use of behavioral strategies, the child receives a highly structured and consistent set of naturalistic conditions to enhance learning and behavior change. The inclusion of both systems in a treatment program seems to maximize the development and maintenance of behavioral improvements.

PROGRAM EVALUATION

Assessment of Parental Behavior Change

The therapeutic effectiveness of parent-training programs has largely been established on the basis of anecdotal and experimental evidence documenting changes in the targeted child's individual behaviors. However, there has been a general lack of details regarding the changes in parental behavior that occur subsequent to training, despite the obvious significance of such data. Measures reflecting changes in parents' skills have been included in only a few instances. Moore and Bailey (1973) provided an analysis of a mothers's behavior after being trained to facilitate her child's preacademic and social behavior using cued instructions. After the cuing procedure was applied, errors in the mother's use of reward and punishment decreased. Greater similarity in performance was found between the mother and the experimenter following the training program. More-over, the mother's behavior remained at consistently high levels even in the absence of the experimenter's cued instructions.

A comparably extensive outcome investigation describing changes in paren-tal behavior was reported by Hemsley et al. (1978). Compared to mothers in an untreated control group, mothers who received home-based parent training showed greater active involvement with their children, made more remarks, and used more praise, corrections, and both gestural and physical prompts. More-over, the trained mothers made more utterances directed toward the child's use of language and fewer general non-language-related utterances than mothers in the control group. Such findings suggest that behavioral parent training is indeed associated with qualitative changes in the educational skills employed by parents when attempting to promote improvements in their children's communication and overall socialization.

An overview of the pattern of change in parental behaviors documented following a speech and language training program is found in a recent account by Harris and Milch (1981). The authors reported that mothers asked fewer yes–no questions, while modeling and rewarding speech with greater frequency, follow-ing the first year of a training program. In their new role as teachers, parents were observed to be more skillful at timing their commands, offering prompts and appropriate rewards, and managing the pace of the session. To the author's credit, data were obtained on both mothers and fathers.

An evaluation of the parent-training component of the TEACCH program described earlier has recently been conducted in an attempt to specify the parameters governing increased treatment effectiveness. Marcus, Lansing, Andrews, and Schopler (1978) compared the task performance of 10 mothers before and 2 months after treatment on nine teaching variables (e.g., organization of material, language use, teaching techniques, behavior control). The results pointed to significant increases for the group in all ratings. Child compliance improved from 2.9% to 51.3% subsequent to the training program. Greatest improvements were observed in older children of low socioeconomic status. Such investigations are needed in order to establish the functional relationship between the application of parent training and childrens' behavioral improvements.

Assessment of the Generalization of Therapeutic Gains to Novel Settings and Behaviors

An issue of primary concern to individuals responsible for the treatment of autistic children concerns the degree to which the changes brought about by behavioral training actually transfer to other important contexts (Koegel and Rincover, 1977). In recent years, evidence has suggested that generalization to different settings and untreated behaviors must be explicitly programmed through specific training efforts (Stokes and Baer, 1977). Indeed, the surge of interest in parent-training applications is, in part, a reflection of the need to promote generalization to the child's natural environment.

The few studies examining the issue of generalization have been primarily concerned with the generalization of the effects of parent training to novel settings, that is, those in which treatment has not been introduced. Wulbert *et al.* (1974) evaluated the extent of generalization of three targeted behaviors (compliance, verbalization, hand slapping) to the child's school and home after preliminary behavioral treatment in a training apartment. A variety of behavioral techniques were employed by the child's parents to gain control over the child's behavior. The results indicated that all three behaviors showed limited generalization to the two novel settings. Generalization to the home occurred only when a particular intervention strategy was implemented in that setting. The authors point out that the parents' teaching behaviors likewise failed to generalize from the apartment to the home.

In the manual sign-language training study reported by Casey (1978), generalization from the laboratory-based parent–child session to the child's classroom was evaluated for four communicative (e.g., manual sign use, spontaneous verbal responses) and four inappropriate behaviors (e.g., self-stimulation, disruptive behavior). In addition to demonstrating the rapid effects of the program, the author presented experimental evidence for the generalization of all behavioral improvements to the classroom, with some variability among the 4-, 6-, and 7-year-old children. Interestingly, the extent of generalization continued to increase throughout the 5 weeks of the training program.

Finally, comparably optimistic findings regarding the generalization of treatment gains to novel settings were obtained by Zifferblatt et al. (1977) working with 12 adolescent autistic children. Parents and teachers applied token reinforcement procedures in the home and school, and generalization of treatment effects occurred in both places, suggesting the feasibility of implementing a training program in either setting. As in the previous study, there was a steady improvement for each behavior as time passed which was more characteristic of some behaviors than of others. The fact that generalization has been found in certain investigations should prompt additional research regarding those training conditions that seem to promote the transfer of behavioral gains to new situations. Studies of stimulus overselectively underscore the need to directly train the autistic child in multiple settings with diverse cues to facilitate generalized responding (Kolko, Anderson, and Campbell, 1980; Rincover and Koegel, 1977).

Assessment of the Maintenance of Therapeutic Gains

An overview of parent-training research would be incomplete without some discussion of the long-term effects associated with behavioral treatment programs (Graziano, 1977; Harris and Milch, 1981). While the majority of research in this area has been concerned with the induction of therapeutic change, a few studies have reported long-term outcome data.

Two studies have reported group follow-up information subsequent to behavioral treatment (Casey, 1978; Hemsley et al., 1978). Casey (1978) assessed follow-up in the classroom for 1 week, 3 months after the termination of a laboratory-based language program. A 25% increase in communicative behaviors and a 70% decrease in inappropriate behaviors were observed for the group on the average. In one of the longest follow-up evaluations to date, Hemsley et al. (1978) showed changes in both childrens' and parents' behaviors 18 months after treatment was initiated. On the basis of an analysis of several mother–child pairs, improvements in the children's communication, ritualistic behavior, and cooperation, and the mothers' activity, speech direction, and gestures were demonstrated. Compared to children in the control group, children whose parents received behavioral training showed greater improvements in the use of comprehensive and socialized utterances. Moreover, children of trained parents were rated as showing more social responsibility and imaginative play and less disruptive and stereotyped behaviors than did untrained parents.

Assessment of Parental Satisfaction with Program Objectives and Outcomes

While the major goal of most parent-training programs is to boost parents' abilities to teach and manage their children at home, an implicit evaluation objective is to determine the role played by the program itself in implementing their increased effectiveness. Of particular importance to program developers and administrators is the degree to which aspects of a training curriculum are believed to be responsible for changes in parent effectiveness and parents' overall satisfaction with the program.

As a means of assessing parental perceptions of the widely acclaimed TEA-CCH program, Schopler, Mesibov, and Baker (1982) sent follow-up questionnaires to 657 families, of which 348 were returned for analysis. Their results bear upon several significant program considerations. Regarding the program's general utility, the average overall evaluation rating of the "helpfulness" of the program was a 4.6 on a 5-point scale. It was found that highest ratings were consistently associated with maximal participation in all three aspects of the program. In terms of the program's impact on different categories of problem behaviors, parents indicated significant changes in the areas of social relationships, motor skills, self-help skills, language and communication, and bizarre behaviors. Finally, the authors report that in a comparison of the rated helpfulness of 17 alternative support systems in the state, the TEACCH program was assigned a higher rating than any other service (3.3 out of 4).

While Schopler *et al.* (1982) point out the limitations inherent in questionnaire-obtained information, they are to be commended for their systematic approach to examining the effectiveness of parent-mediated educational programs and parents' overall satisfaction with program outcomes. The latter concern has only recently been investigated by determining the social validity associated with behavioral interventions for the autistic child (Schreibman, Koegel, Mills, and Burke, 1981). Only through continued systematic investigation can consumer satisfaction with parent-training programs be directly examined to permit improvements in the delivery of professional services.

SUMMARY

The studies reviewed here provide preliminary documentation of the feasibility of training parents to serve as behavior therapists for their autistic children in order to facilitate overall psychosocial adjustment. Concurrent programming of family and educational systems has resulted in progress in social, self-care, language, academic, and imitative behaviors. The fact that training could be conducted efficiently in a short period of time demonstates that behavioral techniques can be used successfully by parents. As noted earlier, however, the methodological adequacy characteristic of these studies as a whole has been less than desirable. To expand the experimental data base of parent-training efforts, greater emphasis must be placed on such empirical concerns as clinical significance, accurate measurement, experimental control through controlled designs, replicability of findings, generalization to novel populations, maintenance, and cost-effectiveness.

REFERENCES

Baker, B. L., Brightman, A. L., Heifetz, L. J., and Murphy, D. M. *Behavior problems*. Champaign, Ill.: Research Press, 1976.

Bristol, M. M., and Wiegernik, R. Parent involvement. In M. Parluzsky (Ed.), *Autism: A professional guide for parents and professionals*. Syracuse, N.Y.: Syracuse University Press, 1979.

Browning, R. M., and Stover, D. O. *Behavior modification in child treatment: An experimental and clinical approach*. Chicago: Aldine-Atherton, 1971.

Casey, L. Development of communicative behavior in autistic children: A parent program using manual signs. *Journal of Autism and Childhood Schizophrenia*, 1978, *8*, 45–59.

Cone, J. D., and Sloop, E. W. Parents as agents of change. In W. N. Spradlin and A. Jacobs (Eds.), *The group as agent of change*. New York: Behavioral Publications, 1974.

Davids, A., and Berenson, J. K. Integration of a behavior modification program into a traditionally oriented residential treatment program. *Journal of Autism and Childhood Schizophrenia*, 1977, *7*, 269–285.

DeMyer, M. K. *Parents and children in autism*. New York: Wiley, 1979.

Freeman, B. J., and Ritvo, E. R. Parents as paraprofessionals. In E. R. Ritvo (Ed.), *Autism: Diagnosis, current research and management*. New York: Spectrum, 1976.

Gardner, J. E., Pearson, D. T., Berkovici, A. N., and Bricker, D. E. Measurement, evaluation, and modification of selected social interactions between a schizophrenic child, his parents, and his therapist. *Journal of Consulting and Clinical Psychology*, 1968, *32*, 537–542.

Graziano, A. M. Parents as behavior therapists. In M. Hersen, R. M. Eisler, and P. M. Miller (Eds.), *Progress in behavior modification* (Vol. 4). New York: Academic Press, 1977.

Harris, S. L., and Milch, R. E. Training parents as behavior therapists for their autistic children. *Clinical Psychology Review*, 1981, *1*, 49–64.

Hemsley, R., Howlin, P., Berger, M., Hersov, L., Holbrook, D., Rutter, M., and Yule, W. In M. Rutter and E. Schopler (Eds.), *Autism: A reappraisal of concepts and treatment*. New York: Plenum, 1978.

Hewett, F. M. Teaching speech to an autistic child through operant conditioning *American Journal of Orthopsychiatry*, 1965, *35*, 927–936.

Howlin, P. A. The effectiveness of operant language training with autistic children. *Journal of Autism and Developmental Disorders*, 1981, *11*, 89–105.

Howlin, P. A., Marchant, R., Rutter, M., Berger, M., Hersov, L., and Yule, W. A home-based approach to the treatment of autistic children. *Journal of Autism and Childhood Schizophrenia*, 1973, *3*, 308–336.

Israel, M. L. Educational approaches at the Behavior Research Institute, Providence, R.I. In E. R. Ritvo (Ed.), *Autism: Diagnosis, current research and management*. New York: Spectrum, 1976.

Koegel, R. L., Glahn, T. J., and Nieminen, G. Generalization of parent-training results. *Journal of Applied Behavior Analysis*, 1978, *11*, 95–109.

Koegel, R. L., and Rincover, A. Research on the difference between generalization and maintenance in extra-therapy responding. *Journal of Applied Behavior Analysis*, 1977, *10*, 1–12.

Kolko, D. J., Anderson, L. T., and Campbell, M. Sensory preference and overselective responding in autistic children. *Journal of Autism and Developmental Disorders*, 1980, *10*, 259–271.

Kozloff, M. A. *Reaching the autistic child: A parent training program.* Champaign, Ill.: Research Press, 1973.

Lansing, M. D., and Schopler, E. Individualized education: A public school model. In M. Rutter and E. Schopler (Eds.), *Autism: A reappraisal of concepts and treatment.* New York: Plenum, 1978.

Lovaas, O. I. Parents as therapists. In M. Rutter and E. Schopler (Eds.), *Autism: A reappraisal of concepts and treatment.* New York: Plenum, 1978.

Lovaas, O. I., Koegel, R. L., Simmons, J. Q., and Long, J. S. Some generalization and follow-up measures on autistic children. *Journal of Applied Behavior Analysis*, 1973, *6*, 131–166.

Marcus, L. M., Lansing, M., Andrews, C. E., and Schopler, E. Improvement of teaching effectiveness in parents of autistic children. *Journal of the American Academy of Child Psychiatry*, 1978, *17*, 625–639.

Margolies, P. Behavioral approaches to the treatment of early infantile autism: A review. *Psychological Bulletin*, 1977, *84*, 249–264.

Moore, B. L., and Bailey, J. S. Social punishment in the modification of a preschool child's autistic-like behavior with a mother as therapist. *Journal of Applied Behavior Analysis*, 1973, *6*, 497–507.

Nordquist, V. M., and Wahler, R. G. Naturalistic treatment of an autistic child. *Journal of Applied Behavior Analysis*, 1973, *6*, 79–87.

O'Dell, S. L., Blackwell, L. J., Larcen, S. W., and Hogan, J. L. Competency-based training for severely behaviorally handicapped children and their parents. *Journal of Autism and Childhood Schizophrenia*, 1977, *7*, 231–243.

Ora, J., and Wiegernik, R. *Regional Intervention Project for parents and children.* Progress Report. Bureau of Education for the Handicapped, U.S. Office of Education, 1970.

Reichler, R. J., and Schopler, E. Developmental therapy: A program model for providing individual services in the community. In E. Schopler and R. J. Reichler (Eds.), *Psychopathology and child development.* New York: Plenum Press, 1976.

Rimm, D. C., and Masters, J. C. *Behavior therapy: Techniques and empirical findings* (2nd ed.). New York: Academic Press, 1979.

Rincover, A., and Koegel, R. L. Research on the education of autistic children: Recent advances and future directions. In B. B. Lahey and A. E. Kazdin (Eds.), *Advances in clinical child psychology* (Vol. 1). New York: Plenum Press, 1977.

Risley, T. R. The effects and side effects of punishing the autistic behaviors of a deviant child. *Journal of Applied Behavior Analysis*, 1968, *1*, 21–34.

Risley, T. R., and Wolf, M. M. Experimental manipulation of autistic behaviors and generalization into the home. In R. Ulrich, T. Strachnik, and J. Mabry (Eds.), *Control of human behaviors.* Glenview, Ill.: Scott, Foresman, 1966.

Schell, R. E., and Adams, W. P. Training parents of a young child with profound behavior deficits to be teacher-therapists. *Journal of Special Education*, 1968, *2*, 439–454.

Schopler, E. Towards reducing behavior problems in autistic children. In L. C. Wing (Ed.), *Early childhood autism* (2nd ed.). Oxford: Pergamon Press, 1976.

Schopler, E. Changing parental involvement in behavioral treatment. In M. Rutter and E. Schopler (Eds.), *Autism: A reappraisal of concepts and treatment.* New York: Plenum, 1978.

Schopler, E., Mesibov, G., and Baker, A. Evaluation of treatment for autistic children and their parents. *Journal of the American Academy of Child Psychiatry*, 1982, *21*, 262–267.

Schopler, E., and Reichler, R. J. Parents as cotherapists in the treatment of psychotic children. *Journal of Autism and Childhood Schizophrenia*, 1971, *1*, 87–102.

Schreibman, L., and Koegel, R. L. A guideline for planning behavior modification programs for autistic children. In S. Turner, K. Calhoun, and H. Adams (Eds.), *Handbook of clinical behavior therapy*. New York: Wiley, 1981.

Schreibman, L., Koegel, R. L., Mills, J. L., and Burke, J. C. Social validation of behavior therapy with autistic children. *Behavior Therapy*, 1981, *12*, 610–624.

Stokes, T. F., and Baer, D. M. An implicit technology of generalization. *Journal of Applied Behavior Analysis*, 1977, *10*, 349–367.

Sullivan, R. C. Autism: Current trends in services. In E. R. Ritvo (Ed.), *Autism: Diagnosis, current research and management*. New York: Spectrum, 1976.

Tramontana, J., and Stimbert, R. Some techniques of behavior modification with autistic children. *Psychological Reports*, 1970, *27*, 498.

Wetzel, R. J., Baker, J., Roney, M., and Martin, M. Outpatient treatment of autistic behavior. *Behaviour Research and Therapy*, 1966, *4*, 169–177.

Wolf, M. M., Risley, T. R., and Mees, H. Application of operant conditioning procedures to the behavior problems of an autistic child. *Behaviour Research and Therapy*, 1964, *1*, 305–312.

Wulbert, M., Barach, R., Perry, M., Straughan, J., Sulzbacher, S., Turner, K., and Wiltz, N. The generalization of newly acquired behaviors by parents and child across three different settings. *Journal of Abnormal Child Psychology*, 1974, *2*, 87–98.

Zifferblatt, S. M., Burton, S. D., Horner, R., and White, T. Establishing generalization effects among autistic children. *Journal of Autism and Childhood Schizophrenia*, 1977, *7*, 337–347.

10

A Training Program for Families of Children with Autism

Responding to Family Needs

MARTIN A. KOZLOFF

INTRODUCTION: A PERSPECTIVE ON NEEDS

Work with families of children with autism is approximately 20 years old. It began in a context in which parents were seen as both partly responsible for their children's condition and perhaps disturbed in their own way. At least three factors, however, provided momentum for the phenomenon of parent training or programs for families. One was criticism of the logic behind and weak empirical evidence for the psychogenic and sociogenic explanations of autism, i.e., that autism constituted the child's defense against, or was the result of, a harsh, conflicting, unrewarding family environment. A number of researchers, including Ornitz (1967a, 1976b), Ornitz, Brown, Mason, and Putnam (1974), Reynolds, Newsom, and Lovaas (1974), Rimland (1964), and Schopler (1965) showed that many of the deviant behaviors and developmental abnormalities of autistic children were associated with and perhaps were accounted for by sensory, perceptual, cognitive, and neurological impairments for which their parents were not responsible. In addition, the work of DeMyer (1979), Eberhardy (1967), Farber (1959), Fowle (1968), Holroyd and McArthur (1976), Kozloff (1979), Schopler (1971), and Schopler and Loftin (1969a, 1969b), suggested not only that the blaming of parents for their children's condition benefited those

MARTIN A. KOZLOFF • Department of Sociology, Boston University, Boston, Massachusetts 02215. The material in this chapter was written with the support of grant number MH 14761, awarded to the Department of Sociology, Boston University, by the National Institute of Mental Health.

who developed and applied the psychogenic and sociogenic explanations, but that much of the anxiety and the apparently disordered behavior of the parents was a result of the painful, draining, and confusing experiences of the parents almost from the time their autistic child was born, not the least of which were experiences with professionals.

A second factor was the passage of Public Law 94-142, which requires that all children be provided with an appropriate education regardless of handicap, and the unceasing advocacy of parents on behalf of their children.

And a third factor was the early, tentative work of those who had the daring and foresight to work with parents more as equals, teaching them principles and methods that might enable them to help their children to learn (Engeln, Knutson, Laughy, and Garlington, 1968; Hamblin, Buckholdt, Ferritor, Kozloff, and Blackwell, 1971; Johnson and Brown, 1969; Risley and Wolf, 1966; Schell and Adams, 1968; Schopler and Reichler, 1971; Walder, 1968). Gradually, a curriculum for teaching parents evolved, followed by a number of studies that demonstrated the effectiveness and the benefits of parent training (Brown, Gamboa, Birkimer, and Brown, 1976; Hemsley, Howlin, Berger, Hersov, Holbrook, Rutter, and Yule, 1978; Kaufman, 1976; Kovitz, 1976; O'Dell, 1974; Peine, 1971). At this point, then, we have what might be called an "approach" (i.e., a shared set of ideas and methods), such that work with families is fairly routinized.

The routinization of work with families has both advantages and disadvantages. Dissemination is perhaps the major advantage. It is easy to teach others (indeed, it is often rather easy for newcomers to the field to figure out for themselves) the basics of how to plan and conduct programs with families, because the main ideas and methods have been around for so long now. However, the farther we (as a field) go in our work with families, the more specific, technical, and potentially narrow the work becomes. More and more, we ask questions about smaller and smaller problems relevant to already-organized programs, or we spend our time thinking of better ways to package our programs. Consequently, it is easy to lose sight of the larger issues and problems faced by families, and of the earlier, enduring needs that got the field of "parent training" started. The danger is that, given the very acceptance of the need to work with families, and the routinization of methods for doing so, programs for families could become just another component or appendage of existing educational or treatment services for the children. In this way, programs could lose their original significance as a setting within which parents can begin to understand and solve their individual and common problems. Moreover, professionals may come to believe that conducting programs for families is a relatively straightforward, predictable, and easy affair, resulting in a decline in expended effort, an oversimplification of methods used in working with families, a lack of program development, and, eventually, a decline in effectiveness.

In my opinion, it is important that work with families be a regular part of the services available to children with autism, but that programs for families not be subsumed under the children's educational needs. For, along with education, there are at least four other sets of needs that must be served by programs for families. Indeed, it may be that unless some of the other needs are served first, parents and siblings may not be able to live with or help to educate the child with autism.

One set of needs consists of family members somehow coming to grips with the fact that they have a child or sibling with a severe and chronic condition, that many of their hopes have been irrevocably dashed, and that family and personal life will never be the same. In other words, we are dealing with the more general problems (potential or actual) of suffering, tragedy, and sacrifice. Here, parents' needs may be voiced with such questions as "What did I (we) do to cause this? What did we do to deserve this? What will life be like for us in the future? What has happened to us? What, if anything, can we do to deal with this?"

A second set of needs concerns the cultural and familial issue of how a child acquires a "place," becomes a member, is perceived by other members, and comes to see himself or herself. This is the broader issue of how members define normality and deviance, how they react to deviant development, the expectations they have of, and the roles they provide for, a deviant member. Here, family members might ask such questions as "How is it appropriate to feel about a child who is so strange and disruptive, and causes us such pain? Who is (i.e., what roles are played by) this child—enemy? alien? clown? cross to bear? my-child-for-better-or-worse? my-increasingly-competent child? What can I expect of my child now and in the future? What can I expect of myself? Am I to be a parent, guardian, disciplinarian, teacher, attendant?"

A third set of needs concerns the family as a social system consisting of individuals with particular strengths and needs, who play roles in a family that is affected by its larger context—the community. Here, family members might ask: "How can I do what I am obligated to do as a family member and still get my personal needs met? How or what do I change in myself or in this family so that things change for the better? If we make some changes here, how do we keep them going? We seem so isolated. How do we get hooked up with others who care or who can help us?"

The final set of needs is the educational one. And with respect to this set, family members may ask: "Just what is wrong with my child? What are her strengths and needs? What, specifically, do we do to teach or change specific behaviors? Where do I start? Where do I go (what do I work on) next? What do I do when there are problems in teaching and/or learning?"

The Goals of Our Programs for Families

Our past work with families of children with autism, as well as with families of children with other chronic disorders of childhood (Kozloff, 1973, 1976,

1977), was primarily behavioral, but in addition to teaching parents to observe and count behavior, to utilize prompting, shaping, and chaining techniques, and to differentially reinforce desirable behaviors, we also taught parents to be mindful of the pervasive patterns of interaction or structured exchange in the home that might complement or conflict with their intentional teaching. For example, although they might not reinforce their children's disruptive behavior during teaching sessions, they might reinforce such behavior at other times of the day or might forget to reinforce desirable behaviors. While our programs were generally successful in teaching parents to teach and interact productively with their autistic children, resulting in substantial change in their children's behaviors, a year-long evaluation of our work, during 1975–1976, indicated that one-third of the families had changed very little if at all. A review of all of the videotapes made each week during home visits, data collected by observers in the homes, parents' logs, notes made during phone calls, and interviews with the parents suggested that most, if not all, of the families had many other needs besides those that might be satisfied by the behavioral and interactional methods that we had provided—that is, the needs described above. Consequently, our current work with families is informed by the literature on all of the broad perspectives noted above and is designed to satisfy the additional needs of individual families and families as a class. Specifically, we attempt to teach family members (1) a set of concepts and principles for understanding how change takes place in both the short run and the long run; (2) methods for assessing the family and their own, their children's, and their children's school's strengths and needs; (3) how to plan a rather comprehensive program of change, including interaction patterns, specific behaviors of members, and relationships with schools and other organizations; (4) how to evaluate the change process and solve the problems that arise; (5) how to maintain a process of beneficial change by upgrading their home programs and by anticipating and avoiding problems; and (6) to become more independent of program staff through membership in and use of existing networks.

Besides addressing and helping to satisfy the specific and general needs of families, work with families can have a number of other benefits. For instance, by teaching family members, we increase the number of people who are skilled at working with, and at making informed decisions regarding the lives of, children with autism. Parents and siblings can also give the autistic child a head start on his or her education or, if necessary, provide a substitute for nonexistent or inadequate services. Moreover, by working with the autistic child, family members can increase the amount or rate of the child's learning and can help to generalize the child's improved or new skills to other settings. And finally, family members are in a natural position to work toward normalization, i.e., to teach the child functional skills that increase the child's chances of competent participation in everyday social contexts and to perform more normal roles than would otherwise be available.

THE DEVELOPMENT OF STRENGTHS AND NEEDS AS SEEN IN THE FAMILY CAREER

By the time we work with families, even families of young autistic children, the families have had a number of experiences that have affected the feelings, thoughts, behaviors, and interactions of members. Certain of the experiences, in some cases, have a strengthening effect; for example, the family members learn to cooperate and support each other a great deal, and may come to identify and utilize beneficial personal and familial traits. Other experiences for many families, however, engender changes that are problematic. For example, interaction patterns designed to cope with the children's problem behaviors may worsen or stabilize the behavior, or the parents may become pessimistic and drained of energy. In order to help families, then, we have found that it is important to see that the particular behavioral-educational and medical problems of the autistic child are only a part of the overall picture of historical and current family life. There are many other aspects of family life that need to be understood in order to help family members to produce beneficial changes—indeed, to even motivate members to make the effort to participate in our programs. The following is a brief description of the typical "career" of families with an autistic child.

Background Factors

The larger environment of the family (i.e., economic, cultural, political, and community factors) not only provides problems for the family but affords certain resources for dealing with problems. In general, the families experience an inadequate distribution of resources for helping themselves and their children, which means that much of their efforts to help their children constitutes trial-and-error behavior. But when or if they do get help, it is often after several years of precious time have gone by. Second, the work life of many people (both the breadwinners and the child-rearers) is often experienced as alien, unpredictable, and not in their control. Consequently, parents' self-esteem may be rather low, and they may require from their spouse a great deal of support. To the extent that both the person who works outside of the family and the person who works in the family (trying to rear and take care of the autistic child) experiences his or her daily work as alien and unsatisfying, each partner may have emotional needs that are so great and emotional reserves that are so low that neither can sufficiently gratify the other, resulting in tension, anger, and possibly discord, which weakens their ability to cope effectively with their child.

The fact that many families are nuclear families, geographically isolated from the extended family, may pose further problems. Since the nuclear family consists of two adults, each adult's role in the family division of labor may contain a large number of tasks, which become especially burdensome in light of the great demands made by the autistic child's behavioral inadequacies and problem behaviors. In addition, the nuclear family structure implies that the two adults are primarily responsible for satisfying each other's needs, which, again, is especially difficult given the excessive demands of their role as parents to an autistic child.

Cultural factors also have an impact on the family. To a great extent, we are treated as members in good standing, are deemed competent and valuable, on the basis of our acquisition of certain socially significant symbols, such as material possessions, skills, and life circumstances. When we fail to acquire, or when we lose, socially significant symbols, others may see us as less than competent, as having less value, and may question our membership in society. One important symbol is one's child. To the extent that a child is handicapped, others may see the parents as perhaps to blame, tainted, objects of pity, different, and living outside the experience of other members of society. Thus, the parents of an autistic child may feel that their social worth and place in society are reduced by virtue of others' reactions to them and to their child.

"Deviant" Behaviors of the Child

The behavioral repertoire of the autistic child is deviant and problematic in at least two ways. On the one hand, the child displays a number of problem behaviors, in too many places, at an excessive rate and/or intensity. Thus, family members are exposed to many aversive stimuli during the day: noise, strange mannerisms, self-injurious behaviors, behavior that disrupts routine family activities (e.g., meals) and even sleep. In addition, the child's repertoire is characterized by a number of behavioral inadequacies; i.e., "appropriate" or expected behaviors occur too seldom, in too few places, or with not enough skill. Thus, in addition to trying to tolerate, keep up with, and clean up after the child's problem behaviors, family members must also try to anticipate the satisfy the child's needs and wants, and to do for the child much of what the child does not do for himself or herself.

Societal Reaction

Whether we intend it to be the case or not, much of our public behavior is like a performance, and those in the vicinity are like an audience, whose reactions express approval or disapproval. Many parents of autistic children experience disapproval when they take their children to public places. They are aware of the stares and whispers; they notice that they are being avoided or that others are uncomfortable in their presence; they are given advice that they have not solicited, which communicates that they are too ignorant to even know that they need it. In part, the societal reaction to them and to their child's deviant behavior in public places helps to lower the parents' self-esteem and increase their feelings of differentness, aloneness, and vulnerability.

Experiences with Professionals

Once they recognize that their child's condition is serious, many families begin a round of experiences with professionals, such as the pediatrician and a host of specialists. In many cases, the parents find that the services are costly and unrewarding. They do not get a definitive or even an unambiguous diagnosis or prognosis. Often, evaluations provide information that is, on the one hand, obvious and, on the other, so specific to a particular test or instrument that its connection to behavior in daily life is questionable. And finally, they are not provided with concrete methods to use to help themselves and their child. As a result, many parents become even more confused, pessimistic, and desperate, and possibly distrustful of professionals in general.

Increased Vulnerability

As time goes by, the usual vulnerabilities to time (mortality), other persons (opinions), and the economic system (job insecurity) may be magnified. The parents begin to realize that as they grow older and their child grows larger, the child's problems become more serious. They worry about what will happen to their child after they die or if the child becomes too large to handle. They also spend a lot of money and time away from the job looking for services. And their sensitivity to messages of rejection from others may increase.

Isolation

Families of autistic children may become isolated in several ways. On the one hand, their isolation may be imposed by others, as when they are not invited to go out or when they have a hard time obtaining respite care or baby-sitters. Isolation can also be self-imposed as a result of past reactions from others in public places or because of their child's disruptive behavior in the homes of others. In time, the family may go out less and less, with or without their autistic child. In this way, they avoid the pain of societal reaction. However, isolation also entails an increasing burden on family members to gratify one another. It also means that the child is exposed to fewer and fewer normal experiences and that the child's energy must be expended within the family often in the form of problem behavior.

Structured Exchanges

All social systems are characterized by a number of interaction patterns or structured exchanges. By a ''structured exchange'' I mean a pattern of interaction between two or more persons, in which each person's behavior constitutes or provides antecedents, consequences (positive reinforcers, aversive stimuli) and possibly prompts for the other, and in a durable, recurrent way, i.e., structure or arrangement. Each person, then, reciprocally modifies the behavior of the other person. Given the particular structure of an exchange, certain rather predictable changes are likely to take place in the feelings and behaviors of each participant and in the exchange itself, both in the short run and in the long run. That is, recurrent exchanges are a context that organizes and guides behavior change. Often, the long-term changes are just the opposite of what the participants might have intended. Thus, some exchanges may be considered productive in that they generate pleasurable feelings and desirable behaviors in the long run. Others are counterproductive in that they generate unpleasant feelings and the acquisition of undesirable behavior, e.g., aggression or helplessness. Finally, structured exchanges gradually mold the behaviors and feelings of participants whether or not they are aware of or can describe the exchanges.

Like all other families, those with an autistic child display both productive and counterproductive exchanges. In families of autistic children, however, the frequency of certain counterproductive exchanges may be higher than in families of normal children since the autistic child engages in a higher frequency of problem behavior and a lower frequency of desirable behavior. The exchanges that characterize a family at a particular time seem to evolve rather slowly as members attempt to cope with the difficulties posed by their autistic child and in the context of the experiences and problems described above.

Coercion–Escape. One predominant counterproductive exchange is coercion–escape. In this exchange, the child emits a behavior (e.g., a tantrum) that is aversive to another family member and, by virtue of its aversiveness, coerces the other person to respond. Typically, in reacting to the child's aversive behavior, the other is trying to escape from it or to stop it. Often, what the other does (e.g., talking, holding, giving something to the child) in order to get the child to stop results in a temporary stoppage of the aversive behavior; i.e., the escape behavior seems to work. This stoppage produces a feeling of relief in the person. Thus, whatever he or she did in response to the aversive behavior of the child has been negatively reinforced: strengthened. Ironically, however, the escape behavior that has just been reinforced by the child's stopping was probably a *positive* reinforcer to the child. Thus, the child has been reinforced for engaging in an aversive, coercive behavior, and the other family member has been reinforced for reinforcing the child. Since both people are reinforced, each will engage in his or her respective behavior more often and with more skill. The exchange will also take place more often and will decrease the likelihood of other productive exchanges. Gradually, family life can become *dominated* by the child's coercive behavior, which other members continually try to stop, but with little long-term success. Indeed, other members may come to see themselves as victims or at least as incompetent.

Placation–Avoidance. In this exchange, also counterproductive, family members have learned that certain events lead up to or are predictors of behaviors that are highly aversive. Instead of waiting for the aversive behavior, they try to short-circuit it by gratifying the child before the aversive behavior occurs (e.g., while the child is "working himself up"), or they simply do not ask the child to do things or take the child places where aversive behaviors are likely to happen. Thus, the family members may use a number of positive reinforcers to prevent the child from "blowing up" or becoming disruptive. The child is learning, however, to engage in mildly aversive, threatening behavior so as to produce the placating reinforcers from the others. In the long run, family members are kept constantly vigilant and the child learns to control the family through threats. The child also fails to learn many desirable behaviors.

Earning Reinforcers or the Differential Reinforcement of Other and/or Incompatible Behavior. An alternative to both the coercion–escape and threat–placation exchanges is an exchange in which the parents do not reinforce the child's coercive behavior or threats of coercive behavior. Instead, the parents first establish a broad context for beneficial change by providing their child with many opportunities during the day to earn reinforcers contingent upon desirable behavior, even weak approximations, instead of for coercive or threatening behavior. For instance, the parents reinforce their child's attention, closer proximity to family activities, cooperation with simple requests, eye contact, attempts to communicate in a more normal fashion, or efforts to occupy himself or herself in more appropriate ways. Second, the parents identify the situations in which coercive or threatening behaviors occur. Then, instead of avoiding those situations altogether, or instead of reinforcing disruptive behaviors in those situations, the parents teach the child alternative responses in those situations. For example, if their child throws tantrums as a way of escaping from or avoiding teaching sessions, the parents might conduct very short sessions at first, followed by the child's favorite activities. Or, if the child becomes aggressive in situations in which he or she is likely to make errors, the parents might teach their child to relax in such situations, to intentionally make errors, or to relax or try again after having made an error, with nonaggressive behavior receiving a great deal of reinforcement.

Multiple Signals. Still another counterproductive exchange involves multiple signals. That is, when a family member makes a request of the child and the child fails to cooperate, the other member may repeat himself or herself over and over. Each repetition, however, may be positively reinforcing to the child; the child is learning that the way to keep people talking is to act as if he or she does not understand, and that it is more reinforcing not to cooperate with their requests. If and when the child finally cooperates, the adult is reinforced for having emitted so many repetitions. The mutual reinforcement then keeps the pattern alive. Eventually, however, the other members may make fewer and fewer requests of the child, resulting in lost opportunities for the child to learn functional skills.

Mutual Positive Reinforcement. This is a major productive exchange that can be used to replace all of the other counterproductive ones. In this exchange, each person's behavior constitutes positive reinforcement for the other. In particular, the child engages in behavior that the other likes, and the other family member responds (reciprocates) in a way that is gratifying to the child. Thus, each person is reinforced for desirable behavior; the frequency and skill of performance of the desirable behaviors increase, as does the frequency of the exchange itself. Moreover, each person begins to have feelings of pleasure at the other's presence and may come to see himself or herself as valuable and competent.

Other Long-Term Changes

Given the experiences and problems described above, a number of changes can take place in the family, some of which pose further problems, and some of which constitute strengths or resources. On the one hand, having gotten little from professionals (and perhaps having experienced rejection from other members of the community), family members may become more self-reliant; they may commit themselves to helping their child in the home; and with luck, creativity, and common sense, they may develop methods for teaching their child many important behaviors. Thus, family bonds and members' self-confidence may grow and the autistic child may be seen as a member of the family with developing competence.

On the other hand, family members, in time, may become fatigued and drained; problems may develop in relationships among the members, such as marital discord; some members may develop "personal" problems, such as depression and anxiety; and members may come to see themselves as excessively and personally responsible for the autistic child's present behavior and future. Moreover, they may develop patterns of fatalistic or pessimistic thinking, become highly distrustful of professionals, and gradually lead lives in which they are barely keeping things organized enough to cope on a day-to-day basis.

As noted earlier, one goal of our programs is to help family members to understand what has happened to them, i.e., the changes that have taken place, many of which resulted from factors over which they had little or no control. Another is to help family members to use a number of methods for remedying some of the problematic aspects of their lives and for generating beneficial change.

ORGANIZATION AND OPERATION OF THE PROGRAM FOR FAMILIES

In general, our programs for families have three stages: preprogram, program, and maintenance/follow-up. Programs vary along several dimensions. We

work with between 5 and 10 families in groups. Most programs are heterogeneous with respect to age of the children and severity of the children's condition, parents' social class, area of residence, ethnicity, and education. Some
programs consist of approximately 12 weekly meetings. Others consist of approximately 20 meetings: the first 6 weekly (to maintain continuity) and the rest
biweekly (to allow time for change to take place) for most of a year.

Preprogram Period

The preprogram period consists of five tasks, which take sometimes a
month to complete. We operate on the assumption that the chances of success in
our work with families are increased by the amount of important information that
is collected and by the number of desirable changes that are produced before the
program period (i.e., meetings and home visits) begins.

Contact. Our programs are conducted either independently of any outside
organization and on the premises of the Boston University Department of Sociology, or under the auspices of and in facilities provided by local school systems.
In either case, prospective parents are contacted or made aware of the availability
of the program through ads, brochures, presentations made to parents' groups, or
indirectly through teachers of their children. Whatever the initial contact, parents
are informed that they must take the next step by writing or calling us, either to
learn more about the program or to schedule an initial interview. Those parents
who do contact us might be given more information about the program, either
over the phone or by means of a brochure that is sent to them. If they are still
interested, an initial interview is scheduled. If parents are not interested, we ask
them if we may remain in contact with them in the future, to see if we can be of
any service to them. By providing such noncontingent contact (and, along with
it, support and advice), we try to strengthen parents' interest and commitment for
a future program.

Strengthening Readiness to Change. Readiness to change is a more
lengthy way of referring to motivation. Often, as a result of their career experiences, parents are not ready to change for at least several reasons. We have found
over the years that the more aspects of readiness to change on which the families
display strength, the more likely they are to be successful in the program.

Readiness to change is defined by the following items (Kozloff, 1979): (1)
trust in the consultant; (2) confidence in what the consultant has to offer; (3) a
recognition of the need to conduct a home educational program; (4) a recognition
that each person in the family mutually affects and is affected by the behavior of
the others; (5) a recognition that for beneficial change to take place in the child,
one needs to change some of one's own behavior, e.g., to learn certain teaching
methods; (6) an expectation of success at changing one's own and the child's
behavior (cautious optimism); (7) the willingness and ability to temporarily
shelve some time and outside interests so that one can participate in meetings and

conduct a home educational program; (8) energy, or the belief that one has energy sufficient to participate in the program and to conduct a home educational program; and (9) a tentative acceptance of the behavioral-educational approach, i.e., some of its basic assumptions and methods.

Readiness to change is assessed and strengthened during the initial interview(s), which are held at times and places convenient to the family. Both parents are expected to participate. Interested siblings are also encouraged to attend. A number of methods are used during the interview(s) to establish rapport, to facilitate the parents' expression or description of behaviors, feelings, and thoughts indicative of the various aspects of readiness to change, to acknowledge those that are strong, and to strengthen those that appear weak. In particular, the interviewer-consultant (1) first asks the parents general questions about their historical experiences, to encourage conversation; (2) is mindful of the emotional meanings of family members' posture, tone of voice, and statements, labels what they seem to be expressing, and empathizes with expressed concerns and feelings; (3) pinpoints instances of desirable thinking, effort, and action and reinforces family members for these, in an effort to build a partial success story to counter an overly negative view held by members; (4) works to build a more behavioral-educational perspective by translating expressed events and processes into behavioral terminology; (5) builds confidence and trust by accurately empathizing with members, by predicting what the family has been through as well as certain events that are likely to have occurred, by pointing out the differences between the interviewer's approach and the less successful approaches of others from whom the family has sought help, and by beginning to suggest alternative methods that family members might use to improve conditions in the family; (6) describes the prospective program in greater detail, including tasks expected of family members and consultants, possible benefits, and possible negative consequences; (7) anticipates and defuses (i.e., voices) a number of misconceptions and hesitations that family members may have about privacy, success versus failure, and time commitments; (8) handles reservations brought up by family members by empathizing with their expressed concerns and by offering alternative interpretations, e.g., reservations about the planned use of reinforcement, about deprivation and punishment, about the "mechanistic" quality of some behavioral approaches, about their ability to give up a certain amount of time, about the program not working, or about teaching not being their job.

If, after one or two initial interviews, it is clear both to the interviewer and to the parents that the program is likely to be of benefit to the family, and that the family members are indeed ready to participate, the program would be made available to the family and the third step of the preprogram period would be taken, as described below. If, on the other hand, it seems that family members are weak on the readiness-to-change items (e.g., they still have rather strong reservations about behavioral-educational methods or they are not sure that they need to conduct a home educational program), then the interviewer would offer them a partial program. That is, the interviewer would offer to work with the family on a more limited basis, e.g., to work on a few selected behaviors of the child, to help the parents to read and understand some written material relevant to their child's condition or education, or to help the parents to evaluate the child. Such a partial program might be continued indefinitely or might be gradually developed into a full-scale (i.e., comprehensive) program.

Formalizing a Working Relationship. We have found that it is best to have a working relationship that balances informality and formality, empathy and a businesslike approach to change. To establish and maintain the businesslike side of the program, both parents and all staff members (family consultants) write and sign a contract that specifies each party's obligations, such as attendance, conducting home visits, providing materials, doing assignments, and protecting various rights. In some of our programs, the major program contract is coupled with a backup reinforcement system in which families earn positive reinforcers, such as college credit, respite care, or additional home visits. In several programs, a negative reinforcement contingency was used, in which all participants (staff and parents) wrote certified checks in small amounts to persons or organizations that they did not like. Unless a certain number of credits was earned in a particular week for having fulfilled the terms of the contract, a check was sent. Although few checks ever had to be sent, it is impossible to say what function was served by the credit-check system, if any. It may be that it merely served to engender a more serious approach to participation in the program.

Assessment. Once the working relationship is formalized, the next task, assessment, is worked on. Assessment is accomplished via *interviews,* which help family members to describe their historical and current experiences, *direct observation* in the home, parents' descriptions of daily events on *logs, videotape* (used both by staff and by family members to record themselves), and more standardized behavior *checklists.* In general, the assessment involves two interviews and approximately three 2-hour observations in the home. Two things are assessed: the behavioral repertoire of the child with autism and all of the aspects of family life that we believe have a bearing on the child's repertoire and on the family's ability to conduct and maintain a successful home educational program.

In the past, assessment of a child's repertoire consisted of observing the child both during short teaching sessions conducted by the parents (e.g., on small motor, imitation, and language tasks) and during "spontaneous" activity. The child's behavior was then scored with the Behavior Evaluation Scale (Kozloff, 1974), which consists of 99 behaviors arranged into seven skill areas. Each behavior can be ordinally scaled according to probability or frequency, duration, and skill. In addition, both the parents and the observer-consultant pinpointed several behaviors to count and chart with greater accuracy, e.g., problem behaviors, cooperation, or speech.

The above approach has been very useful in several ways. First, it is simple for parents and the observer to use. Second, it helps to reduce the parents' confusion about what is "wrong" with their child because it asks concrete questions and requires specific observations. Third, it helps the parents and observer to obtain a more balanced picture of the child, i.e., neither completely incompetent nor completely competent. However, the approach has several shortcomings. It rarely describes the child's performance with respect to a social context. It often treats behaviors as static and abstract. It does not yield a picture of the nature and extent of the child's actual participation in daily affairs. And it does not enable one to discover the organization of the child's repertoire. At this time, while we continue to use, and to teach parents to use, the above method of assessment, we also utilize the following methods, which emphasize functional behavior in routine contexts.

First, parents observe and write logs of daily events—from large units to the smaller activities and tasks that constitute the larger units of family life. Gradually, the logs are synthesized into a picture of a typical day. The question, then, is how the child fits into the routine. To help answer this question, the second addition to our assessment methods is to observe the child's performance of a number of tasks, either alone or in the larger context of an activity. Either the child is videotaped or a record is kept according to a task analysis form. The task analysis form simultaneously allows the observer or parent to note the child's performance on each movement-step of the task sequence and to score the nature of prompt required, if any—e.g., repetition of request to perform task; gesture; template or "jig"; model; instruction; or physical prompt. Later, by comparing videotapes and/or analyses of various tasks, we and the parents can determine the "weak" and "strong" behavioral links in the child's performance and note how general the weaknesses and strengths are to other tasks. In this way, we can begin to determine where it might be best to begin a child's education.

Third, in order to assess the extent and nature of the child's actual participation in daily life, parents (and staff serving as consultants) observe what the child does during routine activities. Thus, for each activity in the family, the observer can note (1) if the child was present in the room where the activity was taking place; (2) if the child was not present, what the child was doing (an alternative, desirable behavior; some type of unproductive, bizarre, or disruptive behavior); (3) if the child was present, what the child was doing (not participating but *attending;* not participating but *available,* i.e., likely to be cooperative if given an opportunity; partially participating; fully integrated, i.e., performing tasks integral to or necessary to the accomplishment of the activity). Information from this method also helps us to determine those activities where it might be best to begin to improve the child's functioning in the family.

As noted, in addition to the child's repertoire and how it fits into or contributes to the round of daily life, we also assess those other aspects of family life that have a bearing on the child and on the success of the program for the family. Information on the various items is obtained through interviews, direct observation, and parents' logs. The following is a list of the items assessed. The first 10 items are, we believe, most important in predicting a family's success at conducting a home educational program during the program period (i.e., the phase when family members attend meetings). The remaining 6 items are predictors of a family's success at persisting at and maintaining a good home educational program once the program for families is faded out.

1. Objectivity: observing, pinpointing, describing, analyzing, evaluating, charting, scaling.
2. Confidence in more general principles and a long-term time perspective.
3. Ability to plan a comprehensive educational program: areas to work on, specific behaviors to work on, educational sequence to follow.
4. Agreeing to try specific methods of teaching or at least accepting responsibility for making own decision, evaluating outcome, and revising plans if indicated.
5. Displaying a response pattern of waiting and planning rather than reacting, i.e., following a problem-solving sequence.
6. Instituting and maintaining productive exchanges, replacing counterproductive exchanges.
7. Skill at using general teaching methods: setting up physical environment so as to facilitate learning and performance of desirable behavior; signaling, prompting, fading, and reinforcing; evaluating progress.
8. Cooperation among parents and/or siblings regarding educational program for autistic child.
9. Organized home life: routine, chores, schedules, noise and activity level.
10. Ability to solve personal problems, e.g., tension, anxiety, depressed mood.
11. Being honest with self, partner, other children, and consultant about feelings, beliefs, behavior, progress.
12. Taking scheduled breaks while maintaining gains.
13. Instituting reinforcement patterns for own and other members' efforts and successes.
14. Being integrated in networks offering support and resources.
15. Ability to generalize own and child's gains to other settings, e.g., in community.
16. Ability to anticipate and solve postprogram problems, e.g., decline of reinforcer effectiveness, learning plateaus.

Information gathered on the above items (as well as on the items defining readiness to change mentioned earlier) is summarized on the Assessment and

Programming Guide (Kozloff, 1979), which describes and allows a scoring of a family's strengths and difficulties with every item.

Organizing Information and Planning the Program. Once the assessment is completed, the family members and the consultant organize and review the information that has been collected. In general, both the strengths and needs of the child, of the family members, and of the family system are noted. A tentative plan is then drawn that is designed to achieve the various short-term and long-term goals of the family by helping family members to use their strengths and to work on the needs pinpointed and described during the assessment stage. In general, the instructional sequence for an individual family or for a group follows the list of 16 items presented above. Improvement on earlier items is seen as facilitating change in later items, all of which contribute to changes in the social environment of the child such that the child learns to be a more competent participant in the family and community.

Program Period

General Considerations. Before describing specific units of instruction, the more common aspects of the program stage might be mentioned. First, most of our work is with groups of families, with an average of about eight families. Both parents are expected to attend all meetings. If that is not possible, a substitute is suggested, e.g., an older sibling or a family friend. In some programs, the children's teachers either have been invited to attend or have been formal participants along with the parents. Other programs have been for the families alone.

Although some programs have been intensive (12 or so weekly meetings) and others extensive (20 or so biweekly meetings), the optimum arrangement seems to be no more than about 16 meetings (not including maintenance or follow-up), of which the first 6 are weekly and the remaining 10 are biweekly.

Participants are provided with written materials, portions of which are assigned for each meeting—*Educating Children with Learning and Behavior Problems* (Kozloff, 1974) and *Unraveling the Special Education Maze* (Cutler, 1981). Additional materials, on such topics as relaxation, language development, or self-help skills, are obtained from other readily available sources. In addition to reading, participants are given weekly (or biweekly) assignments on *data-taking, instituting productive exchanges, and teaching.* Home visits for observation, coaching, and program revision are conducted between meetings by the same consultant. All assignments and the time and date of home visits are written on a weekly contract form, one copy of which is kept by the family and the other of which is kept by the consultant. As much as possible, notes are kept on conversations, teaching program plans, daily events, progress, problems, and occurrences during meetings. All group meetings are, in addition, audiotaped.

Problems that arise during the program that are common to the participants (e.g., fear that change will not take place, lack of cooperation among parents) are often made part of the agenda of future meetings. Individual problems (e.g., one family's continual failure to do agreed-upon assignments) are handled by the consultant with that family.

The various units of instruction during the program period are arranged into three smaller groups of meetings: early meetings, the bulk of the work, and preparation for maintenance.

Early Meetings. The first six or so meetings (generally weekly) focus on the "basics." That is, parents are taught (1) to be more objective in observing and describing family life and their children; (2) to use behavioral and social-exchange concepts and principles to analyze or understand their career experiences and current patterns in the family (e.g., the strength of certain behaviors, anxiety about teaching, the existence of particular exchange patterns and their likely long-term effects); (3) how certain events become signals for behavior, how behaviors are strengthened in frequency, skill, duration, and intensity as a function of particular contingencies of reinforcement; (4) how to use their observing skills and basic behavioral and exchange principles to pinpoint and replace counterproductive exchanges with productive ones; and (5) how to evaluate their child's behavioral repertoire, role, and participation in family life (using the Behavior Evaluation Scale, logs, and task analyses), and how to pinpoint skill areas, target behaviors, and everyday tasks and activities to work on.

The series of early meetings culminates in two major changes. The first is the *early home program.* After the first four or five meetings, parents are taught to apply what they have learned, using a plan such as the following:

1. Make a list of some behaviors that your child can do—even if they are not done perfectly well. Examples include chores, self-help routines, simple tasks, communications.
2. Make a list of specific places and times where your child can do *more* of the behaviors listed in number 1.
3. Make a list of things that are rewards for your child—both new ones that you might not have used and old ones that have been around.
4. Now state some rules about which behaviors get what rewards. For example:
    "As much as possible, when he . . . , then he can (I will give him . . . ; we can. . .)."
   Or, you can state the rule to your child in the form of Grandma's Law:
    "As soon as you . . . , then you can (we can . . . ; I will give you. . .)."
   This is also a good time to tell yourselves what you will try *not* to do. For instance,

"When she (whines; makes messes; makes mistakes),
I will try not to. . . . Instead, I will. . . ."
5. Now select several of the new rules and *use them*.
6. Make sure to keep an eye out for "good" behaviors (behaviors that you want to see more of). Reward them quickly and often.
7. Also keep your eyes open for little chances to have your child learn or do some behavior. Can he put his own plate in the sink? Can she soap her own washcloth? Can she open the door for you? Can he stir the soup? Can she ask for that music? If the answer is "Yes," "Maybe," or "I don't know," find out.
8. Use your signals (such as questions and requests) wisely. Get your child's attention first; use words he or she understands; make it short and to the point.
9. Help your child to perform a behavior correctly. Think of ways to make it easier to do.

The second major change at this time is that the families have a rather comprehensive home educational program plan that can be followed. Their plans, worked out with their consultants, tentatively specify a number of things.

I. Skill areas in which the child needs specific kinds of help.

II. Target behaviors within each skill area that are strong and those that are weak, and the ways that each may need to be changed or further improved.

III. Activities and tasks in the round of daily life where the child's competent participation can be improved (e.g., meals, wake-up time, dressing, shopping, leisure time).

IV. A set of criteria for deciding when to work on which behaviors. (V to follow.)

In the past, the method for selecting behaviors to work on, as described in Chapter 4 of *Educating Children* (Kozloff, 1974), involved the use of a table that listed a number of prerequisite behaviors for each skill area. If the assessment indicated that a child did not adequately perform the prerequisites for a particular skill area, the child by definition was not yet "ready." The parents then backed up to an easier skill area and began with the area for which their child was ready.

With our increasing focus on normalization and functionality, additional criteria have become important. Thus, the list of criteria guiding parents' selection of behaviors to work on now include the following:

A. Feasibility
1. Does the child have the learning readiness skills?
2. Does the child have other obvious prerequisite skills?
3. Do the parents have the teaching skills?
4. Does the desired behavior fit family goals?

B. Least Cost (Economical)
1. Will this behavior change as much as or more than other behaviors, given the same effort?
2. Are the materials required to teach the behavior readily available?
3. Does the parent have to exert reasonable amounts of effort or energy to teach the behavior?
4. Does the behavior create the least interruption of other activities of the child and family?

C. Most Generalizable (Most Applicable in Other Situations of the Day)
1. Is the behavior one that the child will have repeated opportunities to practice and use?
2. Is the behavior part of other significant behaviors or skills?
3. Is it easy to engineer opportunities for this behavior?

D. Functionality
1. Is it useful for the child?
2. If the child doesn't do it, will someone else have to?
3. Is the behavior part of the role of a competent member of the family and community?

E. Change in Family Members' Perception
1. Will success in teaching this behavior improve family members' images of themselves as teachers and of the child as a learner and family member?

F. Change in Child's Perception
1. Will success at learning the behavior make the child feel proud, more competent, less deviant, more helpful, more accepted?

G. Age-Appropriateness
1. Is the behavior one that is typically expected of a person of this age, or is it "beneath" the person?

H. Normativeness of Methods
1. Are the methods that seem to be necessary to teach or maintain the behavior (e.g., reinforcers, prompts) usual or normative, or are they "bizarre," "unnatural," untypical, or coercive?

Using the above list, the parents and consultants can select behaviors to change that are likely to have the biggest payoff, for the least cost.

V. A tentative sequence to follow in moving from one behavior (goal) to another as a child makes progress.

The educational sequence for children is guided by two sets of criteria: *developmental* and *functional*. Developmentally, a child's curriculum is guided by the Skill Sequence Table (Kozloff, 1974), which suggests that learning readiness skills (e.g., attention, cooperation) facilitate the learning of motor skills, which facilitate the learning of chores, self-help skills, and motor imitation, the latter of which facilitates the learning of verbal imitation, which facilitates the learning of functional speech. Thus, as a child improves in each "area," the parents work on harder behaviors within the area and begin to work on easier behaviors in the next area or areas for which the child appears ready. In effect, such a developmental sequence proceeds by the accumulation and synthesis of simpler behaviors into more complex ones. For example, attention to the parent, observation of the parent's mouth movements, and repetition of a word uttered by the parent constitute the more complex behavioral sequence of verbal imitation.

A child's educational sequence also moves according to criteria that are more relevant to functionality, i.e., to the child's competent participation in the round of daily life. For instance, the criterion or dimension of *generalization* encourages parents and consultants to be mindful of other physical settings and action settings in which the child's improved performances can occur. The criterion of *application*, on the other hand, helps parents and consultants to move from practice sessions (e.g., on motor imitation) to appropriate usage (e.g., imitating the method for making a bed). And finally, the criterion of *expansion or chaining* involves adding more and more components to an existing performance, in either a backward or a forward sequence. For instance, once a child can competently participate during meals (the basic performance), the child can be taught either to eat and then help clean the table (forward chaining) or to help to prepare the meal and then eat (backward chaining).

The Bulk of the Work. The second group of approximately eight meetings involves parents actually conducting a number of teaching programs in the home, with weekly or biweekly coaching from their consultants. In this phase of the program parents learn (1) more advanced teaching methods (shaping, prompting, and fading); (2) methods for teaching a variety of behaviors, tasks, and skills (cooperation, attention, small motor, chores and self-help, imitation, verbal imitation, functional speech, relaxation); (3) how to teach in more naturalistic ways (i.e., in the context of routine activities and using everyday reinforcers); (4) how to plan, write, and follow teaching programs for changing particular behaviors; (5) how to cooperate among themselves as a family, reinforce themselves, and take scheduled breaks; (6) how to generalize behavior change to settings outside the family; (7) how to evaluate teaching programs and revise them if necessary; (8) how to replace problem behaviors; and (9) how to be effective advocates for their children.

Several things are worth noting about this phase of the program. First, the families generally work on cooperation with simple requests as one of their first target behaviors. Strengthening cooperation has the benefits of (1) increasing the child's participation in everyday affairs; (2) improving the child's competence in a wide range of areas (i.e., it is highly generalizable); (3) engendering a set of family interaction patterns or exchanges that are productive (e.g., providing the child with opportunities to learn, reinforcing desirable behavior); (4) giving the parents and siblings many opportunities to use basic teaching methods; (5) focusing family members' attention on a basic and desirable behavior, and away from as-yet-unattainable goals and problem behaviors; and (6) facilitating change in family members' conceptions of the child (e.g., from clown or adversary to more competent and likable member.) Shortly after they begin to work on cooperation, however, more diversity appears. That is, the families begin working on different behaviors and change takes place at varying rates. Unless it is extreme, such diversity is actually productive, for the group members then have the chance of describing (and learning) a host of methods for teaching and for solving problems.

Second, as the parents (and siblings) are successful in helping the autistic child to learn and perform new behaviors, they are encouraged to apply the criteria of generalization, application, and expansion, so that the child gradually learns to participate competently in more and more activities in daily life.

Third, this is the point at which difficulties appear with approximately one-fourth to one-third of the families. Typically, the difficulty is not the child's lack of progress but rather the family's change process. In some cases, the parents fail to do their assignments, e.g., reading, data-taking, or teaching. In other cases, the parent or parents may do their assignments but are troubled. They may be pessimistic about the future, feel sad and overwhelmed (''She'll never get better, really better. It's such hard work living with her. Sometimes I just want to leave or I want to put her away''). And in still other cases, the difficulty is that one parent's expectations and plans are different from the other parent's, and they have a hard time planning and conducting a joint home program.

We seem to be successful in resolving perhaps one-half of the above kinds of difficulties, either by working with the family during home visits or, in the case of a general or potentially general problem, by working on it in the group. In most cases, we try to solve problems by helping parents to (1) describe their actions, feelings, and beliefs; (2) correct misconceptions or misperceptions (e.g., about how much or how little their child has progressed or about their being ''bad'' parents if they require their child to earn reinforcers); (3) reassess their goals and perhaps establish those that are more feasible and less costly; (4) use relaxation and self-reinforcement procedures; (5) conduct complementary teaching programs if they cannot agree on which behaviors to teach and on which methods to use.

Preparation for Maintenance. The final group of approximately four meetings is designed to help the families to prepare for the future, when meetings and home visits will gradually be faded out. Topics of meetings include (1) anticipating and avoiding, or solving, postprogram problems, such as fatigue, a decline in the rate of progress, the emergence of problem behaviors, or disagreements with methods being used in the child's school; (2) planning long-term and short-term goals to work on, and some methods to use for achieving those goals; (3) becoming part of and using networks of services and support, such as parents' organizations and the group itself; and (4) helping parents to express their feelings about their experiences in the program and their feelings about the program coming to a close, as well as helping them to assess the progress they have made.

Maintenance/Follow-Up

Once the program period is over, meetings and home visits are gradually faded, from biweekly to monthly, to bimonthly to quarterly. The purpose of such meetings and visits is to review with parents their progress and any problems to date, and to upgrade or revise their home programs.

CONCLUSION: STRENGTHS AND ENDURING NEEDS

At this point, our programs for families of children with autism are effective in several ways. In particular, we are able to (1) assess and strengthen parents' readiness to change; (2) assess the autistic child's needs and strengths in various skill areas, describe the round of family life and the nature and extent of the child's participation in it, and determine the strengths and needs of the family with respect to many aspects of family functioning that have a bearing on instituting and maintaining a process of productive change; (3) use assessment information to plan educational programs for the children and programs of change for the family as a whole; (4) conduct programs for families, individually and in groups, that generate a process of beneficial change and, by helping to alleviate such problems as pessimism, fear of failure, and tension, help families to maintain and generalize change.

Nevertheless, there are two sets of enduring needs that our programs do not sufficiently address. One concerns the chronicity of the problems of the autistic child and the effects of that chronicity on the family. Except in rare cases, inputs from our programs are not enough to help the other family members to deal with many of the likely changes in their child's behavioral needs and strengths, their child's future living and working requirements, and their own relationships and feelings. Despite their skills, the beneficial changes that have taken place in their child's repertoire, and their associations with other parents, many parents continue to feel isolated and vulnerable; they experience difficulties in obtaining an adequate education for their child; and they are concerned about the future. Thus, much work is needed in the provision of continued support for families, perhaps in the form of networks among families, home-visiting educational specialists, advocacy, and respite care.

Second, although our overall rate of success is higher than it was, we are still unable to facilitate more than a minimal amount of change in approximately one-fourth of our families. In some of the cases, it seems that little can be done in the way of instituting an effective home educational program because during the course of the program the parents have had to deal with other, more pressing problems, such as illness. With these families, however, a program that is continuously available (e.g., is an integral part of the child's education) might eventually be able to help when the parents finally become ready enough to use it. In other cases, we simply do not know enough about some aspects of family and personality dynamics to overcome the obstacles to change. For example, some parents (1) seem to have adapted to their own and to their child's condition such that they see no need to change themselves or the child; (2) have such different expectations of themselves and of the child that they constantly undermine each other's efforts (e.g., one parent trying to teach the child new skills and the other trying to maintain old behavior patterns); or (3) seem to have such a strong belief that only professionals can help their child that they do not conduct their own home program. While a behavioral-educational approach to families certainly was useful in the early stages of work with families, instilling optimism and providing concrete methods for engendering change, it does not seem to contain enough concepts to sufficiently describe many of the complexities of family life. Thus, it will be fruitful to incorporate ideas and methods from such fields as family systems theory and therapy.

REFERENCES

Brown, J. H., Gamboa, A. M., Jr., Birkimer, J., and Brown, R. Some possible effects of parent self-control training on parent–child interaction. In E. J. Mash, L. C. Handy, and L. A. Hamerlynck (Eds.), *Behavior modification approaches to parenting*. New York: Brunner/Mazel, 1976. Pp. 180–192.

Cutler, B. *Unraveling the special education maze*. Champaign, Ill.: Research Press, 1981.

DeMyer, M. K. *Parents and children in autism*. Washington, D.C.: Winston, 1979.

Eberhardy, F. The view from the couch. *Journal of Child Psychology and Psychiatry and Allied Disciplines*, 1967, *8*, 257–263.

Engeln, R., Knutson, R., Laughy, L., and Garlington, W. Behavior modification techniques applied to a family unit—A case study. *Journal of Child Psychology and Psychiatry*, 1968, *9*, 245–252.

Farber, B. Effects of a severely mentally retarded child on family interaction. *Monographs of the Society for Research on Child Development*, 1959, *24* (2, Serial No. 71).

Fowle, C. M. The effect of the severely mentally retarded child on his family. *American Journal of Mental Deficiency*, 1968, *73*, 468–473.

Hamblin, R. L., Buckholdt, D., Ferritor, D., Kozloff, M., and Blackwell, L. *The humanization processes*. New York: Wiley, 1971.

Hemsley, R., Howlin, P., Berger, M., Hersov, L., Holbrook, D., Rutter, M., and Yule, W. Treating autistic children in a family context. In M. Rutter and E. Schopler (Eds.), *Autism: A reappraisal of concepts and treatment*. New York: Plenum, 1978.

Holroyd, J., and McArthur, D. Mental retardation and stress on the parents: A contrast between

Down's syndrome and childhood autism. *American Journal of Mental Deficiency,* 1976, *80,* 431–436.

Johnson, S. M., and Brown, R. A. Producing behavior change in parents of disturbed children. *Journal of Child Psychology and Psychiatry,* 1969, *10,* 107–121.

Kaufman, K. F. Teaching parents to teach their children: The behavior modification approach. In B. Feingold and C. Bank (Eds.), *Developmental disabilities of early childhood.* Springfield, Ill.: Charles C Thomas, 1976. Pp. 96–120.

Kovitz, K. E. Comparing group and individual methods for training parents in child management techniques. In E. J. Mash, L. C. Handy, and L. A. Hamerlynk (Eds.), *Behavior modification approaches to parenting.* New York: Brunner/Mazel, 1976. Pp. 124–138.

Kozloff, M. A. *Reaching the autistic child.* Champaign, Ill.: Research Press, 1973.

Kozloff, M. A. *Educating children with learning and behavior problems.* New York: Wiley, 1974.

Kozloff, M. A. Systems of structured exchange: Changing families of severely deviant children. *Sociological Practice,* 1976, *1,* 86–104.

Kozloff, M. A. A comprehensive behavioral training program for parents of autistic children. In D. Upper (Ed.), *Perspectives in behavior therapy.* Kalamazoo, Mich.: Behaviordelia, 1977.

Kozloff, M. A. *A program for families of children with learning and behavior problems.* New York: Wiley, 1979.

O'Dell, S. Training parents in behavior modification. *Psychological Bulletin,* 1974, *81,* 418–433.

Ornitz, E. M. Medical assessment. In E. R. Ritvo (Ed.), *Autism.* New York: Wiley, 1976. Pp. 7–23. (a)

Ornitz, E. M. The modulation of sensory input and motor output in autistic children. In E. Schopler and R. J. Reichler (Eds.), *Psychopathology and child development.* New York: Plenum Press, 1976. Pp. 115–133. (b)

Ornitz, E. M., Brown, M. B., Mason, A., and Putnam, N. H. The effect of visual input on vestibular nystagmus in autistic children. *Archives of General Psychiatry,* 1974, *31,* 369–375.

Peine, H. *Training parents using lecture-demonstration procedures and a contingency-managed program.* Unpublished doctoral dissertation, University of Utah, 1971.

Reynolds, B. S., Newsom, C. D., and Lovaas, O. I. Auditory overselectivity in autistic children. *Journal of Abnormal Child Psychology,* 1974, *2,* 253–263.

Rimland, B. *Early infantile autism.* New York: Appleton-Century-Crofts, 1964.

Risley, T. R., and Wolf, M. N. Experimental manipulation of autistic behavior and generalization into the home. In R. Ulrich, T. Stachnik, and J. Mabry (Eds.), *Control of human behavior.* Glenview, Ill.: Scott, Foresman, 1966.

Schell, R. E., and Adams, W. P. Training parents of a young child with profound behavior deficits to be teacher-therapists. *Journal of Special Education,* 1968, *2,* 439–454.

Schopler, E. Early infantile autism and receptor processes. *Archives of General Psychiatry,* 1965, *13,* 327–335.

Schopler, E. Parents of psychotic children as scapegoats. *Journal of Contemporary Psychology,* 1971, *4,* 17–22.

Schopler, E., and Loftin, J. M. Thinking disorders in parents of young psychotic children. *Journal of Abnormal Psychology,* 1969, *74,* 281–287. (a)

Schopler, E., and Loftin, J. M. Thought disorders in parents of psychotic children: A function of test anxiety. *Archives of General Psychiatry,* 1969, *20,* 174–181. (b)

Schopler, E., and Reichler, R. J. Parents as cotherapists in the treatment of psychotic children. *Journal of Autism and Childhood Schizophrenia,* 1971, *1,* 87–102.

Walder, L. *Teaching parents and others principles of behavioral control for modifying the behavior of children.* Final Report. Silver Spring, Md.: Institute for Behavioral Research, 1968.

11

Training Parent–Child Interactions

LAURA SCHREIBMAN, ROBERT L. KOEGEL,
DEBRA L. MILLS, AND JOHN C. BURKE

Given the severe behavioral deficits and bizarre behavioral excesses so characteristic of autism, it is not surprising that these children present one of the most serious challenges facing child therapists and educators. Many of these children who fail to receive specialized treatment are eventually placed in out-of-home (typically institutional) environments. One major reason for placement out of the home is that most parents simply are unable to cope with their child's behavior. The challenge of autism is certainly most strongly felt by the family. The purpose of this chapter is to discuss and assess the effect that a parent-training program can have on various aspects of family functioning.

Parents of autistic children historically have carried the burden of being implicated in causing, or at least contributing to, their child's disorder. The parents have been described as undemonstrative, unemotional, cold, and perfectionistic (Kanner, 1949). Thus, Bettelheim (1956) has described autism as a reaction of extreme psychopathological mother–infant interactions. However, when parental characteristics have been systematically investigated as causal factors, the results have proven inconclusive. For example, when they are compared with those in the general population, a higher incidence of nonpsychotic affective disturbances has been reported in the families of autistic children (Lot-

LAURA SCHREIBMAN • Psychology Department, University of California, San Diego, La Jolla, California 92093.   ROBERT L. KOEGEL • Social Process Research Institute, University of California, Santa Barbara, California 93106.   DEBRA L. MILLS • Psychology Department, University of California, San Diego, La Jolla, California 92093.   JOHN C. BURKE • Speech Department, University of California, Santa Barbara, California 93106. Preparation of this chapter was supported by U.S.P.H.S. Research Grants MH28231 (Laura Schreibman, Ph.D., principal investigator) and MH28210 (Robert L. Koegel, Ph.D., principal investigator) from the National Institute of Mental Health.

ter, 1967; Wing, O'Connor, and Lotter, 1967). In contrast, other studies have found no reliable differences in parental attitudes, warmth, nurturance, and stimulation of the infant (Cox, Rutter, Newman, and Bartak, 1975; DeMyer, Pontius, Norton, Barton, Allen, and Steele, 1972). In addition to the unnecessary guilt felt by the parents, the emphasis on parental causation has undoubtedly led some clinicians to overlook the parents as potentially effective change agents.

In recent years, however, a growing number of professionals, from a variety of orientations, have advocated the participation of parents in their children's treatment programs (e.g., Kozloff, 1973; Schopler and Reichler, 1971; Watson, 1973; Wing, 1972). The inclusion of parents as treatment providers for their children has several conceivable advantages. First, parents are around their child more than anyone else. Whereas a clinician or teacher may interact with the child for only a few hours a day, parents have the potential to provide a round-the-clock treatment environment. In comparison with clinics and schools, which are geared more toward remediating academic deficiencies, the home treatment environment can be readily amenable for treatment of other aspects of the child's behavioral deficits (e.g., tantrums, compulsive behaviors, and self-stimulatory behaviors). Second, since treatment gains made in one setting are not always transferred to other settings, it has been suggested that generalization of gains could be facilitated by involving the parents (e.g., Rincover and Koegel, 1975; Wahler, 1969). For example, eliminating tantrums in the clinic or classroom does not necessarily mean that the child will not cry and scream for attention at home. Since a trained parent provides the treatment in the home environment, problems of generalization of treatment gains from clinic or school to the home can be greatly reduced. Also, the parent can work in conjunction with the child's teacher or therapist to provide consistency in procedures across all settings. This would help ensure that gains made at school or in the clinic are extended to the home. Third, schools and clinics specializing in the treatment of autistic children are relatively scarce and may not be conveniently located for families living in more isolated or rural communities. The time and expense of traveling to the clinic or relocating near a treatment facility may not be feasible. Since all autistic children have a parent or guardian, parent training, in essence, has the potential to make the treatment more available by bringing the clinic to the child. Fourth, training programs that emphasize general treatment procedures may enable the trained parent to handle any new problem behaviors their child may exhibit. This alleviates the need for additional, and costly, professional intervention. Fifth, after training, parents who may have previously felt excluded from their child's education are actively involved in their child's development. Additionally, it is hypothesized that trained parents will need to spend less time in custodial activities (e.g., bathing, dressing) with their child and can spend more time in leisure activities with the family.

But perhaps the most crucial advantage of parent training was demonstrated in a follow-up study of 20 autistic children who had participated in a behavior modification treatment program (Lovaas, Koegel, Simmons, and Long, 1973). The study demonstrated that although appropriate behaviors were increased and inappropriate behaviors were decreased during the original treatment, prognosis for the children at follow-up 4 years later depended on the postreatment environment. Those children whose parents had been trained in behavior modification continued to improve, whereas children who had been institutionalized or returned to untrained parents had lost their previously acquired skills. The authors concluded that contingencies must be maintained to prevent learned behaviors from being extinguished.

Aside from the formal advantages to training parent–child interactions such as those above, parents of autistic children have typically illustrated the need as they describe their autistic child in the context of the family's daily lives. For instance, one father of a 4-year-old autistic child described his son in the following manner:

> He was neither toilet trained nor could he feed himself; he seldom spoke expressively; his attention span was almost nil; he rarely played with toys at all; he never came when he was called by name; he was almost always lost in a world whose activities consisted solely of thread-pulling, lint-picking, blanket sucking, spontaneous giggling, inexplicable crying, eye-squinting, finger-walking, wall-hugging, circle-walking, bed-bouncing, head-nodding, and body rocking.

Though some of these behaviors can be seen occurring during normal child development, they are for the most part not exhibited to the same degree or extent as by autistic children. The impact of an autistic child is, however, very similar to the impact of a young child on the family's daily lives. It requires more parental supervision and consequently makes it more difficult for the parents to participate in other joint activities (cf. Berk and Berk, 1979; Burke, Note 1).

Research conducted in our laboratories comparing clinic treatment to parent training has also supported these results (Schreibman, Koegel, and Britten, 1982). That study was conducted over a 5-year period, with more than 50 families participating in the program. The children of trained parents, unlike the children receiving treatment only in the clinic, showed improvement over time and in a variety of different environments. The research also indicated that parent training had other positive collateral effects on the family, which will be discussed later in the chapter. Thus, in addition to the obvious advantages of parent training, it appears to be essential in the treatment of autism.

BACKGROUND ON PARENT TRAINING

Parent-training programs did not begin with the treatment of autistic children but, indeed, have been in use for many years. A detailed discussion of the parent-training literature in general is presented below because it foreshadows many of the issues that arise in the field of autism as well. Reviews of the parent-training literature indicate that training parents in the techniques of behavior modification is an efficacious mode for changing many different types of children's behavior (e.g., Berkowitz and Graziano, 1972; Forehand and Atkinson, 1977; Johnson and Katz, 1973; O'Dell, 1974; Resinger, Ora, and Frangia, 1976). The majority of these investigations have been concerned with procedures for reducing undesirable behaviors such as aggression, operant vomiting, irrational fears, and stealing. A recent review paper was devoted entirely to child noncompliance (Wells and Forehand, 1980). Other programs have utilized parent training to increase appropriate behaviors such as toileting, speech, and independent behaviors (e.g., Baker, Brightman, Heifetz, and Murphy, 1976; Hewett, 1965; Risley and Wolf, 1967; Tahmisian and McReynolds, 1971).

The content and methodologies of various training programs have also been reviewed (Berkowitz and Graziano, 1972; Johnson and Katz, 1973; Moreland, Schwebel, Beck, and Wells, 1982; O'Dell, 1974). Training methods have included instructing parents in behavioral principles through discussion or written materials (Arnold, Sturgis, and Forehand, 1977; Barrett, 1969; Fowler, Johnson, Whitman, and Zukotynski, 1978; Johnson, Whitman, and Barloon-Nobel, 1978; Kelly, Embry, and Baer, 1979; McMahon and Forehand, 1978; Tahmisian and McReynolds, 1971; Baker and Heifetz, Note 2). Other programs have utilized behavioral rehearsal and feedback (e.g., Crowley and Armstrong, 1977; Crozier and Katz, 1979; Forehand and King, 1977; Peed, Roberts, and Forehand, 1977), modeling procedures *in vivo* and through videotapes (e.g., Crozier and Katz, 1979; Flanagan, Adams, and Forehand, 1979; Koegel, Glahn, and Nieminen, 1978; O'Dell, Flynn, and Benlolo, 1977; O'Dell, Krug, O'Quin, and Kasnetz, 1980; O'Dell, Mahoney, Horton, and Turner, 1979), and telephone contacts (e.g., Frederiksen, Jenkins, and Carr, 1976; Heifetz, 1977; Baker and Heifetz, Note 2) and the majority of programs cited above have utilized various combinations of these components. Training procedures have also been conducted with groups, as well as with individual families (Kovitz, 1976; Brightman, Baker, Clark, and Ambrose, Note 3).

As noted by Moreland *et al.* (1982) and Taplin (1974), a considerable proportion of the literature has focused only on the child's behavior. This fact, in conjunction with the lack of consistent methodologies and measurement techniques across studies, has made it difficult to compare the effects of the different training procedures on the entire family system.

Investigations studying the effects of different training procedures on parent skills have primarily focused on one target behavior—the correct use of time-out. Typically, modeling procedures, either live or videotaped, have been shown to be superior to other procedures, such as written presentation, lectures, and role-playing (e.g., Flanagan *et al.*, 1979; Nay, 1975; O'Dell *et al.*, 1977, 1979; O'Dell, Krug, O'Quin, and Kasnetz, 1980). However O'Dell, Krug, Patterson, and Faustman (1980) found no significant differences between training groups when the parents' behavior was measured at home.

The last study (O'Dell, Krug, Patterson, and Faustman, 1980) raises the issue that various training procedures may have differential effects on the parents' behavior at home versus in the clinic. It cannot be assumed that skills demonstrated in the clinic will automatically be applied in the home. Zangwill and Kniskern (1982) showed that although there were significant correlations between parents' rates of reinforcement and rates of punishment at home and in the clinic, there were significant differences between settings in the absolute amount of the behaviors observed. Mothers' mean rates of reinforcement and punishment were much higher in the clinic than at home. Although clinic observations may be more economical for the experimenter, the necessity of transfer of skills to the home setting is important enough to warrant home observations.

Other investigators have demonstrated the need to teach general social learning principles in order to generalize parenting skills to the home and/or to handle a wide range of behaviors (Glogower and Sloop, 1976; Koegel et al., 1978; McMahon, Forehand, and Griest, 1981). A recent study (O'Dell, O'Quin, Alford, O'Briant, Bradlyn, and Giebenhain, 1982) compared the effectiveness of four training methods, all of which included training in general learning principles, on parent reinforcement skills. All procedures were superior to a minimal-instructions control group. There were no significant differences among the written, manual, videotaped modeling, or live modeling with rehearsal methods. An audiotaped manual was significantly less effective than the other training methods. And the videotape training was reported to more consistently train a wider range of parents.

The studies comparing different training methods are also problematic in that they rarely measure parent–child interactions. O'Dell et al. (1982) measured child compliance but did not find a significant difference in behavior between the children of trained parents and those in the control group. The lack of effect was attributed to a high base rate of the children's compliance. A test using a variety of responses may have been more sensitive to differences between training procedures. Both Koegel et al. (1978) and McMahon et al. (1981) measured parent–child interactions; however, differences in training methods make comparison of the results difficult in determining which of the components is responsible for the generalized treatment effects (Britten, Note 4).

Finally, the effect of training on parental attitudes, expectations, and confidence has been omitted from the majority of studies. O'Dell et al. (1982) found no differences in parental attitudes toward treatment among various training procedures or the control group. All parents expressed satisfaction with the program. The absence of differences between groups may have been due to the measure itself. Only three questions were asked of the parents. The generality of their content was likely to produce social desirability in responding. Parental expectations were measured by O'Dell *et al.* (1979) but only with reference to differences between groups prior to training. The effect of training on expectations was not investigated. The effect of training on confidence levels was examined by Heifetz (1977) and Baker and Heifetz (Note 2). These studies found that parents trained with a written manual reported less confidence in their abilities than did parents trained with a combination of manual plus phone contact, manual plus group training, or manual group training and home visits. For a more extensive review of the literature comparing various training methods, please refer to Moreland *et al.* (1982) and Britten (Note 4).

Due to differences in experimental procedures and measurement techniques and the dearth of information regarding attitudes, expectations, and confidence levels, there is still a need for systematic analysis of the effectiveness of various training procedures on parent–child interactions and their collateral effects on the family.

OUR PARENT-TRAINING PROGRAM

Our current training program was designed to provide parents with the knowledge and skills necessary to teach a wide variety of new behaviors to their autistic child and to effectively manage behavior problems as they arise. The procedures utilized in the program are based on a behavioral view of autism and have been empirically documented as effective in changing behavior of autistic children (Schreibman and Koegel, 1981).

Training Content

The foundation of the training program lies in teaching the parents the basic principles of behavior modification. This approach is based on a study conducted by Koegel *et al.* (1978). This study showed that after a therapist demonstrated how to teach a specific behavior, parents were able to teach their child that behavior. However, they were unable to teach their child additional behaviors unless the therapist had previously demonstrated the procedure. Thus, these parents did not acquire generalized teaching skills. In contrast, parents who had achieved mastery of general behavioral principles were able to generalize their acquired skills and to teach their child previously untargeted behaviors.

The curriculum encompasses a variety of techniques and how to apply them with autistic children. One of the first skills parents are taught is how to select behaviors they wish to change. Potential target behaviors are categorized into groups of behavioral deficits and excesses. The parents then learn to operationally define the behaviors, select appropriate measurement techniques, and assess the behaviors for functional content.

The next step in the program focuses on structuring the teaching situation. Parents are instructed in the format and correct execution of the components of discrete training trials. The training components include the following: (1) presentation of the instruction or question, (2) prompting and prompt fading, (3) shaping and chaining, (4) reinforcement, extinction, and punishment, (5) intertrial intervals, and (6) assessment of behavior change. Further information is provided on procedures to promote stimulus generalization, response generalization, and maintenance of behavior change. (See Koegel and Schreibman, 1982, for a complete discussion of the procedures trained.)

After the parents are familiarized with the general procedures, specific treatment programs to teach independent living skills (e.g., eating, dressing, bathing, toileting, and speech and language) and to control problem behaviors are addressed according to the individual needs of the parents and the child.

Training Procedures

Based on previous literature regarding training procedures, the parent-training program incorporates a comprehensive package of training materials. First, the parents are given a selection of reading materials encompassing the basic principles of behavior modification (e.g., Baker *et al.*, 1976; Hall, 1971). Additional readings with question-and-answer exercises are provided to show in specific detail how the principles may be applied with autistic children (Koegel and Schreibman, 1982). Second, a videotape is shown to the parents in which correct and incorrect applications of behavioral procedures are demonstrated and discussed. In the third component of the program, the parents are actively involved in structured teaching sessions with their child. During these sessions, the parent-trainer provides brief demonstrations of the various behavioral techniques. The parents then apply these procedures while attempting to teach their child a new behavior. Feedback to the parent regarding his or her performance of therapy skills is provided by the parent-trainer. This training with feedback continues until the parent(s) demonstrate their proficiency by using the specific teaching procedures at 80% correct criterion during a videotaped test session. Fourth, once the parents are able to teach new behaviors (not previously demonstrated) to their child in the structured setting, the training sessions are primarily focused on teaching the parents to design, implement, and evaluate treatment programs for their child. When the parents are independently designing and implementing their own programs, the home visits by the parent-trainer are reduced in frequency to approximately one per month. These visits are supplemented with weekly telephone contacts, and additional visits may be scheduled for special needs.

Data Analysis

In many areas of analysis, the data from the parent-training program are compared to that of a control clinic group. Parents of the children in the control (clinic) group do not receive training and are not involved in providing treatment for their autistic children. However, each child in the clinic group receives 4½ hours of treatment per week for 1 year. This treatment follows the same basic behavior modification guidelines as are taught to the parents in the parent-training group. There are two primary therapists for each child, each having a minimum of two lecture courses and two practicum courses in behavior modification with autistic children. The curriculum employed by the clinicians is the same as that given to the parents in the experimental group. In summary, the two groups receive very similar behavior modification treatments; the difference is that the parents in the experimental parent-training group become trained in the use of the procedures and then become their child's primary treatment provider, instead of having a clinician implement the treatment.

Assessment Procedures

In order to determine the impact of the training program on the family, indices are taken to reflect changes in the child's behavior, parent–child interactions, general family interactions, parent psychological and marital adjustment, parental expectations for their child, and parent satisfaction with the program.

Child measures are obtained through observations of the child's behavior and standardized questionnaires. Assessment measures are conducted prior to the time the child's parents enter the program, at 6 months into training to assess the child's progress, at 1 year as a posttest assessment, and at follow-up 3 months after the completion of the program.

Observations of the child are conducted in a *structured laboratory setting* to assess the child's behavior in a free-play situation. Videotapes of each session are made through equipment concealed behind a one-way mirror. A multiple-response recording procedure is utilized to analyze the proportion of appropriate behaviors (play with toys, social nonverbal behaviors, and appropriate speech) relative to inappropriate behaviors (psychotic speech, noncooperation, tantrums, and self-stimulation). For a more detailed description of the observation and reliability procedures, please refer to Schreibman *et al.* (in press) An additional measure obtained is the Vineland Social Maturity Scale.

Observations of *parent–child teaching interactions* are videotaped in a structured teaching situation in the clinic. These measures are carried out prior to training, after the parents complete the home feedback sessions, and at follow-up. The structured teaching sessions involve having each parent attempt to teach a new task to their child in a 10-minute session. The task chosen is discrete and nonambiguous, and is one that the child does not currently know but that is within his or her abilities at the time of the session. A multi-response scoring procedure is used to assess both the parent's and the child's behavior. The parent's behavior is analyzed for the correct or incorrect delivery of discriminative stimuli, prompts, shaping procedures, and consequences according to the criteria established by Koegel and his colleagues (Koegel *et al.*, 1978; Koegel, Russo, and Rincover, 1977). The child's performance of the target behavior is measured to determine if the parent's actions have any affect on their child's learning. Each trial is scored for a correct versus incorrect response, whether the response was prompted, or if it was an approximation of the target behavior.

Unstructured observations taken in the home provide a measure of the parent–child interactions at home. Videotapes are made of the family at the dinner hour since the entire family tends to be around at this time. Data are collected on child compliance with parental question and commands. This scoring scheme is adapted from Koegel *et al.* (1977).

A *general measure of family interaction* is provided by the Family Environment Scale (FES) (Moos, Insel, and Humphrey, 1974). This instrument is a self-report scale yielding 10 scale sums in areas of interest such as conflict, organization, and control. The scale is administered separately to each parent.

Parent adjustment measures are taken in response to the hypothesis that parental psychopathology plays an important role in the etiology of autism. The *Minnesota Multiphasic Personality Inventory* (MMPI) is administered because it is a widely accepted index of personality adjustment. To determine the impact of the training program on the marital relationship, the Dyadic Adjustment Scale (Spanier, 1976) is given to the parents. The scale is used because it is based on an empirical composite of the most widely used measures of marital adjustment (e.g., Burgess and Cottrell, 1939; Locke and Wallace, 1959; Nye and Mac-Dougall, 1959; Orden and Bradburn, 1968). In addition, the measure has good validity and high scale reliability, is very brief, and can be administered in a minimum amount of time (Spanier, 1976).

Another measure, the 24-hour Diary (Burke, Note 1) (or Time Activity Budget), was employed to provide information about how the parents spent their time during the day. The parents were asked to list each activity they engaged in during 1 weekday and 1 weekend day. This information allowed for the assessment of possible effects of the parent-training program on various aspects of daily interactions between parents and children.

Parental expectation prior to treatment and *satisfaction* with the program after treatment are also measured. The questionnaire regarding the expectations is designed to reflect the parents' specific expectations regarding the treatment process, such as the number of hours required of them, types of changes they expect in their child's behavior, and the magnitude of the changes. Previous work in the area of psychopathology (Goldstein, Heller, and Sechrist, 1966) has indicated that expectation is related to satisfaction of clients in a treatment program. Therefore, an index is needed to examine how realistic parental expectations are, and what relationship exists between these expectations and consumer satisfaction with the treatment intervention.

The satisfaction questionnaire measures parental satisfaction with the program in seven domains: (1) the staff's ability to provide treatment, (2) relevance of the treatment to the child's future, (3) child's improvement, (4) parent's commitment to provide treatment to the child, (5) parents' ability to provide treatment to the child, (6) the staff's commitment to provide treatment to the child, and (7) overall satisfaction with the child. We feel such measures are necessary because no matter how effective a program is by behavioral criteria, if the parents do not like it, they will be less likely to use it.

Results

The particular analyses presented below have been conducted on a preliminary corpus of data obtained from a total of 31 families that participated in the first part of our research program. This facilitates a comprehensive discussion of the influence that parent training has on a wide variety of both global and specific parent–child interactions.

Child Measures

Global Measure: Vineland Social Maturity Scale. The results from the Vineland Social Maturity Scale showed that the children who were involved in the parent-training program and those in the control clinic group demonstrated significant and similar pre- to posttreatment gains in their Social Quotient (social age divided by chronological age). Furthermore, both groups of children maintained their gains at the time of follow-up. These data are based upon interviews conducted with numerous significant people in the children's daily lives (e.g., parents, teachers, and clinicians) and includes reported information covering several broad areas of child development (e.g., independent functioning, communication abilities, locomotion, and socialization). On the basis of these data, it appears that both intervention programs (i.e., parent training and direct clinic intervention) can produce similar positive "global" changes in the children's overall development. However, since this measure is based upon a composite of information derived from many interviews, it does not give specific information about the relative amount of change taking place in any one specific environment in comparison to the other environments. Therefore, it is interesting to examine the results from the more specific behavioral measures described below.

Specific Measure: Structured Laboratory Observations. Unlike the findings from the Vineland Social Maturity Scale, the data from the structured laboratory observations showed mixed results in terms of child improvement. Specifically, the results indicated that while the children were with their treatment providers (i.e., parent-training group with mother, clinic group with therapist), they showed similar and significant gains from pre- to posttreatment and from posttreatment to follow-up. However, when the children were interacting with nontreatment providers (unfamiliar adult for both groups, as well as mothers for the clinic treatment group), they exhibited no differential improvement at either posttreatment or follow-up. The improvement seen in the parent-training group children while interacting with their mothers appears to be a direct result of having their mother as their treatment provider. As a consequence, it appears that parent training may be superior to clinic treatment in that the treatment provider (the parent) is present in many different settings (e.g., home) and thus (as previously noted in this chapter) could have a greater impact on the child's gains.

Specific Measure: Unstructured Home Observations. The results from the unstructured home observations provide additional data showing the impact of parent training on the children's appropriate responding while with their mothers. Specifically, the results show that by the time of follow-up, the children in the parent-training group had significantly improved in responding to their parents' instructions and commands. In contrast, the children in the clinic group evidenced no improvement in their appropriate responding at follow-up. These results are highly consistent with those reported above from the structured laboratory observations in that both measures indicate that the children do not evidence their gains when a treatment provider is not present.

In summary, while the results of the Vineland Social Maturity Scale suggest that the children in both groups "globally" improved, the results observed in the structured laboratory observations and unstructured home observations indicated that the children demonstrated the improvements only when interacting with their treatment provider (parent-training group with mother, clinic group with therapist). Thus, these data seem to indicate that additional research on methods of promoting generalization to nontreatment-providing adults is still greatly needed and should be considered a primary area for future research efforts. Such work is currently a major focus of the research efforts in our own laboratories.*

*This work was supported by grants from the National Institute of Mental Health (MH28231 and MH29210) and from the Office of Special Education No. 300-82-0362 in collaboration with Drs. Glen Dunlap, Thomas Bellamy, and Robert Horner.

Parent Parameters

Global Measure: MMPI. The results from the MMPI show that the parents scored well within the normal range on all the subscales both before and after their involvement in the parent-training program. A similar result was found for the parents whose children were involved in the clinic group in that they also scored well within the normal range before and after their children's involvement. These results are highly consistent with those reported in the literature on families with autistic children (cf. McAdoo and DeMyer, 1978). However, while numerous authors did not find any statistically significant differences between parents of autistic children and their "normal" counterparts, there seems to be a tendency for some authors (e.g., McAdoo and DeMyer, 1978; Wolff and Morris, 1971) also to mention that the direction of their results is consistent with the parental stress reaction hypothesis. This hypothesis states that parents with autistic children are in a general state of psychological stress as a result of having a handicapped child, and that this stress is reflected in their general personality. While McAdoo and DeMyer (1978) and Wolff and Morris (1971) have suggested that a generally high level of stress may be present in these families, some investigators (e.g., Schopler and Loftin, 1969; Burke, Note 1; Koegel, Schreibman, O'Neill, and Burke, 1983) have suggested that the stress may be more specific to certain types of situations (e.g., shopping with a tantrumous child) and have begun to systematically investigate this possibility. Some of these results are presented in later portions of this chapter.

Global Measure: Spanier Dyadic Adjustment Scale. The pre- and posttreatment data from the Spanier Dyadic Adjustment Scale indicate that the parents in both groups (parent training and direct clinic intervention) scored similar to each other and well within the range of Spanier's happily married normative group. These data are consistent with the MMPI results in that both the parents' general personality characteristics and their marital adjustment do not seem to be influenced as a function of their involvement in the parent-training program.

The above measures all relate to global types of functioning rather than to specific problematic areas. However, several specific areas of functioning may merit a closer examination. These include anecdotal reports of lack of leisure time, and requirements of large amounts of custodial care needed for autistic children. While some investigators have begun to isolate and define these areas more precisely, little research has directly sought to assess the influence of a training program on these measures that were employed to assess the occurrence of certain types of changes across several types of parent–child interactions.

Specific Measure: Parent–Child Teaching Interactions. Posttreatment observation data on the mothers' correct use of the five teaching procedures (taught in the parent-training program) indicate that in addition to learning to use the techniques during structured teaching situations, the parents in the parent-training program also scored significantly higher than the parents in the control group during the structured laboratory observations. These were relatively less formal than the teaching sessions since they primarily involved play. Further, when the trained parents employed these techniques correctly, the autistic children demonstrated significantly more appropriate responding than the children in the control clinic group. Specifically, the average score for the children in the parent-training group was twice as a high as the average for the children in the control clinic group.

These data suggest that the parents in the parent-training group are able to generalize their ability to effectively teach their children in unstructured situations and consequently have a greater positive influence on the autistic children's performance in such settings. In contrast, if one considers these results from the perspective of the clinic treatment group, one might suspect that their lack of ability to effectively teach the children in unstructured settings might negatively influence other areas, such as the amount of time devoted to leisure versus custodial care activities. These areas are, therefore, discussed in detail below.

Specific Measure: 24-Hour Home Diary (Time Activity Budget) Data. As previously mentioned, the 24-hour home diary was employed to assess possible effects of the parent-training program on certain important types of daily interactions between the parents and their children. For instance, Burke (Note 1) systematically tabulated the amount of time the parents in the parent-training program and those in the control clinic group were involved in two types of activities: (1) *teaching activities* and (2) *direct custodial care activities*. The results from the investigation showed that at posttreatment the parents in the parent-training group reported twice the amount of time used for teaching their children various behaviors (e.g., self-care, dressing, bathing, educational games, school-related work) as compared to the parents in the control clinic group. In addition, Burke (Note 1) found that the parents in the training program reported significantly less time involved in providing custodial care for their children than the parents in the control clinic group. Burke (Note 1) suggested that as the parents acquire and transfer their skills to home situations, they are able to teach their children many necessary daily behaviors and consequently spend less time performing the same behaviors in a custodial care manner.

In addition to the effects that parent training has on the amount of time the parents spend in teaching and custodial care activities, preliminary data have also been gathered on other collateral effects. Koegel et al. (1983) reported that families who were involved in the parent-training program reported a significant increase in the amount of time they participated in *leisure and recreation activities*. These activities included going on outings, having friends over to their home, and quiet leisure time alone in the home. These investigators focused on these types of family activities as a result of anecdotal reports from parents who prior to their involvement often felt ''chained to their children'' or ''trapped in their house," which resulted in an unusually small amount of time spent in leisure and recreational activities for the entire family. Their results indicated that the parents in both groups (parent training and direct clinic intervention) reported almost identical amounts of time spent in leisure and recreational activities at pretreatment. By posttreatment, however, the parents in the parent-training program averaged approximately seven times more per sample than the control group.

Consistent with these results are data obtained on the MOOS Family Environment Scale. The three subscales on this measure that showed the greatest difference between the two groups of parents were Expression, Intellectual-Cultural Orientation, and Active Recreation Orientation. These data greatly favored the parent-training group in that, while the two groups scored well below the normal level at pretreatment, only the parent-training group had posttreatment scores that were very near to the standardized scores for normal families (cf. Koegel *et al.*, 1983).

Parent Satisfaction Measures

Consistent with the outcome results reported above are the results from the parent satisfaction measures. Klaila (Note 5) employed the parent satisfaction questionnaire as described earlier in the chapter and, in part, found that the parents in the parent-training group reported more overall satisfaction with their children and a greater commitment to provide treatment. In addition, and seemingly contradictory to the observation results presented above, the parents in the training program reported a decrease in their ability to work with their children after 1 year of treatment. Klaila suggested that this latter finding could have been a result of a self-report bias on the intake questionnaire (i.e., the parents at intake could have possibly overrated their actual ability before receiving training).

In a further attempt to isolate variables that might influence parental satisfaction with parent training versus direct clinic treatment, Schreibman, Koegel, Klaila, Burke, Webb, and Parker (Note 6) conducted an investigation that focused on measuring parent satisfaction after having sequentially participated in both programs (in a random order across families). The results from this additional assessment are presented below.

Program Preference (Parent Training vs. Direct Clinic Intervention). Of the 15 parents, 38% preferred the parent-training program while 62% preferred the clinic program. The parents who preferred the clinic treatment intervention program often stated that it was a result of feeling more confident in the professionals' ability to provide the children's treatment. While these parents were provided with free treatment services for their children, most parents are unable to locate these types of services at no cost. Therefore, additional questions were also posed to these parents. For example, given a $35 an hour charge, what would their program preference be? The results from this question showed that only 8% preferred the clinic program. Also, 0% preferred the parenting program; however, the remaining 92% of the parents reported a preference for a new "combination program," which would include both parent training and the "professional" service.

Parent Ratings of Amount of Contact Time with Project Personnel. The parents rated the adequacy of the amount of contact time for both programs as being very positive, with the parent-training program receiving a 5.4 and the clinic program a 5.5 on a 7-point rating scale (1 = not enough time and 7 = a more than adequate amount of time).

Parent Ratings of Programs' Influence on Autistic Children's Functioning. Mean parent ratings were determined for the programs' influence on the following eight subareas of child functioning: (1) communicative abilities, (2) interactions with family, (3) interactions with strangers, (4) socially acceptable behavior at home, (5) socially acceptable behavior in public, (6) ability to follow instructions given by parents, (7) ability to follow instructions given by others, and (8) reduction of self-stimulatory behavior. In general, the parents rated both programs as having positively influenced their children's development. However, the degree to which a program influenced a child in specific areas differed. For instance, the clinic program was viewed as having influenced the children's communicative abilities to a greater extent. This finding is consistent with anecdotal comments from parents who reported that clinic intervention is superior for the child in the acquisition of speech. In the subarea of socially acceptable behavior, parent-training intervention was more beneficial and *necessary* for promoting their children's gains as well as improving their families' overall functioning.

CONCLUSION

Overall, these results on family interactions suggest that parent training is superior to clinic treatment (which does not involve parent training). That is, parent training promoted widespread improvements in family interactions and child functioning across a variety of settings, resulting in numerous improvements in behavior and in more normalized daily family routines. Further, rather than altering any underlying mental process or personality traits, it appears that parent training influences only specific abilities of the parents to correctly use well-established teaching procedures while interacting with their autistic children. Consequently, the parents are able to facilitate the child's development and help promote the generalization of gains to both the home and other leisure and training environments. Further research, however, seems very important in the areas of identifying variables influencing parent satisfaction with different subareas of the programs, and in identifying variables important for promoting generalization of treatment gains to untrained individuals in the children's environments.

REFERENCE NOTES

1. Burke, J. C. *Collateral effects of parent-training on the daily interactions of families with autistic children.* Unpublished master's thesis, University of California, Santa Barbara, 1982.
2. Baker, B. L., and Heifetz, L. J. *Manpower and methodology in behavior modification: Parents as teachers one year after training.* Paper presented at the meeting of the Association for the Advancement of Behavior Therapy, San Francisco, December 1976.
3. Brightman, R. P., Baker, B. L., Clark, D. C., and Ambrose, S. A. *Effectiveness of alternative parent training formats.* Unpublished manuscript, University of California, Los Angeles, 1980.
4. Britten, K. R. *A two part review of parent training: The comparison of operant parent-training procedures and the social validation of parent training.* Unpublished manuscript, University of Kansas, 1982.
5. Klaila, D. A. *Parental satisfaction with clinic treatment and parent training in the treatment of autistic children.* Unpublished master's thesis, Claremont Graduate School, 1982.
6. Schreibman, L., Koegel, R. L., Klaila, D. A., Burke, J. C., Webb, J., and Parker, S. Parent satisfaction of parent-training as a treatment for autistic children. *Sixteenth Annual Convention of the Association for Advancement of Behavior Therapy,* Los Angeles, 1982.

REFERENCES

Arnold, S., Sturgis, E., and Forehand, R. Training a parent to teach communication skills: A case study. *Behavior Modification,* 1977, *1,* 259–276.

Baker, B. L., Brightman, A. L., Heifetz, L. J., and Murphy, D. M. *Steps to independence—A skills training series for children with special needs: Early self-help skills.* Champaign, Ill.: Research Press, 1976.

Barrett, B. Behavior modification in the home: Parents adapt laboratory-developed tactics to bowel-training a 5.5 year-old *Psychotherapy: Theory, Research and Practice,* 1969, *6,* 172–176.

Berk, R. A., and Berk, S. F. *Labor and leisure at home: Content and organization of the household day.* Beverly Hills: Sage, 1979.

Berkowitz, B. P., and Graziano, A. M. Training parents as behavior therapists: A review. *Behaviour Research and Therapy,* 1972, *10,* 297–317.

Bettelheim, B. Childhood schizophrenia as a reaction to extreme situations. *American Journal of Orthopsychiatry,* 1956, *26,* 507–518.

Burgess, E. W., and Cottrell, L., Jr. *Predicting success or failure in marriage.* New York: Prentice-Hall, 1939.

Cox, A., Rutter, M., Newman, S., and Bartak, L. A comparative study of infantile autism and a specific developmental receptive language disorder. II Parental characteristics. *British Journal of Psychiatry,* 1975, *126,* 146–159.

Crowley, C. P., and Armstrong, P. M. Positive practice, over correction, and behavior rehearsal in the treatment of three cases of encopresis. *Journal of Behavior Therapy and Experimental Psychiatry,* 1977, *8,* 411–416.

Crozier, J., and Katz, R. C. Social learning treatment of child abuse. *Journal of Behavior Therapy and Experimental Psychiatry*, 1979, *10*, 213–220.

DeMyer, M., Pontius, W., Norton, J. Barton, S., Allen, J., and Steele, R. Parental practices and innate activity in autistic and brain-damaged infants. *Journal of Autism and Childhood Schizophrenia*, 1972, *2*, 49–66.

Flanagan, S., Adams, H. E., and Forehand, R. A comparison of four instructional techniques for teaching parents to use time-out. *Behavior Therapy*, 1979, *10*, 94–102.

Forehand, R., and Atkinson, B. M. Generality of treatment effects with parents as therapists: A review of assessment and implementation procedures. *Behavior Therapy*, 1977, *8*, 575–593.

Forehand, R., and King, H. E. Noncompliant children: Effects of parent training on behavior and attitude change. *Behavior Modification*, 1977, *1*, 93–108.

Fowler, S. A., Johnson, M. R., Whitman, T. L., and Zukotynski, G. Teaching a parent in the home to train self-help skills and increase compliance in her profoundly retarded adult daughter. *AAESPH Review*, 1978, 3, 151–161.

Frederiksen, L. W., Jenkins, J. O., and Carr, C. R. Indirect modification of adolescent drug abuse using contingency contracting. *Journal of Behavior Therapy and Experimental Psychiatry*, 1976, *7*, 377–378.

Glogower, F., and Sloop, W. E. Two strategies of group training of parents as effective behavior modifiers. *Behavior Therapy*, 1976, *7*, 177–184.

Goldstein, A., Heller, K., and Sechrist, C. *Psychotherapy and the psychology of behavior change.* New York: Wiley, 1966.

Hall, R. V. *Managing behavior*, (Vols. a, b, and c). Lawrence, Kans.: H & H Enterprises, 1971.

Heifetz, L. J. Behavioral training for parents of retarded children: Alternative formats based on instructional manuals. *American Journal of Mental Deficiency*, 1977, *82*, 194–203.

Hewett, F. M. Teaching speech to an autistic child through operant conditioning. *American Journal of Orthopsychiatry*, 1965, *35*, 927–936.

Johnson, C. A., and Katz, R. C. Using parents as change agents for their children: A review. *Journal of Child Psychology and Psychiatry*, 1973, *14*, 181–200.

Johnson, M. R., Whitman, T. L., and Barloon-Nobel, R. A home-based program for a preschool behaviorally disturbed child with parents as therapists. *Journal of Behavior Therapy and Experimental Psychiatry*, 1978, *9*, 65–70.

Kanner, L. Problems of nosology and psychodynamics of early infantile autism. *American Journal of Orthopsychiatry*, 1949, *19*, 416–426.

Kelly, M. L., Embry, L. H., and Baer, D. M. Skills for child management and family support: Training parents for maintenance. *Behavior Modification*, 1979, *3*, 373–396.

Koegel, R. L., and Schreibman, L. *How to teach autistic and other severely handicapped children.* Lawrence, Kans.: H & H Enterprises, 1982.

Koegel, R. L., Glahn, T. J., and Nieminen, G. S. Generalization of parent training results. *Journal of Applied Behavior Analysis*, 1978, *11*, 95–109.

Koegel, R. L., Russo, D. C., and Rincover, A. Assessing and training teachers in the generalized use of behavior modification with autistic children. *Journal of Applied Behavior Analysis*, 1977, *10*, 197–205.

Koegel, R. L., Schreibman, L., O'Neill, R. E., and Burke, J. C. *Personality and family interaction characteristics of families with autistic children. Journal of Consulting and Clinical Psychology*, 1983, *51*, 683–692.

Kovitz, K. E. Comparing group and individual methods for training parents in child management techniques. In E. J. Mash, L. C. Handy, and Hamerlynck (Eds.), *Behavior modification approaches to parenting.* New York: Brunner/Mazel, 1976.

Kozloff, M. *Reaching the autistic child: A parent training program.* Champaign, Ill.: Research Press, 1973.

Locke, H. J., and Wallace, K. M. Short marital adjustment prediction tests: Their reliability and validity. *Marriage and Family Living*, 1959, *21*, 251–255.

Lotter, V. Epidemiology of autistic conditions in young children II. Some characteristics of the parents and children. *Social Psychiatry*, 1967, *1*, 163–173.

Lovaas, O. I., Koegel, R. L., Simmons, J. Q., and Long, J. S. Some generalization and follow-up measures on autistic children in behavior therapy. *Journal of Applied Behavior Analysis*, 1973, *6*, 131–166.

McAdoo, G. W., and DeMyer, M. K. Personality characteristics of parents. In M. Rutter and E. Schopler (Eds.), *Autism: A reappraisal of concepts and treatment*. New York: Plenum, 1978.

McMahon, R. J., and Forehand, R. Nonprescription behavior therapy: Effectiveness of a brochure in teaching mothers to correct their children's inappropriate mealtime behaviors. *Behavior Therapy*, 1978, *9*, 814–820.

McMahon, R. J., Forehand, R., and Griest, D. L. Effects of knowledge of social learning principles on enhancing treatment outcome and generalization in a parent training program. *Journal of Consulting and Clinical Psychology*, 1981, *49*, 526–532.

Moos, R. H., Insel, P. M., and Humphrey, B. *Combined preliminary manual for the family, work, and group environment scales*. Palo Alto: Consulting Psychologists Press, 1974.

Moreland, J. R., Schwebel, A. I., Beck, S., and Wells, R. Parents as therapists: A review of the behavior therapy parent training literature—1975 to 1981. *Behavior Modification*, 1982, *6*, 250–275.

Nay, W. R. A systematic comparison of instructional techniques for parents. *Behavior Therapy*, 1975, *6*, 14–21.

Nye, F. I., and MacDougall, E. The dependent variable in marital research. *Pacific Sociological Review*, 1959, *2*, 67–70.

O'Dell, S. Training parents in behavior modification: A review. *Psychological Bulletin*, 1974, *81*, 418–433.

O'Dell, S., Flynn, J., and Benlolo, L. A comparison of parent training techniques in child behavior modification. *Journal of Behavior Therapy and Experimental Psychiatry*, 1977, *8*, 261–268.

O'Dell, S. L., Krug, W. W., O'Quin, J. A., and Kasnetz, M. Media-assisted parent training—A further analysis. *Behavior Therapist*, 1980, *3*, 19–21.

O'Dell, S. L., Krug, W. W., Patterson, J. N., and Faustman, W. O. An assessment of methods for training parents on the use of time-out. *Journal of Behavior Therapy and Experimental Psychiatry*, 1980, *11*, 21–25.

O'Dell, S. L., Mahoney, N. D., Horton, W. G., and Turner, P. E. Media-assisted parent training: Alternative models. *Behavior Therapy*, 1979, *16*, 103–110.

O'Dell, S. L., O'Quin, J. A., Alford, B. A., O'Briant, A. L., Bradlyn, A. S., and Giebenhain, J. E. Predicting the acquisition of parenting skills via four training methods. *Behavior Therapy*, 1982, *13*, 194–208.

Orden, S., & Bradburn, N. Dimensions of marriage happiness. *American Journal of Sociology*, 1968, *23*, 715–731.

Peed, S., Roberts, M., and Forehand, R. Evaluation of the effectiveness of a standardized parent training program in altering the interaction of mothers and their noncompliant children. *Behavior Modification*, 1977, *1*, 323–350.

Resinger, J. J., Ora, J. P., and Frangia, G. W. Parents as change agents for their children: A review. *Journal of Community Psychology*, 1976, *4*, 103–123.

Rincover, A., and Koegel, R. L. Setting generality and stimulus control in autistic children. *Journal of Applied Behavior Analysis*, 1975, *8*, 235–246.

Risley, T. R., and Wolf, M. Establishing functional speech in echolalic children. *Behaviour Research and Therapy*, 1967, *5*, 73–88.

Schopler, E., and Loftin, J. Thought disorders in parents of psychotic children: A function of test anxiety. *Archives of General Psychiatry,* 1969, *20,* 174–181.

Schopler, E., and Reichler, R. J. Developmental therapy by parents with their own autistic child. In M. Rutter (Ed.), *Infantile autism: Concepts, characteristics, and treatment.* London: Churchill-Livingstone, 1971.

Schreibman, L., and Koegel, R. A guideline for planning behavior modification programs for autistic children. In S. Turner, K. Calhoun, and H. Adams (Eds.), *Handbook of clinical behavior therapy.* New York: Wiley, 1981.

Schreibman, L., Koegel, R. L., and Britten, K. R. Parent intervention in the treatment of autistic children: A preliminary report. *Proceedings of the XIIth Banff International Conference on Behavior Sciences: Essentials of behavior treatment for families.* New York: Brunner/Mazel, in press.

Spanier, G. B. Measuring dyadic adjustment: New scales for assessing the quality of marriage and similar dyads. *Journal of Marriage and the Family,* 1976, *38,* 15–30.

Tahmisian, J., and McReynolds, W. Use of parents as behavioral engineers in the treatment of a school phobic girl. *Journal of Counselling Psychology,* 1971, *18,* 225–228.

Taplin, P. *Changes in parental consequences as a function of intervention.* Unpublished doctoral thesis, University of Wisconsin, 1974.

Wahler, R. G. Setting generality: Some specific and general effects of child behavior therapy. *Journal of Applied Behavior Analysis,* 1969, *2,* 239–246.

Watson, L. S. *Child behavior modification: A manual for teachers, nurses and parents.* New York: Pergamon Press, 1973.

Wells, K. C., and Forehand, R. Child behavior problems in the home. In S. M. Turner, K. Calhoun, and H. E. Adams (Eds.), *Handbook of behavior therapy.* New York: Wiley, 1980.

Wing, J. K., O'Conner, N., and Lotter, V. Autistic conditions in early childhood: A survey in Middlesex. *British Medical Journal,* 1967, *3,* 389–392.

Wing, L. *Autistic children: A guide for parents.* New York: Brunner/Mazel, 1972.

Wolff, W. M., and Morris, L. A. Intellectual and personality characteristics of parents of autistic children. *Journal of Abnormal Psychology,* 1971, *2,* 155–161.

Zangwill, W. M., and Kniskern, J. R. Comparison of problem families in the clinic and at home. *Behavior Therapy,* 1982, *13,* 145–152.

12

Behavior Therapists Look at the Impact of an Autistic Child on the Family System

SANDRA L. HARRIS and MICHAEL D. POWERS

A CASE HISTORY

A child is born. He is the first son of a man and a woman who were married for 3 years before they planned this conception, and who were delighted when the wife became pregnant. Throughout the pregnancy the husband and wife shared their dreams of what life in a family would be like and the multitude of happy possibilities for the child's future. They decorated a room—in pale yellow and green so that it would suit a boy or a girl—and began the process of rearranging their lives to accommodate a third person. As they envisioned their life with a child, the couple found themselves drawn even closer than in the past. This infant was to be a tangible sign of the bond of love that held them together. The man, sometimes still impatient with the failings of his own parents, found himself mellowing as he began to contemplate his role as a father. The woman, feeling herself now well beyond the separation process of adolescence, was able to enjoy her parents more than she had in years.

The infant was born following an uneventful labor of 10 hours. The mother was fully conscious and the father an active participant in the birth process. The boy appeared healthy at birth, nursed well, slept well, and evidenced all the technical signs of a normal infant during his brief stay in the hospital. A process

SANDRA L. HARRIS and MICHAEL D. POWERS • Graduate School of Applied and Professional Psychology, Rutgers University, Piscataway, and Douglass Developmental Disabilities Center, New Brunswick, New Jersey 08903.

of emotional attachment, which had started in pregnancy, was further strengthened during the period just after birth. Mother and father felt a deep tenderness
for the infant and found their connections with one another further enhanced by
sharing the experience of their son's birth.

Everything went smoothly for the next few months. He was an easy baby to
care for, his parents enjoyed him, the grandparents were thrilled, and aside from
the inevitable fatigue of late-night feedings, life went well. It was not, of course,
idyllic. The parents growled at one another from time to time. This was the
inevitable friction of three people living together and adapting to one another's
needs in a more complicated pattern than had existed when there was just a
couple. Nonetheless, both the man and the woman felt good about their lives in
this family.

In spite of this sense of goodwill, as time passed the first nibbling of
concern began to grow, first in the mother and then in the father. There was
something inexplicably not right about their son. When they came into his room
to pick him up he did not reach out his arms to be picked up. He seemed to care
little about their presence, to be indifferent to their cuddling. However, both
parents pushed aside their doubts, and the pediatrician who saw the baby every
few months reported that he was developing normally.

By the time the boy was 18 months old it was impossible to turn away from
the problem; he was not developing as he should. There were no indications that
he was going to talk, he seemed quite indifferent to other people, and he appeared content to be left alone. At first, his parents wondered if he were deaf, but
since he would respond to the soft rustling of a candy wrapper this hardly seemed
likely. By the time the child was 24 months of age, their anxiety was acute, and
they began to push their pediatrician for more information. It was at that point
that they were referred for a complete assessment at a special child evaluation
center of the local hospital. Shortly before their son was 30 months of age, the
parents received a definitive diagnosis: Their boy was autistic.

His parents recall vividly the sickening impact of that first conference in the
pediatric neurologist's office. A feeling in the stomach of dread and fear that
remained for weeks and that still, after all these years, returns when they talk
about that day.

Abruptly, the woman and the man underwent a transformation in their view
of themselves and their child. They were the parents of a defective child. This
child, made of their body and their love, was irreversibly damaged. A child who
would never be normal. A child whose future was radically different from all
they had envisioned. Their sense of normalcy, of belonging in a snug niche in the
community around them, was rudely shaken. They were different, and life would
never be the same for them. Their dreams were shattered and they hardly knew
what to do.

Meeting the First Crisis

In this case history the family of an autistic boy have confronted the first of many crises they will endure. We have written no ending to this hypothetical case because we have witnessed many endings to such tragic events. The outcome will depend upon the resources of the parents as individuals and as an interactive unit, the community in which they live, the support system available to them from extended family, friends, and neighbors, and other factors. If the parents blame one another, are abandoned by their own parents, find professional services unavailable or unresponsive, the end result may be far different from what will ensue if they comfort one another, are supported by their families, and find appropriate community resources for their child. In the pages that follow we will consider some of these issues in detail.

INTRODUCTION

We know a fair amount about the needs of autistic children.* For example, it is hard to overestimate the importance of a good educational experience for the autistic child. There is a substantial literature demonstrating that the autistic child and his or her parents can benefit in important ways from parent training in behavior modification techniques and from the intensive education of the child. Nonetheless, such interventions are not a complete answer to the needs of a family. Relatively little attention has been paid to the question of the impact of the child upon his or her family and how the feelings of the parents can affect their ability to care for their child. What does it do to a family when parents must function as teachers? How does one adapt to knowing that a child will never be self-sufficient? What are the effects on a family unit when a trip to the country must be curtailed because an autistic child is having a tantrum? How do brothers and sisters react to the "special privileges" of their handicapped sibling? We need to understand more about these daily realities in the life of the family of an autistic child.

When a healthy family is confronted by a crisis, there may well follow a period of time during which they appear dysfunctional. They are searching for a solution to a problem, and their definitions of themselves and how they can or should behave have been badly shaken by a life experience. Until they can

*Our thanks to Norbert Wetzel, who taught us both a great deal about family therapy; JoLynn Powers and Han van den Blink, who read portions of the manuscript while it was in preparation; and Linda Hoffman, for her secretarial work. Support for this research came in part from a grant from the National Institute of Mental Health (MH29897-94) to the first author.

establish a new equilibrium and a new functional pattern of behavior, they are likely to experience considerable stress. We see this repeatedly in families of a recently diagnosed autistic child. Such stressful conditions may produce a variety of maladaptive behaviors in the family. The behavior therapist can ill afford to overlook this distressed family context when attempting behavioral intervention.

It is the purpose of the present chapter to consider some ways in which the presence of an autistic child can affect the normal family as they move through the life cycle and to examine ways in which the clinician might be helpful to parents as they attempt to resolve these problems. Although much of what we describe here has relevance for the family that functions in a pathological fashion, the primary focus is upon ordinary people who might never have come to our professional attention were it not for the gravity of their child's problems and the consequent stress this creates within the family system.

In examining the impact of the autistic child upon his or her family and of that family upon the child, we will adopt a life cycle framework, looking at the activities a family performs over time and how these functions may be altered by the presence of a handicapped child. For purposes of simplicity, we will consider an intact, middle-class family with a mother, a father, and children. Nevertheless, these same basic considerations should be valid for the single-parent family, a low-income family, a multiproblem family living in a chaotic environment, and other variations in living style.

FAMILY SYSTEMS IN BEHAVIOR THERAPY

It is important to put the writing of this chapter in proper perspective. We are both behavior therapists who have done considerable work training parents of autistic children to work as behavior therapists for their own children. Both clinically and empirically (Harris, Wolchik, and Milch, 1982; Harris, Wolchik, and Weitz, 1981; Weitz, 1982) we have seen direct evidence that parents of autistic children can learn to be skillful teachers for their children. We have seen this effect replicated in dozens of families and have witnessed the improved child behavior, calmer family life, and enhanced sense of parental self-efficacy that follows from these interventions. We both are committed to the importance of this kind of didactic training for parents of developmentally disabled children.

In spite of our satisfaction with the impressive track record of parent training as a viable treatment modality for autistic children, we have felt a gnawing sense of incompleteness in some of our interventions with families. We noted, both informally and in conjunction with our research (Harris *et al.*, 1981), that parents, no matter how skillful they might be as behavior change agents, were not always able to follow through on their home programming efforts with their children. There appeared to be obstacles to the effective maintenance of parent teaching behavior that did not yield to simple pep talks or the renegotiation of treatment contracts.

Having encountered this problem, we reviewed some of the work that has been done in training parents as behavior modifiers in various clinical contexts. We discovered that we were not alone in finding that while it is relatively easy to teach parents the behavioral skills they need, it is not always possible to ensure that they will continue to use these skills once training ends. For example, in 1977 Heifetz studied a variety of modalities for training parents to work with their mentally retarded children at home. When Baker, Heifetz, and Murphy (1980) revisited these families, they found that although the parents still remembered the behavioral techniques and the children had not forgotten how to perform the skills their parents taught them, most of the parents were no longer engaged in formal teaching. Among the reasons they gave for this change were lack of time, the child's limited ability to learn, the parents' perceived limits as teachers, and the lack of professional support. Such findings point compellingly to the importance of examining more closely the context in which one trains parents as teachers.

Compatible with this view, Mealiea (1976) noted with concern the tendency of some behavior therapists to adopt a narrow framework for change. He argues that the failure to be sensitive to the impact of one's behavioral interventions can sometimes lead to a deterioration in the overall functioning of the family. We cannot expect to change the behavior of a child without having an effect upon everyone else in the family. For example, if a parent is recording episodes of self-injury, making bathroom checks every half hour, and demanding speech during every encounter with his or her autistic child, there will be less time for meal preparation, PTA meetings for the other siblings, or an evening out. These shifts in the allocation of energy will have a direct, often negative, impact on every member of the family. Unless our interventions are planned with sensitivity, Mealiea (1976) suggests that the changes may possibly be harmful rather than beneficial to the members of the unit.

Such concern is consistent with the extensive work of Gerald Patterson and his colleagues, pioneers in training parents to work with their aggressive children at home. For example, Patterson, Reid, Jones, and Conger (1975) note that their standard package for behavioral intervention is not sufficient to help every family who consults them. Approximately two-thirds of their clients required some measure of help beyond this package, including consideration of marital conflict or more extensive parental support within the home. Aware of the importance of considering the needs of the entire family, Patterson and Fleischman (1979) suggest that the right interventions can have a beneficial effect not only upon the child but upon the family as a whole. They urge that research be directed toward the question of reciprocal change among family members.

When Bernal, Klinnert, and Schultz (1980) failed to find that parents trained in behavior modification techniques were any more effective in the long run than parents trained in client-centered techniques, they examined their subject population with care. They note that their subjects were unselected in terms of degree of parental motivation to work with their child and that some of the subjects suffered from severe marital or personal problems. It seems entirely reasonable to anticipate that such subjects would have a difficult time mobilizing themselves to focus upon a behavioral program for their child and that their performance is therefore not a valid test of the efficacy of parent training *per se*.

The direct impact of the social system upon the ability of parents to work effectively with their children was documented by Robert Wahler (1980) in his work with lower-income mothers and their oppositional children. Wahler (1980) reports that although the mothers mastered the behavioral techniques and were able to bring about change in their children's problem behaviors, at a 1-year follow-up there was a return to baseline levels of behavior. It is important to note that Wahler found those mothers who had a more extensive network of friends to be better able to sustain the task of effective parenting than those who did not. The support system of friends may act as a form of extended family and may serve a facilitative function for the mother–child duo (see Bristol, Chapter 17, this volume). Alternatively, women who are capable of sustained friendship may have better interpersonal skills in general and thus may be more adept at child-rearing. Wahler (1980) argues on behalf of the notion that if one could help the isolated women change their friendship patterns to provide them with greater interpersonal gratification, their ability to deal more consistently with their children might be enhanced. Such support may be especially important in single-parent families containing an autistic child.

Thus, there exist in the parent training literature a number of studies that have suggested in one fashion or another that behavioral parent-training procedures do sometimes fail, that the reasons for this failure may lie within the interpersonal context of marital, family, or social relationships, and that aiming our interventions at these interpersonal phenomena may increase our ability to help parents be effective child managers.

Do Parents Cause Autism?

In deciding to consider the family context in which parents and autistic children operate, we need to stress two things. First, it is not our belief that the family environment causes autism. Far from it. We are firmly committed to the notion that autism, like mental retardation, cerebral palsy, or blindness, is a tragic physical flaw. There is increasing evidence to support us in this biological view.

Second, we are not suggesting that these families are pathological in their functioning. Rather, it is our contention that even healthy families can suffer from the experience of having to deal with inordinate stress (discussed by Marcus in Chapter 18). Many people doubtless resolve this stress by themselves over time. Nonetheless, if we could facilitate this resolution during the course of working with them, we might speed the process of adaptation and thereby bring direct benefits to everyone.

Neither are we suggesting that every family requires some sort of family intervention in order to function effectively with their autistic child. Indeed, some families, even when they have problems in other areas, are able to set aside their difficulties and focus their effort upon their child. We have seen this happen often enough to know that it is a very real phenomenon. Oltmanns, Broderick, and O'Leary (1977), examining the status of families coming to an outpatient clinic with complaints about their children's behavior, noted that pretreatment levels of marital disorder were not always related to the successful treatment of the child.

Thus, even in some families where tangible problems exist, the parents may be able to concentrate their energy upon their child's needs. We have seen many families who, when given concrete help about what to do for their child, implemented the program with success and followed through after training ended. Nonetheless, there do remain families who, in spite of love and concern for their child, are so stressed by the problem of integrating the autistic child's needs into their life that they find themselves unable to function effectively with their child.

As we examined these empirical and clinical findings, we realized that we could not assume that all the families are in need of help, but neither could we rule this strategy out before we looked carefully at the family. It is important to tailor our interventions to the needs of the family and to have available a repertoire of responses that will meet a range of needs. Teaching parents behavior modification techniques, while helpful in many instances, may sometimes be too narrow an approach and may have to be supplemented with other forms of intervention.

THE FAMILY LIFE CYCLE

The concept of the family life cycle is an important one to many therapists who work with families (Carter and McGoldrick, 1980a). Within this view, families participate in an ongoing cycle of developmental stages, each stage presenting a set of challenges as well as the potential for new sources of gratification. Thus, a young couple marry, go through the adjustment process of leaving their families of origin and building a new unit. This task accomplished, they can comfortably advance to having a child and learning how to integrate this new person into their lives. When the children leave toddlerhood and enter school, there are once again shifts in family function as the time demands upon the mother to be a full-time caretaker begin to lessen. The adolescence of the children is often a time of major challenge for the family since new ideas, new people, and major shifts in parent–child interactions are likely to occur; the child emerges as a young adult. With the ending of adolescence comes a point when the children leave home, setting off to build their own families. The parents are confronted by the need to reexamine their own relationship and to build new sources of gratification beyond child-rearing. In later years there come problems of parental dependence upon children, illness, and the confrontation with death. This cycle continues in its endless round; we change our roles, but the basic story remains.

A variety of events can intrude upon the resolution of the conflicts that arise during the transition from one phase of the family life cycle to the next. Some families get stuck at a particular phase and are unable to move, showing instead a serious problem of dysfunction. Other families, although they ultimately surmount the problems, may experience considerable discomfort in making these essential shifts. The presence of a handicapped child can intensify the problems of going through these transitional phases and can work against a comfortable solution.

The Birth of a Child

In the hypothetical case that introduced this chapter, we met a young couple who learned when their boy was 30 months old that he was autistic. As one thinks about that family a number of themes become evident. First, this is a couple who had done a reasonably good job of differentiating themselves from their families of origin (Bowen, 1978). They were sufficiently mature to enter into an intimate marital relationship without being swallowed up by one another or shutting the other person out (McGoldrick, 1980). Rather, through a process of mutual accommodation, they settled the numerous problems, small and large, that must be resolved for a couple to live together comfortably (Minuchin, 1974). Once their negotiating style was established, this woman and man felt ready to have children.

During the course of the pregnancy a shift began within the marital relationship. They began to think about themselves as a threesome—if asked, they might say they were "really going to be a family." Such a shift requires that one's self-concept as a wife or husband grow to include that of mother or father. If work and marriage have encompassed all of one's life and made that life richly satisfying, how does one expand to include a new person and still retain the old pleasures? How can a woman and a man protect the boundaries of their marital relationship and still become a family of three or more? Most people are able to work out this task, but it requires effort and generates at least transient stress.

In the case we reviewed at the beginning of the chapter, the young couple had satisfactorily negotiated the challenges of the initial integration of a child into their lives and saw their son as a full member of the family unit. Both parents had expanded their self-definition to include the role of parent of an infant. Life was running relatively smoothly when, abruptly, the machinery of daily functioning was jammed by the realization that their son was autistic. The family unit was now confronted by the gravest challenge of its career. How well they met that challenge would influence every day of the rest of their lives.

The first tasks confronted by this family were to accept the reality of their son's handicap, redefine themselves as the parents of a child with a handicap, and figure out how to integrate their son's special needs into the routine of their lives. They needed training in behavior modification techniques to teach them how to help their son. Although other issues will arise over the years, these initial problems are the most acutely disruptive difficulties they will face as the family of an autistic child. This is consistent with Waisbren's (1980) report that parents of young developmentally disabled children view themselves and their child more negatively than do other parents.

Parents have a variety of reactions when they find out that their child has a handicap. As both DeMyer (1979) and Featherstone (1980) describe, these emotional responses include depression, guilt, and anger. For example, Greenfeld (1973) writes of his sense of guilt when he learned that his son Noah might be handicapped. He also notes the depth of his bond with Noah, saying, "I will not love him a mite less, and he will even more be my son" (Greenfeld, 1973, p. 29).

Coping with these intense emotional reactions is enough to create stress in even the best of relationships. When one considers that parents may be angry at one another, at the child, or at professional consultants, may feel guilty about these angry feelings, may feel guilt about their imagined failures in relation to their child, and may be depressed about the child's future and their own, the potential for disruptive patterns of interaction becomes obvious. We know several couples who separated shortly after their child was diagnosed as autistic. In most cases, one spouse was unable to accept the reality that he or she had a handicapped child and was unwilling to make the sacrifice of time, sharing, and caring demanded by the child. Although these marriages were somewhat immature before the identification of the child's handicap, at least some of them might have survived without this added stress. At at a time when mutual support may be vital, individuals may withdraw from one another or turn their pain outward and become hurtful to each other. The family ferment may be further heightened by the reactions of grandparents and other members of the extended family.

Indeed, the behavior therapist would do well to consider involving grandparents and other extended family members in didactic behavioral training and to explore the reactions of these people to the child's handicap.

Few of us are heroic when confronted by such painful problems in life. We flail about, looking for answers, feeling deeply conflicted, experiencing moments of aloneness and pain as we struggle for a solution. Under such conditions parents need the opportunity to sort out their feelings and to distinguish objective problems from their own fears. It is hard enough to be angry for a protracted period; the stress is made more intense when one feels guilty about the anger, recognizes the emotion as "irrational," and yet feels helpless to resolve the conflict. Such events can pose serious problems to the stability of the relationship between husband and wife. Thus, Greenfeld (1973) describes the stress in his marriage when he and his wife learned about their son's handicap, noting that "the good fortune of our marriage seems to have dissipated" (Greenfeld, 1973, p. 64). Their "failure" as parents shakes their confidence in themselves and each other. More generally, Gath (1977) found greater marital discord among the families of Down's syndrome babies than among normal controls.

The behavior therapist encountering the family of an autistic child at this early point has a great deal to offer. First, there is the obvious contribution of helping the parents work with their child so that the acquisition of speech and self-help and social skills may be facilitated. We have good methods for training parents in these skills, and most families benefit rapidly and directly from such intervention.

A somewhat less obvious but at least as important contribution can be made by helping the parents come to terms with their feelings about the child. For example, it may be helpful for the parents to examine their feelings of guilt and consider their realistic and unrealistic sense of responsibility for their child. The therapist may help the parents acknowledge and become comfortable with their feelings of anger and disappointment that this child is handicapped. We have been repeatedly impressed with how well people can use relatively brief interventions to work through some of these issues. Often, meeting once a week for a couple of months can make a substantial difference in helping parents cope. The parents may begin to come to terms with their lost dreams for the child's future.

In addition, the husband and wife can be helped to examine how their reactions to the child's handicap have influenced their relationship with one another and how they might be able to help one another cope with the stress they have encountered. Parents can be assisted in recognizing the importance of maintaining the boundaries of their marital relationship (Bradt, 1980; Minuchin, 1974) and not sacrificing their relationship to child care. For example, we specifically advise parents to get out of the house together at least once a week, even if only for a few hours. We also put a high priority on the treatment of behavior problems such as the child's insisting on sleeping in the parent's bedroom or wandering into their room at night. Such behaviors can be seriously disruptive to the marital relationship. Fortunately, they usually respond to systematic intervention. In as many ways as possible we work to remind a couple of the importance of the bond between them. Sensitivity to these issues, coupled with training the parents in behavior modification skills, may speed the process of coming to terms with the child's handicap and may allow the couple to turn their energy toward the important things that can be done to help their child. As they begin to work with the child and observe progress, there is likely to follow some increased sense of hope that the child can learn to function as a member of the family and that the parents need not abandon their life dreams to care for the child.

We have previously discussed a family in which the mother viewed the autistic son as too "sick" to be responsible, while the father had essentially withdrawn from family transactions (Harris,1982). During the course of parent training in behavior modification, we attempted, through educational activities and modeling by other parents, to help the mother see how valuable it was to make demands upon her son for appropriate behavior. We also reengaged the father in child care by pointing out his special contributions. Both parents were gradually helped to form a more realistic view of their child and, with their combined efforts, to facilitate his development. This had a beneficial spillover effect in their marriage.

It is worth noting that the presence of the young autistic child with his or her extensive needs for child care is in some ways less disruptive of family function than may be true later in the life of the family. Specifically, the parents of very young children expect to devote considerable time to their children. Parents know there will be diapers to change, some sleepless nights, the need for close attention to the child—in short, a job demanding time and physical exertion. Thus, once they can mobilize their resources, the actual demands upon the parents of young autistic children may not be radically different from those of parents of normal preschoolers. Of course, in the case of some autistic children who pose major management problems, the child's needs can grow beyond the parents' capacity to respond.

In sum, the initial task for the family with a young autistic child may be to come to terms with the child's handicap and work out a pattern of interaction that allows them to do the work that has to be done with the child while still reserving time and space for the marital relationship.

The School-Age Child

When the autistic child reaches school age and his or her peers go off to kindergarten, there gradually begins another period of transition for the family.

This process, not as abrupt as the adjustment required when the parents first learned the child was handicapped, is a subtle transition that may pose problems at varying points throughout middle childhood (Carter and McGoldrick, 1980b).

Thanks to contemporary views of special education, the autistic child is likely to spend the school day away from home, and thus provide the parents some respite from child care, as well as expanding the available network of community support. Nonetheless, it is during middle childhood that parents become increasingly aware of the unrelenting nature of their autistic child's needs. Although they had expected to meet substantial needs for an infant and a toddler, they had not bargained for this demand to be a ceaseless one. The autistic child may be slow to be toilet-trained, may not sleep well at night, or may exhibit self-injurious behavior that requires close monitoring. All of these problems demand extensive time from the parents—time that must be taken away from other activities. Although the child grows older, there is little respite from the role of total care (Featherstone, 1980).

When a family functions well, it is characterized by ongoing change (Minuchin, 1974). As the members mature, they take on new and different responsibilities in relation to themselves and to one another. The presence of an autistic child may impede this process and lead the family in the direction of maintaining the status quo rather than growth. For the traditional family structure, where mother is the primary caretaker for young children, and father the source of financial support, the impact of this may be more visible for the mother than for the father. Our own experience has been that while most fathers are concerned and caring, it is mothers who spend the most time with their autistic children.

The mother of a young autistic child finds that demands for basic physical care limit her ability to expand her own activities (Birenbaum, 1971). Although she might have been able to go to the park with her 4-year-old autistic child, who would sit passively and twiddle leaves or sift sand through his fingers while she chatted with other mothers of 4-year-olds, these opportunities decline as the child grows older. The parents of a normal preschooler are not likely to be at ease with the presence of a self-stimulating, nonverbal 8-year-old on the playground, and the 8-year-olds, out playing ball, are not likely to know quite how to respond to their handicapped peer. Thus, the mother may find her lot an increasingly lonely one as her child grows in size and years and she can neither relate comfortably to the mothers of young children who require the same extensive physical care nor integrate her child into the world of his or her chronological age peers. Over the years a number of mothers have shared with us their sense of entrapment about their lives. They fear that they will never be free to define the space of their own existence. This sense of helplessness and burden can produce feelings of depression.

As the mother experiences this increasing isolation in her role, she may turn to her husband for greater support. His capacity to provide companionship, to relieve her of some of the burdens of child care, and to share with her the process of integrating their growing child into the larger community may largely determine how well the family is able to move through this stage of development. The importance of the role of the father in relation to the mother and child illustrates why one must consider the family as a whole and not a single component. It would not be sufficient to educate the autistic child or treat the mother's depression without looking at the father's role as well and the effect all three family members have on one another.

Another family factor that emerges during the years of middle childhood is the presence of siblings (Bradt, 1980). With the birth of another child, parents are given the opportunity to reexperience parenthood and to be able to verify that they can function competently as the parents of a normal child. This offers a new source of pride and pleasure; it also poses new challenges. Time once available for the autistic child must now be divided into smaller units in order to care for a new family member. Siblings have to learn how to cope with their handicapped brother or sister, to handle the negative reactions of outsiders to their brother or sister's handicap, and to deal with their own ambivalent feelings. Greenfeld (1973), describing the potential impact of their autistic son, Noah, on their older boy, Karl, writes of how remarkable Karl will have to be to bear the burden of his brother's handicap.

An example of a potential hazard that may befall the sibling of an autistic child is found in the role of the "parental child" (Minuchin, 1974). Although it is reasonable for siblings to have responsibilities for one another, such arrangements when carried to excess can intrude upon the freedom that is so important in childhood. We described such a case in our discussion of a family where the mother and daughter shared an extensive overinvolvement with the autistic boy while the father had withdrawn from the family to his work (Harris, 1982). In this family, we helped the parents to free the daughter from some of the demands that were made upon her and worked to strengthen the involvement of the father with the children as well as to help the couple reestablish a more satisfying relationship with one another.

The family of three becomes a family of four (or five . . .) and the patterns that once worked to keep the triadic unit functioning have to be revised to accept a new member (Bradt, 1980). New alliances will be formed, new demands posed, new possibilities developed. The parents have available an important new source of pleasure, the siblings can learn to love and value their handicapped brother or sister and emerge from childhood as richer people as a result, and the autistic child has more models from whom to learn. Thus, if handled with some wisdom, the increasing size of the family offers the opportunity for the enhancement of the entire family and not a diminishing of the quality of anyone's life.

Adolescence

Adolescence is a time of rich ferment and possibility in family life (Acker-man, 1980). Teenagers are in a process of reaching out to the world and examining new possibilities and ideas. As they do so, they expose their parents to these new experiences, and parents too are forced to grow if they wish to sustain a good relationship with the young person. Little of this opportunity will accrue to the parents of the autistic adolescent. Rather, the parents will find themselves still providing a great deal of basic care for the child and beginning to confront the realization that their autistic child could be forever dependent upon them. If this child is to leave home, very special preparations must be made to permit the separation (Mesibov, 1983). As Mesibov, Schopler, and Sloan (1983) comment, "By the time their autistic child reaches adolescence the parents have grown older and tired, while the child grows stronger but not much more independent" (p. 419).

The discrepancy between the autistic child and his or her peers that began to emerge during middle childhood becomes conspicuous during adolescence. While other young people are striking off on their own, the autistic adolescent remains at home, indifferent to social events, career plans, or the struggle for independence. If there are other children in the family, the parents may find their own growth facilitated by these youngsters. Otherwise, the impetus for growth will have to come largely from themselves and their wish to develop as individuals and as a unit rather than from the energizing push and pull of a home with an adolescent. Parents are left the poorer for this lack of pressure to move along in their own development (Ackerman, 1980). At a point when they could begin to rethink their relationship to one another and the possibilities that await them as their children leave home, they may instead remain locked in a day-to-day routine that has changed little in basic substance since the autistic child was young. The endless, unvarying texture of their days may leave the family with little sense of joy or hope. Some parents appear resigned to a life at the service of the autistic child and find it difficult to consider that they, as well as the child, could benefit from another arrangement.

The therapist working with the family of an autistic adolescent can be useful to that family by helping them to think about the changes such as vocational training and advanced self-help skills that need to occur for the child to move out of the family home and into a community living unit for young autistic adults (Mesibov, 1983). Some families of autistic children have difficulty coming to terms with the idea that their child can leave home. Although they expect their other children to establish independent lives, they have come to see the autistic child as so dependent upon them that a separation is not possible. As long as the child remains with them, the parents may be deprived of some of the most difficult but also most satisfying aspects of the mature years of adulthood. They may also deny the autistic child the level of independence and self-satisfaction that is potentially available to that youngster. Thus, we believe it is in the best interests of parent and child to challenge such reluctance and prepare the family for separation.

Helping the family to define their functions in relation to their autistic child as an adolescent, to deal with issues of separation, and to redefine their own roles as parents of grown children becomes an important task as the autistic child grows up.

The Adult Years

We are confronted by a number of conspicuous events in the family life cycle as our children become adults. Prime among these are the movement of the young adult child into a new unit with his or her spouse, the birth of grand-children, our own physical decline, dependence upon our adult children, and ultimate death (McCullough, 1980; Walsh, 1980). If we are lucky, these events, even coming to terms with our own death and that of our spouse, can push us to new, if painful, growth and enrich relationships within the family as a whole.

One of the important things that happens when our children strike off on their own is that we are left to redefine our relationship with our spouse (McCullough, 1980). This process begins during adolescence, but since there are still extensive demands involved in being the parents of an adolescent, many couples postpone the question of their relationship until the last of the children leaves home. What if that last child never leaves? What if he or she is an autistic child who remains at home until parental illness or death forces a new arrangement?

Under such conditions the parents may be denied the opportunity to move closer to one another as they reexamine their dyadic relationship independent of their role as parents. In some marriages, of course, these bonds may be so tenuous that the loss of the children might be the end of the marriage. Under such conditions parents may cling to their handicapped child as the force that stabilizes their marriage (McCullough, 1980). Should that occur, it can be counterproductive to the child, who will never be pushed to develop as fully as he or she can until the parents are dead. At that point, the kind of gradual separation that might have allowed the child to learn skills of independent living may be nearly impossible, and the child may be plunged into the life of an institution because no alternatives were arranged for his or her care.

Mesibov (1983) wisely argues that we cannot impose upon the parents of the autistic adolescent or adult the same expectations for time and commitment that were appropriate when the young adult was a child. Even if parents were willing and able to sustain such effort, it could be maladaptive to do so. Parental energy can, however, be channeled toward estate planning, establishment of community programs, and a general advocacy role that works toward a realistic separation of parent and child.

It is important for the autistic adult and his or her family that they consider carefully the long-term plans for the young adult. Where shall he or she live? What skills are needed for the move toward increasing independence? If these changes create stress for the rest of the family, the therapist can turn his or her attention to these problems and help the parents deal with issues that lie between them, without holding back the young adult who needs help in setting out on a semiindependent course.

A Word about Intervention

We have not discussed specific techniques for intervening with a family when problems develop in resolving the tasks of the family life cycle. In an earlier paper (Harris, 1982) we described in some detail methods of intervention with the family of a young autistic child. Essentially, we argued that in doing behavioral training with parents one must be alert to the impact of this training upon the family as a whole and able to recognize when one's help must extend beyond the didactic training to include a sensitive examination of the experience of the family. Our behavioral interventions must be offered in a way that can facilitate the growth of all the family members rather than depleting the resources of some individuals in a misguided effort to help others.

Summary

We have provided an overview of the kinds of issues that may arise for autistic children and their families as they grow together through the life cycle. Although we identified some important issues, space prohibited examining these in detail, nor were we able to enumerate all the issues that arise at different stages. For example, we said little about the impact of the autistic child upon his or her grandparents and the reaction of these senior members of the family to their own children and grandchildren. Nor did we discuss how a family functions when the mother works outside the home rather than engaging in full-time child care. Rather, we tried to present the reader with a broad sense of the tasks that confront all of us through our lives and how the presence of an autistic child may hinder movement through these stages.

We pointed to several themes that emerge over the years. One of these is change in role definitions as one grows older. As children grow up, parents normally broaden their own roles since they have increased time and energy to take on new activities. The effort that was once largely devoted to child-rearing can be redistributed across other tasks. This is most conspicuous in traditional homes where the mother is released from being a primary caretaker to being someone who has time for activities beyond the confines of the home. As the mother's definition of herself changes, that of the father does also. The presence of an autistic child can hinder this transition and keep the mother tied to the role of caretaker.

Another theme that emerges is the impact of separation upon parents and child. As children mature there is an ongoing process of healthy separation that encourages the growth of adults as well as children. This is seen most clearly in late adolescence and early adulthood as children move off to establish their own homes. For the parents of the autistic child this process of separation may be avoided or delayed because of the child's needs. As a result, unless parents push for change, they may never become free of their role as caretaker and the child may remain so dependent that when the parents die there is little choice but institutional care.

The presence of an autistic child may serve to maintain the status quo within a family since the needs of these children are so extensive. Thus, the parents of the autistic child may be denied the opportunity to grow from some of life's most exciting challenges. As a result, they may lose important sources of gratification, and ultimately the child as well as the parents may suffer since the state of total dependence cannot continue indefinitely.

Being helpful to the families of autistic people as they all struggle to cope with the formidable challenge life has presented to them merits the best of our clinical and scientific efforts.

REFERENCES

Ackerman, N. J. The family with adolescents. In E. A. Carter and M. McGoldrick (Eds.), *The family life cycle: A framework for family therapy.* New York: Gardner Press, 1980.

Baker, B. L., Heifetz, L. J., and Murphy, D. M. Behavioral training for parents of mentally retarded children: One-year follow-up. *American Journal of Mental Deficiency,* 1980, *85,* 31–38.

Bernal, M. E., Klinnert, M. D., and Schultz, L. A. Outcome evaluation of behavioral parent training and client-centered parent counseling for children with conduct problems. *Journal of Applied Behavior Analysis,* 1980, *13,* 677–691.

Birenbaum, A. The mentally retarded child in the home and the family cycle. *Journal of Health and Social Behavior,* 1971, *12,* 55–65.

Bowen, M. *Family therapy in clinical practice.* New York: Jason Aronson, 1978.

Bradt, J. O. The family with young children. In E. A. Carter and M. McGoldrick (Eds.), *The family life cycle: A framework for family therapy.* New York: Gardner Press, 1980.

Carter, E. A., and McGoldrick, M. (Eds.). *The family life cycle: A framework for family therapy.* New York: Gardner Press, 1980. (a)

Carter, E. A., and McGoldrick, M. The family life cycle and family therapy: An overview. In E. A. Carter and M. McGoldrick (Eds.), *The family life cycle: A framework for family therapy*. New York: Gardner Press, 1980. (b)

DeMyer, M. K. *Parents and children in autism*. New York: Wiley, 1979.

Featherstone, H. *A difference in the family*. New York: Basic Books, 1980.

Gath, A. The impact of an abnormal child on the family. *British Journal of Psychiatry*, 1977, *130*, 405–410.

Greenfeld, J. *A child called Noah*. New York: Warner, 1973.

Harris, S. L. A family systems approach to behavioral training with parents of autistic children. *Child and Family Behavior Therapy*, 1982, *4*, 21–35.

Harris, S. L., Wolchik, S. A., and Milch, R. E. Changing the speech of autistic children and their parents. *Child and Family Behavior Therapy*, 1982, *4*, 151–173.

Harris, S. L., Wolchick, S. A., and Weitz, S. The acquisition of language skills by autistic children: Can parents do the job? *Journal of Autism and Developmental Disorders*, 1981, *11*, 373–384.

Heifetz, L. J. Behavioral training for parents of retarded children: Alternative formats based on instructional manuals. *American Journal of Mental Deficiency*, 1977, *82*, 194–203.

McCullough, P. Launching children and moving on. In E. A. Carter and M. McGoldrick (Eds.), *The family life cycle: A framework for family therapy*. New York: Gardner Press, 1980.

McGoldrick, M. The joining of families through marriage: The new couple. In E. A. Carter and M. McGoldrick (Eds.), *The family life cycle: A framework for family therapy*. New York: Gardner Press, 1980.

Mealiea, W. L. Conjoint-behavior therapy: The modification of family constellations. In E. J. Mash, L. C. Handy, and L. A. Hammerlynck (Eds.), *Behavior modification approaches to parenting*. New York: Brunner/Mazel, 1976.

Mesibov, G. B. Current perspectives and issues in autism and adolescence. In E. Schopler and G. B. Mesibov (Eds.), *Autism in adolescents and adults*. New York: Plenum, 1983.

Mesibov, G. B., Schopler, E., and Sloan, J. L. Service development for adolescents and adults in North Carolina's TEACCH program. In E. Schopler and G. B. Mesibov (Eds.), *Autism in adolescents and adults*. New York: Plenum, 1983.

Minuchin, S. *Families and family therapy*. Cambridge: Harvard University Press, 1974.

Oltmanns, T. F., Broderick, J. E., and O'Leary, K. D. Marital adjustment and the efficacy of behavior therapy with children. *Journal of Consulting and Clinical Psychology*, 1977, *45*, 724–729.

Patterson, G. R., and Fleischman, M. J. Maintenance of treatment effects: Some considerations concerning family systems and follow up data. *Behavior Therapy*, 1979, *10*, 168–185.

Patterson, G. R., Reid, J. B., Jones, R. R., and Conger, R. E. *A social learning approach to family intervention* (Vol. 1). *Families with aggressive children*. Eugene, Oreg.: Castalia, 1975.

Wahler, R. G. The insular mother: Her problems in parent–child treatment. *Journal of Applied Behavior Analysis*, 1980, *13*, 207–219.

Waisbren, S. E. Parents' reactions after the birth of a developmentally disabled child. *American Journal of Mental Deficiency*, 1980, *84*, 345–351.

Walsh, F. The family in later life. In E. A. Carter and M. McGoldrick (Eds.), *The family life cycle: A framework for family therapy*. New York: Gardner Press, 1980.

Weitz, S. A code for assessing teaching skills of parents of developmentally disabled children. *Journal of Autism and Developmental Disorders*, 1982, *12*, 13–24.

V

Parents as Trainers

13

My Great Teachers

ERIC SCHOPLER

Most of the chapters in this volume are tied to published empirical research. This is not just a requirement of scholarship, it is also one of the few approaches to avoid the oft-repeated mischief and confusion triggered by unsubstantiated theory and opinion. We believe in rationality and the rules of evidence, as the fragile levers by which progress in the understanding and treatment of autism are advanced. Most of the contributors to this volume, including myself, have spent a significant portion of their professional careers dedicated to empirical research conducted with scientific methodology.

Therefore, it may well be heresy for me to admit that the most important contribution to the development of my own knowledge about autism came less from such research than from some of the great teachers I encountered along the way. Although these teachers also were primarily empiricists, I have become convinced that it may be the mysterious chemistry of the teaching–learning interaction with great teachers that generates the most durable understanding and knowledge.

Most of my life has been devoted to being a student and a teacher—about half obtaining a formal education and the other half teaching. This background has made me something of an expert on the topic of "What makes a great teacher?" I will try to clarify this question in this chapter, and I regard it as a proper introduction to this section of parents as trainers.

There are three aspects to a first-rate teacher. The first is the subject matter. How well does he or she know it? How long has she been studying it? How effectively can she relate it to other subjects? Second is teaching style. How

ERIC SCHOPLER • Division TEACCH, University of North Carolina, Chapel Hill, North Carolina 27514. The substance of this chapter was presented at the NCSAAC Meeting, 1978.

clearly is the subject communicated? Is it a lively and straightforward presentation? This is partly a matter of personality. Is she able to make us think and feel about the subject rather than put us to sleep? The third and most important aspect is how well does she relate that subject matter to the student's own life and teach him how to use the information?

When you have been a student as many years as I have, you are bound to meet quite a few outstanding teachers. Below is a summary of the three most impressive aspects of their performance: (1) knowledge of their subject matter, (2) teaching style, and (3) relevance to my own experience.

CHILD TEACHER

The first sample of an outstanding teacher for me was Ellen, whom I met in September of 1960. Her subject matter was autism. As a college student at the University of Chicago, I had the good fortune to meet some very fine teachers in anthropology, biology, philosophy, psychology, and English literature. They were among the best in their field. However, none of them managed to get me hooked into their subject matter. And so I didn't meet my first great teacher until I met Ellen. I was working in a treatment center for autistic and schizophrenic children. My subject matter was autism and Ellen was a 7-year-old autistic child.

I won't go into the question of how or why people select the subjects they study, an important and complex issue by itself. In my case, it started with being fascinated by Ellen and gradually being drawn further into the many questions about her: What was wrong with her? What does it mean that she is called autistic? Can she be cured? What do her problems mean for her family, her schooling, and the community in which she lives? Once I became interested in these questions, there was no denying that Ellen was a great teacher.

She had been autistic all her life, and she had very concrete and simple ways of teaching autism. When she entered a room with me, she acted as if I was not there. She wandered around aimlessly but with a persistence and determination as strong as my motivation to study autism. She taught some important language lessons—she did not talk. Her mother said she could say a few words, but Ellen didn't say them to me. A third topic Ellen wanted to teach me about was her persistent preoccupation with the telephone. Her circling around the room usually ended at the phone. She would pick up the receiver, hold it by its wire, and spin it round and round 'til the operator could be heard to say, "Number please." So there you have it.

She had been familiar with autism for 7 more years than I had. She had, in fact, a longer acquaintance with it than anyone else I knew. She could express the problem of relating to people, a basic problem in many fields, more clearly than anyone I had met before; same for the lack of speech or communication. She was also very persistent in demonstrating the importance of becoming competent at twirling a telephone receiver. She had developed a specialized interest, a major, long before I had. She had a few other topics too, but during the year I studied with her, I was most affected by her abiding commitment to these basic human concerns: interpersonal relations, language, and special interest.

During that year I learned a very interesting lesson from her. I learned how to teach her some new words by stopping her from circling around the room. I would hold her struggling on my lap and keep her there until she repeated the phrase "Let me down." In the same manner, I taught her a number of other phrases while holding her. They included "Get the doll" and "See Mommy," phrases that earned her release from me after she used them appropriately.

Some critics will say that this was a very modest lesson to learn for a student at one of our great and costly universities. But I was quite proud of it because for me it compared favorably with the hundreds of lectures I had sat through by then.

Still, a year of the same curriculum is a long time. And as happens so often, the student–teacher relationship began to change. Our session changed too, but slowly. I began to see the great teacher's clay feet. She had little choice in how she taught me. Her repetition became boring, and I began to feel too limited in my role as her student. I'm not proud of how I felt about her. After all, her teaching style with me was fairly constant. The main change had been in me. Nevertheless, she had instilled in me a strong desire to continue my study of autism. I met many more such children, quite different from each other, including some fine teachers among them, but they all left me feeling that I wasn't learning all I wanted to know about autism, about the cause of this disability, and how to teach the children who suffered from it. Nevertheless, these children were good enough teachers to make me continue with my autism studies.

When I talked to my professional colleagues about my frustrations with these children, they all told me that the real problem was with the parents: They rejected their kids; they were preoccupied with the details of their own lives; they had an unconscious wish to keep them handicapped; they were teaching them those endless repetitive behaviors. I began to realize that if these parents had the power, the will, and the ability to produce these complicated, difficult, fascinating children, then I should be studying and learning from them.

PARENT TEACHERS

At this point I found some new teachers: parents of autistic children. They were among the best I ever met. They were too many to acknowledge here, but I do want to give some indication of what they taught me, using the three previously mentioned elements of teaching: (1) knowledge of subject matter, (2) teaching style, and (3) relevance to their student's life.

Knowledge of Subject Matter

Teaching Family Problems

On the subject matter of autism, I had learned a great deal from Ellen and her colleagues. But from my parent teachers, whole new vistas were opened. They had taken a crash course in autism extending over days, nights, weeks, and years. If the child couldn't talk or understand, some of these parent teachers took on the uncomfortable burden of anticipating the child's meaning. When the child couldn't express his love and attachment to them, they learned how to care for him with little reciprocity. They adapted the family's eating habits to meet their child's strange food preferences. They extended their toilet-training efforts years beyond the time needed for their normal children, and they patiently washed the traces of the slowed training from the never-ending laundry. They taught their other children to protect their belongings from the handicapped brother. They taught them, by modeling, how to take more than their share of responsibility for the handicapped child, and they taught compassion even while their own patience ran thin. Their studies went past bedtime daily, and they often gave sleepless nights to the understanding of autism.

Often the child was difficult to manage in public, unresponsive to usual parental guidance. One father could not get his son to stop sniffing gasoline while he settled up with the attendant. The father was criticized for his ineffective efforts to get the boy into his car, and he explained lamely, "My boy is autistic." The attendant replied, "I don't care how talented he is, you should discipline him more strictly." When neighbors and even relatives criticized and misunderstood, these parent teachers maintained their sense of humor and continued to look for better ways of managing.

And when their best efforts failed to have their child become normal and as well adjusted as most other children, their disappointment and frustration did not turn to chronic despair. They met with other parents and mounted a joint effort to patiently educate their friends and community, without rancor, on how their child and they could be helped so that they could continue to keep him at home with his family and in their community.

Teaching Problem Solving

To teach the community about their children's needs and to develop services that had not been provided required financial, political, social, and professional support. In solving these many problems, my parent teachers provided a broad range of skills. Some parents gave of their political and organizational skills. They formed a parents' group that could formulate service needs and through their consensus sounded a politically audible voice with the state legislature. Others used their intellectual and artistic abilities to write books, articles, and newsletters that were easily understood. They made pictures, gave and organized benefit performances to raise revenues. They organized auctions, ran bake sales, and sold Christmas cards. Some parents developed special teaching skills effective with their own child, but also usable by others. Some found new ways of teaching their own child, or adjusted their own thoughts and feelings. The range of what they had to teach was great, and as different as people are different. These parents drew on their reserve of thought, feeling, and spirit, in a way other parents are rarely required to do.

Unlike researchers, these parents could not ignore questions for which they had no established methodology. Unlike clinicians, they could not transfer the child because they were unprepared for these severe problems. It was because they sustained their studies in spite of failures, frustrations, and defeat that so many became great teachers.

Teaching Style and Relevance

I have tried to give a thumbnail sketch of some observations and lessons I learned from my great parent teachers. Knowledge that could not be as readily obtained from scientific research was generated by the mysterious chemistry of the teacher–student interaction. This chemistry includes not only commitment to subject matter but also teaching style and relevance.

What was their teaching style? They told me about their efforts modestly. More important, they demonstrated them in their daily lives. They were eager to have me learn, but it was clear that they could continue with their efforts even if I did not understand, just like any fine teacher committed to his subject matter.

What did their teaching efforts mean to me personally? Well, there are many different facets to that. As a psychologist, I was taught to change my understanding of assessment and of psychotherapy, from expressing feelings to solving problems. As a teacher, I learned about the value of demonstration rather than rhetoric and lectures. Some extensions of these lessons into clinical procedures are discussed in Chapter 4 (TEACCH). But most important was what they taught me as a human being.

Parents taught me that it was possible to have an ordinary expectation—like bringing a normal child into this world and raising it—thwarted for no apparent reason, and to live with that disappointment day in and day out. That there is not just one way of appropriately raising a child, even with serious handicaps, but a good many different ways. These depend on the form and extent of the child's handicap, the resources and aspirations of the family into which the child was born. There is room for great individual variation within the available childrearing norms. Parents have shown me that it is possible to find faith when formal religion is not always available. They have taught me cheer, humor, and the ability to get on with it regardless of obstacles.

These lessons are basic for all of us who do not have a handicapped child. To the parents who taught me these valuable lessons I will be eternally grateful.

14

Parents as Trainers of Legislators, Other Parents, and Researchers

RUTH CHRIST SULLIVAN

Parents of autistic children learn early in their child's life how little professionals know about autism. Trained by their culture to trust the experts, they are soon dismayed and unsettled to learn that the "experts" know as little as they do, or less. Alone, especially at first, and faced with an extremely atypical child, many exhaust themselves in finding information that might help. They soon realize that the service providers will not provide unless there is a better understanding of autistic children and the urgency of their needs. With the fervor of desperation they read articles, study references, write to authors, call authorities in the field, exchange information with more knowledgeable parents. They will often deluge a professional with material from their latest search. Their files become fat, their wallets thin from copying at the local libraries.

Their role of petitioner-for-services becomes, sometimes with little awareness of the change, petitioner-for-attention-to-new-information. Without setting out to do it, these parents become trainers.

Though it is a rare parent who is well-informed about this severe, low-incidence disorder at the time of their child's diagnosis, it is *common* to find parents of older children who are highly informed. They are often invited to speak before college and university classes; they appear on conference programs; they serve on policy-making, fact-finding, advisory, and planning commissions at local, state, and federal levels of government. They write articles and books for the popular and professional press. Sometimes they return to school for advanced degrees and professional training and often enter a field related to autism, e.g., special education, psychology, hearing and speech science, or law

RUTH CHRIST SULLIVAN • Autism Services Center, Huntington, West Virginia 25702.

school. Some decide they can help by running for public office, like school boards and the legislature.

It is this growing number of well-informed, activist parents who have been and continue to be instrumental in raising the level of knowledge and awareness of autism. They are largely self-taught, and some dedicate their energies and long segments of their lives to the job of getting services for their own and other autistic children. Clara Claiborne Park, who typifies the above described parent, sums it up in the introduction of her book, *You Are Not Alone* (1976, p. xii): "We have learned how to get things done now, and begun to work for the future. We have had the happiness of discovering new friends where trouble was deepest, and of finding that even more often than anger, we share laughter. We have shared the pride of knowing that our work was making new things happen."

LEGISLATORS

I've been at this "training" business for over 20 years and I can see no end in sight. Even as I begin to put my thoughts together for this chapter I'm distracted by an urgent matter that must be settled today. A key legislator has not returned my call, and I wonder if I have been resourceful enough in trying to reach him. A week-long autism project with 10 autistic children finishes up in 2 days and I want him to see them, meet them, sense them. I want him to be with 11-year-old David, who, like a wound-up spring, tensely glances everywhere but at your eyes, repeats long television commercials when you ask him his name, darts from one chair to the next, bites the back of his hand in frustration, seems not to hear or understand when spoken to, strains against a teacher's hold on his arm. I want this man to see the frustration of the insufficiently trained, though dedicated teachers who, try hard as they might, do not settle David well enough to teach him. Because the teacher does not have the proper techniques to teach, she cannot get David to participate in a learning activity. She struggles to find a reinforcer which would encourage the behavior she wants from him. She is energetic, conscientious and *wants* to help David. As his negative behavior escalates, so does hers, with a loud series of don'ts and threats, plus physical restraint. Now there are tears in David's eyes. His mother says she has rarely seen him cry. Are these tears of anger at injustice, like Victor's in the *Wild Boy of Aveyron* when Jean Marc Itard, his gifted teacher, tested the boy's sense of justice by deliberately punishing him when he'd done well at a task for which he'd received praise before? Itard writes:

> [He] flew at my hand, leaving there the deep trace of his teeth. It would have been sweet to me at that moment could I have spoken to my pupil to make him understand how the pain of his bite filled my heart with satisfaction and made amends for all my labor. How could I be other than delighted? It was a legitimate act of vengeance; it was an incontestable proof that the feeling of justice and injustice, that external basis of social order, was no longer foreign to the heart of my pupil. (1962, p. 95)

I want this legislator to see the poignant beauty of that slim, fair-haired young boy on whose brain nature has visited some cruel disarrangement—"a Nature I never really noticed until it bungled" (West, 1978, p. 31). It is the Davids I'm talking about when I go before this man's legislative committee in the grandly furnished, high-ceilinged rooms of the state capital. Except for a film I showed him once, he's never seen an autistic child.

It's easier to forget the hardships of a large family whose home has just burned down if that family lives across town and you've never heard of them. If you're their neighbor and experience the drama—the flames, the excitement, the tears—you feel much closer to the problem and your responsibility to it. I want this legislator to feel the heat of the autism drama. Until he does, his committee will hold up the teacher-training bill. Until I can get his attention, our bill will never get out of his committee. David's life depends, literally, on what his teachers can teach him, *now*. He's already lost precious years, though he's had a few good teachers. It's teacher-training funds I'm after. We need help from the legislature.

Getting a key legislator's attention, then his* commitment to our cause, takes a combination of luck, good timing, hard work, and persistence.

Luck. Luck includes such things as a similar handicapping condition in someone close to him. One of the most sensitive and helpful legislators in our state has lovingly cared for his mother, who is a stroke victim. He recognizes her in some of the descriptions we give him of our autistic children. Another legislator had clubfoot as a child and is very supportive of "handicapped" legislation. One man, representing a far corner of the state, stopped me as I began to describe life in a state institution for the retarded, where our children are headed unless we get help. His daughter has been there for 12 years (if I'd done my homework thoroughly, I'd have known that before I saw him). U.S. Senator Lowell Weicker of Connecticut became the parent of a Down's syndrome child a few years ago and is now an outstanding advocate for the nation's handicapped population. In 1969 when I began to lobby for autism in Washington, D.C., the minority leader of the Senate knew about autism—his best friend back home had an autistic child.

In one state whose governor was especially insensitive to the needs of the handicapped, advocates tell the story of the handicapped community's reaction to the announcement that his wife was pregnant. There was a constant temptation to speculate about what would happen to his attitude if his child were born with a developmental disability, especially one for which his state had no' services.

Another category of "luck" is having some pleasant connection with key legislators in some other setting, like being fraternity brothers while in law

---

*Because the English language does not yet have a single neutral word for *him* and/or *her*, I will use the masculine pronoun for simplicity's sake, though I am happily aware that, increasingly, members of legislatures are female.

school, serving together on a board or committee, or having you, the "trainer," referred to positively by someone from out of state whom he admires—the farther out of state the better. From abroad is best.

You are in luck if your key legislator is from your area, especially if you are acquainted and he already trusts your integrity, shortening the time it takes for him to accept you, your cause, and your information as serious and legitimate.

It is also "luck" when your request for legislation happens also to be important to the key legislator. In human services, however, one doesn't have that kind of luck very often.

Good Timing. Good timing is essential. Chance encounters in the halls and lobbies of capitol buildings are not usually good occasions to introduce a lengthy new subject. It *can* be a useful opportunity, however, to introduce yourself and your interests and to request an appointment to discuss your concerns with him, after which encounter you can go immediately to his appointments secretary and work out a good time to meet. Most legislators take their appointments seriously, but be aware that during the session situations can change dramatically. Even the best-laid plans to see your key legislator may be put aside if, for instance, there is a sudden roll call and he must rush to the chamber, or a committee on which he serves has scheduled an extra meeting at your time. Over the years I have traveled to the capitol through snow, ice, sleet, darkness, and shenanigans with guards at the visitors' parking lot only to be greeted with "he's in session," when a simple phone call could have saved me a 100-mile trip. The better you know his secretary, the less likely this is to happen, though there is no guarantee. The more conscientious legislators and staff will not want it to happen often.

It is important to know the sequence in which legislation is prepared. You cannot expect much if your legislator does not know about your concern until a few days before the deadline for filing a bill. Sometimes it is best to "train" a legislator when he is back home and not under so much pressure. This is usually a good time to introduce him to autistic children, but not always. For instance, if he is self-employed, your taking his time at his office or place of business could mean you are cutting down on his opportunity for profits. Such legislators sometimes prefer to meet their constituents at the state capital. "Trainers" need to find out which location and schedule best suit their legislators.

Good timing takes good planning. If during the legislative session you sponsor a brunch at 10:00 A.M. and almost no legislators show up, it probably means you didn't do enough homework. Do you know what time the committees meet? (Most of the legislative work is done in committees.) Was that the day a political party caucus was scheduled? Did another more affluent and powerful group have an event planned for the same time?

An excellent example of timing took place in the early days of the North Carolina Society for Autistic Children and the beginning of TEACCH. The parents decided that the best way for the legislators to be trained in autism was to have them meet autistic children. They arranged a breakfast early enough not to compete with daily legislative activities. Every attending legislator sat beside an autistic child throughout breakfast. The bill that funded TEACCH was passed.

Hard Work. Luck and timing play a role, but nothing can substitute for hard work. Parents as trainers must have good information, must know it well, must be able to synthesize and summarize it, must develop the skill of knowing how and when to pull out the essentials and expand on any part. It means reading reports, budgets, studies, plans, laws, regulations, briefs, court decisions, journals, newsletters. It means going, going, and going to meetings. It means working with coalitions, serving on committees, staying in touch with families. It means seemingly unending hours on the phone, night and day. And writing letters—to persuade, dissuade, encourage, cajole, inquire, acquire (information), and *train.*

Parents of handicapped children are writing letters to legislators more now than ever in the history of our country, and it is paying off. With a new federal administration wanting to weaken or dismantle PL 94-142 and Section 504, thereby seriously threatening to undo the work on which we older activist parents (trainers) spent two decades of our lives, there clearly can be no letup of the assault-by-letter. For the foreseeable future it must become an accepted way of life for parents. ("A letter a day keeps the institution away"?)

Yet, as U.S. Senator Morris K. Udall writes, "Perhaps 90% of our citizens live and die without ever expressing a single opinion to the man [sic] who represents them in Congress—a man whose vote may decide what price they pay for the acts of government, either in dollars or human lives" (1982, p. 15). It's these human lives—our children's—that these letters are all about. A "trainer" needs to motivate parents to send in their stories, to personalize the problem.

Persistence. Luck, good timing, and hard work are excellent attributes for a trainer, but without persistence, change may never come at all. Of all the important features a systems-changer needs, none is so essential, so hard to maintain, or so costly to the trainer as persistence, especially for parent trainers because they're usually volunteers.

There is a high burnout rate. As volunteers they don't usually have secretaries, funds for long distance calls, travel money, cash for copying services, or an income that goes on while they're "training." In fact, it might make an interesting study to investigate the cost to companies and agencies with copy machines of the noncompany/agency copying that goes on. I wager they are donating more to private causes than most executives or members of boards of trustees ever suspect. I know of one autism volunteer-trainer who got permission from a county commissioner to use the courthouse Xerox machine. The volunteer was there so frequently that most staff assumed she was one of them, an assumption she carefully did not challenge. She learned how to put in a new paper supply and even to make minor repairs on the large console copier. That county's "donated" copying services did a great deal to advance the cause of autism. Since there were yet no services for autistic children in that state, the volunteer felt the "donation" was justified.

Additionally, by definition, these trainers have an autistic child, usually living at home—which means child care arrangements and costs while they're away training legislators. As one can surmise, a large percentage of these autism trainers are mothers. Most I know do not have full-time paid employment outside the home—which means most must have intact marriages with working husbands in order for them to be lobbyists. These days it is often necessary for both parents to work in order to make ends meet. Some "autistic" families have chosen to live on one income, meaning sometimes a lower standard of living, so the mother can continue the lobbying, without which, these parents know, very little will get done for their own or anyone else's autistic child. Should the husband's support get interrupted (e.g., illness, loss of job, death, or divorce), most mother-lobbyists will have to leave that activity to get a job, usually paying a penalty for having been out of the job market for a period of time. Their "training" activities, then, can put them at risk. For this reason the cost of persistence is high; legislatures are not overrun with autism "trainers."

A final anecdote on persistence. In the early 1970s a group of "trainers" from various developmental disability groups in West Virginia had, after several years' effort, been successful in getting a bill passed on the last day of the session that would have made education mandatory for handicapped children as young as 3 years old. There was much self-congratulation and we all went home. As the session was coming to a close at midnight, a secretary was typing up the bill for the governor's signature. A legislator (so the story goes—I've never learned who) leaned over her shoulder and said, "That's '*five* years old,' not 'three.' West Virginia's mandate is only for five and up." The secretary typed "five"; the governor signed it. Many weeks passed before we learned what had happened. To this day, in spite of similar bills introduced during the last three legislative sessions, West Virginia advocates have not again been successful in getting another 3-year-old bill passed.

If we'd stayed until midnight persistently following the bill until the very end, we would have our law by now.

Legislators train us too, of course. Those who want to can give us advance notice of meetings, can tell us who is most likely to vote yes or no on our bill, can introduce us to other legislators who can help, can give us cues that will advance our cause, can place us on a tight agenda at a public hearing, can educate us on how to win approval from other legislators.

(They can also make our lobbying life a good deal more comfortable, for instance, by inviting us to store our overcoats, hats, gloves, umbrellas, and boots in one of their closets so we don't have to lug them around all day. In fact, in some capitols the privilege of being free of one's outside gear during the day is more prestigious among lobbyists than a permit for the capitol parking lot.)

I've discussed mainly state legislators, but there are others who are to be trained: members of Congress, officials of county and city governments, and those who administer the agencies you are trying to influence. In fact, as much, if not more, training must go on in these agencies. It has been my experience that getting a bill through a legislative body is generally much simpler, quicker, and less frustrating than its implementation.

PARENTS TRAIN THEMSELVES, THEN OTHER PARENTS

The parents' situation calls first for self-training because, even now, few professionals can help. Parents soon understand they are dealing with a human being whose behavior is so strikingly different from all others in their experience that they often feel compelled to keep good records and learn more. This seems a natural enough response to a dramatic and unique adventure. They are in good company: Christopher Columbus, Marco Polo, Lewis and Clark, Anne Frank, and Jean Marc Itard kept detailed journals. When one perceives that his or her experience is highly unusual, it is intelligent and logical that salient features should be noted. An American fighter pilot who was shot down over North Vietnam and held prisoner for 2,552 days—mostly in solitary confinement—was able to recall his experience in detail. Once liberated, he was able, as he flew out of Hanoi, to dictate the names of 459 fellow POWs (Roddy, 1982, p. 5).

But Leo Kanner, who first wrote about autistic children, called these parents obsessive, a pejorative term in psychiatric circles. He says:

> This much is certain, that there is a great deal of obsessiveness in the family background. The very detailed diaries and reports and the frequent remembrance, after several years, that the children had learned to recite twenty-five questions and answers of the Presbyterian Catechism, to sing thirty-seven nursery songs, or to discriminate between eighteen symphonies, furnish a telling illustration of parental obsessiveness. (1943, p. 250)

Yet when *he* is struck by the same phenomena and writes 33 pages of detailed description of these children's unusual behavior *based on those mothers' notes and good recall* (Kanner, 1943), he is called the "father of autism" and hailed as a gifted observer, which, of course, he was. It is to his credit, however, that in his only address to the National Society for Autistic Children he said, "I especially acquit you people as parents" (Kanner, Note 1).

Because there are not many of us, it is only natural that we see the advantages of meeting with others, collecting, sharing, and disseminating information, and organizing to change laws and get services.

Informed, experienced parents then become natural trainers for those who are new. Some of the most outstanding programs for autistic children were parent-initiated or heavily parent-supported. Benhaven in New Haven, Connecticut, was founded by Amy Ladin Lettick when no school would take her son, Ben; Jay Nolan Center in Newhall, California, was named for the autistic son of actor Lloyd Nolan and his wife, Mell, and was started by a group of Los Angeles parents with the active participation of Mr. Nolan; TEACCH in North Carolina (founded by Eric Schopler), the first statewide, state-supported educational program for autistic children in the United States, had heavy parent support; NSAC's national Information and Referral Service, organized in 1970, was a consequence of this author's years of information collection.

There would probably not be a Developmental Disabilities Act or PL 94-142 if parents (of *all* handicaps) hadn't trained others to take a position and fight for passage. Training other parents is one of the most important tasks of the National Society for Children and Adults with Autism* and of the Autism Hotline operated by Autism Services Center.† It is the ripple effect of parents training parents that makes effective consumer group advocacy. One parent, alone, assaulting the service system may get services for her or his child but is not likely to make an impact on changing the system's policy (though that can, and sometimes does, happen if the parent is energetic and skillful enough).

A large number of parents meet "the system" early in their autism careers, usually when their child is about 2 or 2½, not yet talking, and acting increasingly odd. When they can no longer believe that "he's just slow," their pediatrician is often the first professional to whom they confide their concerns. Until recently, the parents were commonly told they were just overanxious and "let's wait and see." Nowadays, most pediatricians have heard of autism and are more likely to pay attention to the cardinal autistic symptoms. However, making helpful suggestions about what to do is still in the primitive stages. Professionals still do not routinely refer to organized parent groups, still do not have autism literature, still do not seem to know where to refer parents after a diagnosis is made.

Some parents are doing something about that. In West Virginia, Marie Decker, a parent officer of the the state chapter of the National Society for Autistic Children, sought out and got funds from a local private foundation to establish a lending library. She organized a mailout to 500 doctors (psychiatrists, hearing specialists, general practitioners, pediatricians, and others thought likely to be consulted by parents of autistic children), her material boldly headlined: "The next child who walks into your office may be autistic. What will you tell the family?"

---

*NSAC can be contacted at 1234 Massachusetts Avenue, N.W., Washington, D.C., 20005; telephone (202) 783-0125.
†ASC can be contacted at 101 Richmond Street, Huntington, West Virginia, 25702; telephone (304) 523-8269.

Subsequently, NSAC, working through Daniel and Constance Torisky, from Pittsburg, and with funds from the National Football League, established several autism library centers around the United States so that students, faculty, and other professionals will have access to up-to-date information on the state of the art in education, legislation, research, housing, and other aspects of autism.

Like the others, the library project is satisfying. But I believe the sweetest reward of being a parent trainer is seeing a hurt, scared, timid, frustrated, despondent, or angry parent blossom into an articulate, well-informed, assertive, energetic, and successful advocate for her child.

Alice P.'s son Matthew, a fraternal twin, one of five children, is autistic. When he was 3, all the above unhappy adjectives described this mother. She lived isolated in a rural area; there was no nearby program for her extremely hyperactive Matthew or any respite provided by relatives, who believed Matthew just needed some good old-fashioned discipline. A center in a city 20 miles away would take him for a half a day if she'd provide transportation *and* pay a fee, since her postman husband's income was too high for them to meet the criteria for free services. Needless to say, Matthew did not enter the center program.

When at age 3 Matthew was diagnosed autistic, Mrs. P. was shocked and sad. However, she had seen a local mother of an older autistic boy on a television program, so she called her and received a package of helpful information. A short while later the pediatrician phoned to say that, by chance, another autistic child had come to his office. He put the two mothers in touch with each other. Within 2 weeks of diagnosis this young mother was already in communication with two "parent trainers"—experienced, informed mothers. She learned that she could, under permissive legislation, request the county school to take her child into its kindergarten program. Bolstered by her new knowledge of her and her child's rights, and with the active support of the two mothers, she approached the director of special education. Matthew was accepted. Within a few months she and her husband participated in a weekend parent advocacy training workshop, referred and recommended to it by the two mother parent trainers.

By today, less than 2 years later, this mother has served on a state autism task force, been featured along with Matthew in a major local newspaper story on autism (which won a national award), joined the state autism parent group, helped with a large chapter project, appeared at a public hearing at the state capital on a bill for the handicapped during the last legislative session, written her first letter to her congressman, helped several other new parents, distributed literature to professionals in her school district, and contacted her county PTA, which accepted her suggestion of a program on autism. She forced herself to practice driving so she would have confidence enough to drive herself to meetings.

As I write, I call her for an update. Her school system has not yet notified her about transportation, which has been a problem. No longer timid, no longer fearful that Matthew might be pulled out of school (he has just turned 5 and his right to education is no longer permissive but mandatory), she is nudging the system so appropriate transportation will be in place by the time school starts in a few weeks. She has been a good "trainee," though at first she had her doubts. "I'm just a high school graduate, with no experience in the work world, much less in the hallowed halls of state government or even local government," she had said. The result of her "training" is a dramatically improved Matthew, who has become immensely easier to live with, thereby lowering tensions at home. His being in school has given her free time to be a better advocate for him and others. Instead of facing a fearsome and dark outlook for her son, she now knows that by hard work and by joining other parents to fight for their children's rights, she can give Matthew a decent chance at an appropriate program when he is an adult. About a year ago she got a stylish new hairdo and went on a diet. She is happier about herself, laughs more easily, and feels a great deal more *in charge* of her and Matthew's lives.

In spite of cases like this, repeated across the country thousands of times, government agencies are still frustratingly reluctant to spend funds to train parents. Instead, parents, outside the system, often with few resources other than sheer determination and desperate ingenuity, must somehow manage to get changes so their children can have a decent life, with some dignity. How much easier it would be if they had a *fraction* of the resources of those in agencies *whose job it is* to provide services, but who often don't.

The picture is not all gloomy, however. Since the passage of the Developmental Disabilities Act in 1970 and PL 94-142 in 1975, parent training is an activity eligible for funding by state agencies. Some states have provided extensive parent-training projects. Some state DD planning councils and departments of health, education, welfare, and vocational rehabilitation have allocated funds for autism conferences sponsored by the state Society for Autistic Children. Some have special statewide parent-training workshops for advocacy, stressing laws, rights, and how to deal with "the system." These workshops are often run or staffed by trainers who are experienced parents.

PARENTS TRAIN RESEARCHERS

Some might say it's reaching to claim that parents train researchers. The graduate schools (at least most of them) where biochemists, psychologists, neurologists, pediatricians, teachers, and others receive their education almost certainly do not tell their students-bound-for-research that they will receive training from parents of autistic children. But researchers are often surprised at the level at which these parents deal with new and sophisticated information.

I like to tell the story of a researcher from a big-name medical school who was making his first presentation at the annual conference of the National Society for Autistic Children about a decade ago when autism and NSAC were new. He hooked up his microphone and began his lecture delicately, obviously conscious he was addressing nonprofessionals, wanting to make sure he was not speaking above their heads. "Now stop me if you have a question," he said in the same tone one would use to speak to children. The auditorium was packed (parents at NSAC meetings always flock to research presentations).

After only a few minutes a hand went up, and the lecturer stopped. Acknowledged by the speaker, the parent-questioner asked, "What about the 5-hydroxytryptamine efflux from blood platelets as reported recently by Dr. Mary Coleman?" The speaker seemed surprised but answered pleasantly. After a few other such questions, the speaker announced, "Let's hold the questions. I don't get inquiries like this from my medical students and interns!" The whole tenor of his lecture changed. The "training" he got from that and subsequent encounters with NSAC audiences led him to respect the level of parents' knowledge, and in turn gained for him the respect of parents, with whom he now works closely.

Another training story comes from Chris Griffith of Atlanta. When her autistic son was about 9, he was fond of finger-painting with his blood—on his clothes, the living room curtains, a visitor's shirt. He had learned to find old glass in their yard and cut himself with it in order to get his favorite painting material. One day he cut himself so badly his parents couldn't stop the bleeding, so they rushed him to an emergency room. The child had numerous scars over his body and the intern looked at the parents *very* suspiciously. He sutured the wound and was wrapping it carefully with great amounts of bandage, gauze, and adhesive tape. The parents suggested he need not be so elaborate since their son would probably rip it off as soon as they got in the car. Coolly ignoring the parents, the intern finished the job. As he turned around to put away some equipment, the boy not only ripped off the bandages but tore out the sutures. The intern had just received some autism training.

Here's another anecdote, taken from the recently published West Virginia state plan for autism (Sullivan and Mabee, 1982, p. 55):

> The summer my autistic son was nine, he was reluctantly allowed in a communications disorders class operated by the county school system. His regular-school-year teacher was busy in some other part of the building when I arrived with my son that first day.
>
> An older woman was leading the singing of several smiling children with Down's Syndrome who were obediently sitting at a table. She said politely, "Miss _____ will be right back; just leave your son here," pointing to the table of singers. I was holding my extremely hyperactive son securely by one arm, not daring to let him go until there was a second adult in the room.
>
> Seeing my hesitance, the woman said, "I've taught school for over 30 years, dear. Leave him. He'll be all right. Miss _____ will be here soon."
>
> When she told me the third time about her 30 years' experience her tone implied,

"You're just an overanxious mother," so I released the hold on my son and went home.

Within one-half hour the phone rang. It was the principal saying I was to come get my son immediately. The aide in the classroom couldn't manage him and had gone home with a headache.

Parent from Huntington

A few years back, at another NSAC conference, a researcher (let's call him Dr. A.) was reporting some of his recent findings on what many parents feel is some of the most promising and exciting work in the field. His is nonintrusive, observational research. Another researcher (he'll be Dr. B.) had just finished a presentation on biochemical investigations in a highly related field, and was headed for the hotel lobby and the airport. He said he knew little about Dr. A.'s work and had not read his published studies. Two parents convinced him that it was important that he hear Dr. A.'s report. He canceled his reservations and sat almost literally on the edge of his seat as Dr. A. gave his talk, rushing up to the microphone in the auditorium center aisle to ask questions when the speech was over. Long after the audience left, Drs. A. and B. were animatedly discussing their work, exchanging ideas, information, telephone numbers. Except for two parent "trainers" . . .

A veteran mother "trainer" who went back to school asked her professor, a researcher in hearing and speech science, to read a paper she'd written in a graduate psychology course. She had pulled together information from several disciplines—cognitive and developmental psychology, biochemistry, neuroanatomy, embryology—and related what she knew in autism to a set of probing questions about auditory dysfunction and its possible implications for the etiology of autism. He said he read it on the plane as he traveled to San Francisco for a meeting. "I almost fell out of my seat," he exclaimed, and has since begun to study BSERs (brainstem-evoked responses) in autistic children.

Bernard Rimland, authority on and outspoken advocate of vitamin therapy (especially B_6) for autistic children, says he began with all the general prejudices about the efficacy of vitamins. But as letters began to come in from parents who had, on their own, used megadoses of vitamins, and repeatedly reported improved behavior, he decided to lay aside his biases and study the matter.

Researchers (at least the *good* ones) in education and the other "hands-on" professional disciplines have known all along the importance of listening to parents and engaging them as partners (Schopler and Reichler, 1971) in the education (or "treatment"*) of their children. That parents often have new and useful information and ideas to share is a relatively new concept in professional

---

Treatment is a term copied from the medical model and is not, in my opinion, a precise or useful term when speaking of programs for autistic individuals. Since there is at this time no known successful medical treatment for autism, and since the main form of amelioration is a good, structured educational environment, I would opt for using the words *education* or *program*.

training schools, which traditionally have viewed parents as a necessary evil. I have seen signs at a principal's office that read, "No parents allowed beyond this point." Negative attitudes toward parents are clearly demonstrated by a report of a national survey of institutions that admit autistic individual: "Some residential facilities do not allow parents in their children's sleeping quarters. A number of day facilities stipulate, 'No parents allowed on premises without permission' " (Sullivan, 1976, p. 297), and "Some residential programs do not allow parent visitation for as long as six months after admission; one facility prohibits visitation for one year!" (p. 297).

Some of these attitudinal barriers are slowly breaking down as federal and state laws mandate participation of parents in the planning of their children's program, as well as their representation on policy-making boards and commissions.

Researchers and parents share a serious responsibility toward each other to sensitively observe and to report what they find. A parent's intensive "autism experience" can lead to suggested clues that may be missed by a researcher who only occasionally sees the child. The first reported connection (Goodwin, Cowen, and Goodwin, 1971) between autism and celiac disease came from a chance encounter of a pediatrician (Mary Stewart Goodwin) and the (typically) odoriferous celiac stool that was being carried to the utility room of a hospital ward. Dr. Goodwin's experienced nose knew the celiac smell, but her autism background had not prepared her to look for it in autism. No doubt the mother of the child on that ward had known her son's stools had a peculiar smell long before he was hospitalized. Did she never mention it to a physician? Or did she offer the information only to have it dismissed?

CONCLUSION

Parents as trainers will be playing that role for a long time if we are to continue to make progress for our children. In 1969 (Sullivan, Note 2) I wrote the following to the scattered few valiant parents who were fighting for the acknowledgment that autism even existed. The message is not very different from that of today:

> You are about to venture on a project which will profoundly affect the lives of many persons—the mentally ill children [autism was classified as a mental illness then] in your community, their parents and families, and above all, *you*.
>
> In bringing together these individuals—at first mostly parents who have endured the community's degrading neglect of its mentally ill children—you will work long hours, spend your energy, strain your talents, and quite possibly your family treasury. Your telephone will be forever at your ear, and the empty space on your desk will burgeon with files, reports, lists, and letters.
>
> It will all be worth it when, because of pressure from your new Chapter, the first

mentally ill child in your community is admitted to the public school, or the superintendent of your school district invites you to join his advisory committee on special education, or when you see lonely, isolated parents meeting other parents for the first time.

Like others before you, you have been through the preliminary stages of appalling diagnosis, grief, frustration, and anger. Now you are set for ACTION. You could find no more noble a cause or more neglected a minority. Go straight to your work. Be knowledgeable, articulate, energetic, fierce, charitable, militant and persistent.

We can be no less if our children are to get help in our lifetime. NSAC is here to help you.

Best of luck.

Ruth Christ Sullivan
Second President
National Society for Autistic Children

REFERENCE NOTES

1. Kanner, L. Dr. Leo Kanner accepts a citation presented during NSAC's first annual meeting and conference, July 17–19, 1969. Transcribed from a tape recording and edited by Dr. Kanner. Distributed by NSAC's Information and Referral Service, 1969.
2. Sullivan, R. C. A message to organizers of new NSAC chapters. National Society for Autistic Children, 1969.

REFERENCES

Goodwin, M. S., Cowen, M. A., and Goodwin, T. C. Malabsorption and cerebral dysfunction: A multivariate and comparative study of autistic children. *Journal of Autism and Childhood Schizophrenia*, 1971, *1*, 48–62.

Itard, J. *The wild boy of Aveyron*. New York: Appleton-Century-Crofts, 1962.

Kanner, L. Autistic disturbances of affective contact. *Nervous Child*, 1943, 2, 217–250.

Park, C. *You are not alone*. Boston: Little, Brown, 1976.

Roddy, E. Vietnam POW writes saga on survival. A book review of *The Hanoi Commitment* by James A. Mulligan. *The Pilot*, Boston, August 6, 1982.

Schopler, E., and Reichler, R. J. Parents as cotherapists in the treatment of psychotic children. *Journal of Autism and Childhood Schizophrenia*, 1971, *1*, 87–102.

Sullivan, R. C. Autism: Current trends in services. In E. R. Ritvo (Ed.), *Autism: Diagnosis, current research and management*. New York: Spectrum, 1976.

Sullivan, R. C., and Mabee, B. K. *Opening doors for West Virginians with autism: A comprehensive state plan*. Charleston, W.Va.: West Virginia DD Planning Council, Department of Health, June 1982.

Udall, M. Quoted in Association for Children with Learning Disabilities *Newsletter*, Cleveland, O., March 1982.

West, P. *Words for a deaf daughter*. New York: Harper & Row, 1978.

15

The Parent as Trainer of Professionals

Attitudes and Acceptance

BARBARA COYNE CUTLER

A number of factors, including political movements, legal actions, advances in the technology of teaching, and a still-growing understanding of the causes and treatments of autism, have combined to produce a major reversal in professional attitudes toward parents, described in Chapter 1.

In those early decades when autism was first defined and treated through psychodynamically oriented therapies (Bettelheim, 1967; Kanner, 1943), parents were at best viewed by professionals as objects of pity for their parental inadequacies, which were the presumed cause of the profound autistic withdrawal of their potentially normal children. Yet today not only can we discuss the critical importance of involving parents in training to be teachers and managers of their autistic children but we are also ready to address the special contributions that parents can bring to disciplines relevant to autism.

During the 1960s the civil rights movement fostered the growth of consumer advocacy groups, including those parent and citizen networks that would promote educational rights for all handicapped children. The civil rights movement and parent groups combined to achieve those educational rights (Biklen, 1974; Des Jardins, 1969, 1971), first through the courts, then through state and federal laws (Abeson, Bolick, and Hass, 1976).

BARBARA COYNE CUTLER • School of Education, Division of Counseling, Reading, Language Development and Special Education, Boston University, Boston, Massachusetts 02215. This chapter was written with the support of grant number MH 14761, awarded to the Department of Sociology, Boston University, by the National Institute of Mental Health.

PL 94-142 required a major change in the role of parents (Martin, 1979). From hopeful, grateful-for-anything bystanders, parents were advanced to major participants. Recognized by the federal government as partners in the educational process, parents were given both contributing and monitoring functions. New to the task, many were awed by such responsibilities; yet this was preferable to their former submissive and helpless state. The assumption of this burden offered new hope for their children's existence and growth.

Parents of autistic children played an important role in advocating for their children's rights. Nevertheless, their effectiveness as advocates would have been substantially diminished without a simultaneous advance in professional knowledge regarding autism's causes and treatments.

The 1960s and 1970s saw an increase in research that questioned earlier hypotheses (Kozloff, 1973; Rimland, 1964; Rutter, 1971; Schopler & Reichler, 1971; J. K. Wing, 1966; L. Wing, 1975; Schopler, Note 1) and produced evidence that parents were indeed innocent of the charge of generating autism. When Leo Kanner publicly pronounced the acquittal of such charges at the annual conference of the National Society for Autistic Children in Washington, D.C., in 1969, it was a major event for parents. He was, after all, the clinician who had first defined autism and probed for its roots. This professional reversal allowed parents to set aside the old undeserved yoke of guilt, regain their feelings of self-worth, begin to actively engage in advocacy for education and services, and participate in the new educational technology.

Behavior modification surfaced in the 1970s as an appropriate treatment and even the treatment of choice for autistic children (Kozloff, 1973; Risley & Wolf, 1966; Walder, 1968). Initially parents were not seen as resources. In the search for cheap labor to sustain the early gains of their young clients, behaviorists first exhausted their supply of graduate students, undergraduates, and even high school students, as well as the available funds, before they realized that the handiest and least costly resources were the parents, who had the time, opportunity, commitment, and (with training) capacity to modify their children's behavior (Neufeld, Note 2). Parent training soon became an established tool for intervention with children with autism and other disabilities.

The relationships of professionals to parents have undergone drastic changes in the last 15 years. Some of those changes were forced, i.e., judicial and legislative; some were fortuitous, e.g., the discovery of parents as effective trainers; and some were brought about by concerned and questioning professionals who were not satisfied with the state of the art.

Both parents and professionals are experiencing varying degrees of success in adjusting to their new roles and responsibilities. This more balanced association still maintains the useful elements of the expert–client relationship: the parent sharing his or her extensive knowledge of the child (perhaps more effectively and with greater reception than before), and the professional helping the parent to articulate that knowledge through his or her specialized skills (Kyne, 1980).

Now comes a new participant—the parent turned professional. Whereas in the past parent-professionals tended to be secretive about their parent status for fear that they would be taken less seriously by their professional colleagues, today's parents, coming from the recent rights/parent/consumer movements, see their special experience and perspective as assets in their respective fields. The old assumption that being a parent means being emotional and lacking in objectivity is being revised.

Acceptance of the "otherwise qualified" professional, i.e., the parent with academic credentials, may still be a hurdle to be overcome by some professionals and parents. Being a parent of a child with autism has been a handicap of sorts. Like the "otherwise qualified" handicapped person (as defined in Section 504, the 1974 amendment to PL 93-112, the Rehabilitation Act of 1923, which specifies that people with handicaps should not be excluded solely on the basis of their handicaps), parents should also be accepted on the basis of their skills and not discriminated against through lingering and prejudicial assumptions.

How will people deal with parent-professionals, and with the special contributions that they can bring to the field?

What follows is the story of one parent's experiences, first as a parent seeking services, and finally as a professional delivering services to both parents and professionals. The lessons learned from these experiences will be presented as ways to improve the nature of the parent–professional relationship and to develop a true partnership between parents and professionals.

THE MAKING OF A TRAINER

For this writer, the road begun as a "pathological" and helpless parent was uphill and strewn with obstacles, fears, small and major achievements and setbacks, choices, and demands. Along the way I found other parents with whom I could identify, and later I met professionals who provided practical help and support and ultimately served as models for a professional career I would not have dreamed of in the early days of being a parent of a child with autism.

Phase I—The Early Days

Left by divorce with two young children aged 4 years and 18 months, a new home in a strange neighborhood, and a psychiatrist to advise me, I faced grief, isolation, guilt, and the need to search for the fatal flaw in me that was responsible for my son's extreme rejection of the world around him. My older son, Rob, had been a good baby, easy to care for, and responsive to both parents. He sat and stood early, and walked on schedule. At 2, however, he was still not talking and his behavior began to deteriorate—he was easily upset by changes in routine, perseverative, and increasingly withdrawn. He soon acquired the diagnostic labels of atypical and severely emotionally disturbed. The label "autism" would be assigned much later. George, my other son, was as outgoing and assertive as Rob was withdrawn. At 18 months, he was (thank God!) beginning to talk. Rob would not say his first word until he was almost 5. Against the backdrop of divorce, I accepted the hypothesis that I was a defective mother. In odd and frequent moments looking at my two beautiful children, I would wonder what was wrong with me. How could I have produced such a devastating result as autism? In desperation we embarked on an expensive 6-year course of psychotherapy involving five weekly visits with two psychiatrists. When the therapy was finally concluded there was even less hope for Rob.

Other parents have told their stories of frustration, grief, and fear (Akerley, 1978; Park, 1967; Warren, 1978). We have shared a common history under the "benevolent" dictatorship of traditional psychiatrists who, though meaning well, promoted our anxiety and vulnerability. This was done at great cost— financial, emotional, and, in the case of our autistic children, possibly intellectual as well. Certainly all of our children, with and without autism, were to some extent deprived by our constrained and anxious parenting, exacerbated by the treatment process and its faulty assumptions, the effects of which we would not understand until years later.

There was no effort to bring parents together, even when our children shared the same programs. However, the practical details of life such as programs and car pools brought us together. We found each other in parking lots and at doors of programs, and we began, hesitantly, to share our common problems and grief.

Alike in our pain and problems, were we also alike in sharing the destructive flaw? I saw all types of parents, different in size, shape, age, socioeconomic status, personal style. Where was the flaw? As I began to question the basic assumptions of the therapists, I finally concluded that these good and caring parents, including me, were not flawed, but rather misunderstood, misdirected, and cruelly mislabeled. If we were to be blamed for anything, it should be for our vulnerability and for our tolerance of the psychological abuse caused by inappropriate professional assumptions.

Here was the first lesson: Professional "objectivity" was based on assumptions that could and should be questioned. Shaped to believe that professionals were objective, we did not know that, regarding autism, the professionals were as ignorant as we were. But we learned that the experts listened selectively, sometimes ignoring the issues and information we wanted to share. We also learned about the labeling of parents: refrigerator, symbiotic, abusive, or neglectful. Designated the symbiotic type because my son tended to cling to me, I saw the one thing we had going for us somehow turned into a defect. I learned that my son's future depended on my ability to "separate" myself from him. Tickling and holding were to be discouraged. I followed all the rules, and still he lagged in development. Slowly I became aware that he was being deprived by these rules, as I was of my chance to be a warm and affectionate parent. When I realized that he got less physical contact from me than his brother did, I decided that the therapist's assumptions were wrong. My solitary child was being even more isolated. What personal bias, problem, or attitude was the therapist bringing to the treatment that hindered my parenting? What set of norms and values that denied my own? Unresolved conflicts with his own parents? Comparisons with mothers who abused children? Faith in the therapist gave way to doubt and the suspicion that we had become victims of his bias.

This was the second lesson: Parents were not the only people emotionally involved; they had not cornered the market on bias. Professionals too were biased, particularly against parents, by their years of training and practice (if they were wrong now, they would have to accept the responsibility for the harm done in the past), by their professional membership (to differ was to risk becoming a professional outcast), and possibly by their own personal experiences and unresolved conflicts. But psychotherapists were not answerable to parents. Since the therapeutic relationship was an authoritarian one, they continued to label us.

Other professionals, e.g., administrators, school psychologists, and teachers, took their signals from the psychotherapists and too often treated parents as incompetent, unreliable, and interfering.

When, Rob, aged 9, was suddenly without a program, I was desperate enough to try to teach him myself. Drawing on some basic educational principles, I taught Rob to read in about three days. Using words that were important to him, I helped him learn to discriminate 80 words and read simple sentences in less than a week. He was so ready to learn, it was amazing. How had the "objective" educators missed this readiness? When the school called us in for preplacement assessment, we went armed with the 200 vocabulary cards to show the psychologist what Rob had learned. She provided some perfunctory testing (block placement and copying figures) for a somewhat anxious and uncooperative Rob and dismissed my attempts to show her Rob's reading. She had no time for our demonstration and advised me to stop teaching and just be Rob's mother. Rob was assigned to the trainable class for the mentally retarded.

I was so desperate for a placement that I did exactly what she said—I went home and taught no more, although I knew that Rob was at least educable and capable of more than the trainable class could provide. Once again, progress was postponed because of professional prejudice and assumptions.

This was the third lesson: Parents *can* be effective teachers, especially if they have the support and guidance of competent and caring professionals.

In spite of these lessons, learned slowly and at great cost, I felt powerless to apply them. Our situation worsened when Rob, at 12 and full size, became frighteningly and unpredictably hard to manage, and we found ourselves without service of any kind. Exhausted and frightened, I turned at last to the institution for an emergency admission. Once again we were rejected. However, I was told that on the edge of the institution was a clinic with a morning class and a young teacher who might provide some immediate assistance. Still the compliant parent, I was led down the hall to yet another professional from whom I expected more grief and little help. My expectations were to prove wrong.

Phase II—My First Parent–Professional Partnership

I was not prepared for Bobbie Bruno, then a young teacher, 1 year out of her master's program. She offered genuine sympathy for our difficult situation and some help. Rob could come to her morning class, which was only 2½ hours long, but it was at least a start. More important, would I work with her to establish a home program for Rob? I agreed, but without hope. She then rapidly began to put forth ideas and recommendations. Since Rob's behavior worsened when he was anxious, we should try to provide a totally predictable environment through a rigidly scheduled program of daily activities, using rewards for good behaviors. We discussed skills, materials, times, and data, and came up with a plan. Since we should stay in close contact, would I mind if she called me regularly to check on progress? Would I mind! Where before, calling professionals outside of scheduled times had always made me feel that I was imposing, here was someone asking *my* permission to be called.

This first meeting lasted about an hour, but it was unlike any other professional meeting I had experienced. I was treated not as the incompetent, pathetic parent with unrealistic expectations and erroneous observations, but as an equal partner in helping my son through a severe crisis. Our partnership was based on two new (to me) assumptions: that Rob was capable of being helped and that *I* was capable of delivering that help. When I left the meeting, I felt only the slightest ray of hope. Rob deserved at least one last chance and so I committed fully to the home program for a month. If there was no change by then, I would have to push harder for institutionalization.

That month was the most emotionally and physically grueling of my life. Every half hour was programmed by the clock. There was puzzle time, reading time, gross motor time, fine motor time, and an occasional half hour of television or music when the need for collecting data and delivering rewards was less. Wake-up, mealtimes, bath, and bedtime were religiously scheduled. Life was never so organized or predictable. I did not go out that first month except for morning grocery shopping. The only social contacts were grandparents' visit on

Sunday, a Friday night visit from a friend carrying a well-deserved bottle of wine, and Bobbie's frequent and supportive phone calls.

"This is the pest calling again. Have you time to talk to me?" At first, I was speechless. Calls from teachers were generally to inform me of Rob's most recent transgressions—nothing so helpful or friendly as this. She would ask how things were going and she would listen, sometimes offering a suggestion and other times enthusiastically congratulating me on one of my ideas, which she might also institute in the classroom next week. My earlier parent career had not prepared me for this kind of acceptance and equality.

In the first 10 days the aggressions increased and hope diminished. "That's to be expected," Bobbie assured me. "Hang in a bit longer. It will start to decrease." In the beginning I would drag or wrestle Rob to his room for time-out after an aggressive episode. Sometimes I would have to hold him down to keep him there. He would cry; I would cry. I'd think that I could end this by going to the police for a court-ordered admission to the state school. But the promised 30 days was not over.

The specific programs for chores and skill-building activities went well from the start. Rob was a learner and happy to be developing new skills. He liked to see the checks go up on his wall charts and he very seriously watched the x's on the aggression chart. At 2 weeks the aggression had peaked and had begun to decline. Bobbie cheered from the sidelines by phone and shared her own classroom combat stories. I continued consistently and relentlessly until the month was up. Rob was coming under control, learning, and becoming a happier child. Most parents care more deeply about their children's happiness than about skills or competencies. I was fortunate to see that happiness can come from skills and competencies developed in a carefully controlled but caring environment. If the cost had seemed high initially, the rewards were even greater.

The home program continued, but with success it became easier. Bobbie and I continued our partnership by phone and through home and classroom visits. I was comfortable now in the give and take she had established. Both of us could offer ideas to be accepted, shaped, or rejected without the intrusion of status.

At the end of the year Rob was appropriately transferred to a public school educable MR class, Bobbie was setting up a special class in a nearby town, and I was unwinding from a year of heavy home programming. Bobbie's calls continued, and when in late October she offered me the chance to become her student teacher, I was overwhelmed. If I had any residual doubts of my competence, her offer was strong evidence that her support and praise were not merely a subtle professional technique for working with fragile parents and that she truly valued my ideas and skills. Having recently accomplished the "impossible" with Rob's rehabilitation, I did not hesitate to apply to Harvard's Master of Education program, which allowed the student to design a curriculum to meet individual professional needs. I was admitted in January and found myself in

Bobbie's classroom in April. She was the teacher and I was clearly the student, but our partnership continued. Although she was a highly competent behaviorist, skilled diagnostician, and creative and responsive teacher, she continued to listen to my ideas and suggestions.

I was a fortunate parent to have met this young woman in a desperate time at the gate of a desperate place—the state institution. Had she been instrumental only in reversing Rob's decline, that in itself would have been an extraordinary gift. But she met me with compassion and respect, and thereby enlisted me as an equal partner in a great enterprise. She recognized and nurtured strengths and skills in a frightened and overwhelmed parent and allowed me to develop my own critical and evaluative competencies. Our relationship would later become the model and measure of the parent–professional relationship in my work with families.

Phase III—Developing Professional Competence

In the next few years I started a recreation program for autistic adolescents, founded a private day school for autistic adolescents, and developed respite care programs; Rob entered the educable class for the mentally retarded in the local public school system, where he'd continued to make progress. During this period, Martin Kozloff came to Boston. Through our mutual interest in autism and behavioral training, and in developing programs to support autistic children and their families, we became good friends. There were few behavioral programs in the Boston area then and even fewer programs that focused on building appropriate skills through behavioral education. My programs were a resource for Marty's students at Boston University, and he became a personal resource for my staff and me. As a parent I was extra appreciative of his commitment to parent training and his comprehensive understanding of the parents' experience in dealing with their children, the professional community, and society. He offered practical help to parents in changing their children's behavior and in improving their chances for a better life. As a parent I knew how important this help could be.

In 1977 Marty asked me to work with him on a National Institute of Mental Health grant to develop innovative and improved models of training for parents and professionals. Here was a model I believed in and could practice (see Chapter 10); yet the old doubts taunted me. Would I be objective in my work with parents? Would I become too emotionally involved with parents to be effective? I knew that my parent experience had given me insights and a special perspective that would be valuable, but would they be valued? Would others, parents and professionals, doubt my credibility because I was a parent, even though I'd earned degrees and established programs? Furthermore, Rob had not been "cured"; he was still autistic and facing a substantial change in services, which would later prove inadequate and damaging. What if he regressed? Then what of my credibility?

Marty answered my questions with sympathy and clarity: "If it was in your power, you would give Rob all the programs and stability he needs. In spite of being a good advocate and parent, you cannot be responsible for everything that happens. If Rob gets into a bad program and regresses, you will still be a good parent and a good parent trainer. So let's get to work."

Training Parents. In my first year as a parent trainer, I worked with two families whose individual situations allowed me to test some of my own assumptions.

One family, the "Hallorans," proved that though parents may appear resistant to professional offers of help, they may be highly motivated in seeking help for their children. Parents are potentially competent if the professional can empathize with the parents' feelings and respect their concerns. The Hallorans were the aging parents of an adolescent boy with Down's syndrome and with a number of autistic-like behaviors. These parents were defiantly resistant at our introductory meeting, almost challenging us to talk about punishment. When we answered, "No punishment," they obviously did not believe us. But they agreed to an initial interview to take place in their home. To minimize the differences between the staff and the family, I volunteered to work with this family because I was the oldest staff member (there was still a 25-year difference) and, more important, the parent of a handicapped adolescent son.

In the first interview, Mrs. Halloran freely discussed her son's past history and present level of functioning, which seemed dismally low. Other professionals had told her that her son could not learn. She saw the future as a choice between making his few remaining years at home happy or making them miserable by attempting to teach him things he could not learn. I told her I had a son of similar age and handicap who had been helped by the methods we were offering to teach her, and that I understood her concerns. She began to open up, but she was a long way from conviction. Trust would be established slowly.

Although our project offered a comprehensive training program with ordered steps from 1 to 99 (Kozloff, 1974), it was obvious that this woman could continue only if she selected behaviors that she felt were important. Eye contact was not an important behavior to her, but making a sandwich was. She got support and instruction in teaching sandwich-making, and experienced immediate success. She went on to develop an intensive home program, which rapidly led to her son's achievement of many daily living skills and, within a year, to functional reading.

By respecting this mother's needs and priorities and by working to establish a trusting and empathetic relationship, we were able to move beyond this parent's initial resistance and overprotectiveness to help her achieve dramatic progress in her son's performance, i.e., from seemingly profoundly mentally retarded to highly educable. Had we been more dogmatic, we would have lost a valuable professional opportunity to test our initial assumptions and improve our approach with parents.

Another family, the "Reeds," taught us how to keep the door open for other professionals. Unlike the Hallorans, this family was young and eager. During the program, the Reeds had many interruptions in their training because of operations for their mentally retarded son, travel, and moving to a new home. Though they cared deeply for their son, it was clear that these parents were not in one place long enough to implement a program. Should I drive home that they had not upheld their end of the training program? As a parent, I too had experienced the feelings of professional judgment and rejection. I wanted this family to reach out for help in the future, so I told them all the good things I had observed about them and their child, and that, because of almost constant movement, this was not the time to institute a training program. Once settled, they should start again, either with the Kozloff book (1974) or with another program or professional in their new neighborhood to give them the help they would continue to need.

Training Parent and Teacher Teams. Next we took our program to a suburban school system, where we jointly trained volunteer parents and teachers of moderately handicapped children. This program included both home and classroom visits, with the goal of creating effective parent–teacher teams, hoping that teachers might themselves become good trainers of parents. We found that capable teachers could team effectively with both strong and weak parents, but that poor teachers tended to be defensive with parents. If the parents were weak, they tended to go along with the teacher, perhaps making modest gains. If the parents were strong, they were likely to be in conflict with the teacher.

We learned several things from this program.

1. Effective teacher–parent collaboration was possible.
2. Even the strong, supportive teachers who were capable of developing good classroom programs and guiding parents in home programs did not have sufficient time or energy to run parent groups on their own.
3. Parents and teachers might have different goals for the child's behaviors and needed to understand that school and home programs could differ and still benefit the child.
4. Weak parents who assumed that "teacher knows best" had difficulty in developing skills and critical judgment in dealing with poor, defensive teachers.

"Teacher knows best" is the prevailing attitude among both teachers and parents. The nonthreatened teacher could understand that goals might differ for parents and professionals and still be appropriate and compatible. The threatened teacher tended to be more dogmatic and to diminish or disregard the value of parents' suggestions; failure was justified by the complaint "How can I possibly do anything for this child when the parents don't follow my instructions?"

Because we were in the schools by administrative invitation, we felt constrained in our remarks in both group meetings and home and classroom visits. While it was easy to support the good teacher, it was difficult to criticize or openly evaluate the poor one. Most of our parent–teacher teams were effective; some were stellar; but for the all-trusting parent or two, we could only hint and hope. As a parent, I felt this limitation keenly, understanding as I did the destructive effects of subservience to educators.

In those first two training programs, I also worked with two special education directors and a school psychologist, who used my professional skills and occasionally drew on my combined skills and parent experience when they were dealing with a difficult placement or family situation.

Expanding the Training Model. During the third year of the project we developed some significant additions to the training model in the areas of normalization and advocacy.

We had accumulated enough collective experience to know that we wanted to incorporate normalization principles (Wolfensberger, 1972) into our training program. It was consistent with Marty's view of parents as partners that he invited previously trained parents to assist us in integrating normalization into the training model. Mrs. Halloran and other parents had earlier shown us the value of age-appropriate and more normative program objectives for their children. We began to focus on the child's competencies rather than on his deficits. A model was developed that is described in Chapter 10 of this book.

At the same time, we moved to develop an advocacy component when we realized that parents who became skilled home teachers of their children also became better evaluators of the education programs their children were receiving. However, they needed help in using the special education laws to deal with school systems. Marty, insisting that I had some specialized knowledge of systems to share, urged me to write a book. *Unraveling the Special Education Maze* (Cutler, 1981) was developed and became part of our training package. Parents who become skilled home teachers can learn the necessary advocacy skills to influence their children's school programs. The success of the book was sadly balanced by Rob's increasing difficulties. Marty's support was constant and reassuring while I dealt once again with the old issue of my credibility and competence as I watched Rob deteriorate physically and behaviorally in inappropriate and inadequate programs.

Training Professionals. In our fourth year we turned to training professionals (Kozloff, 1979) from neighborhood health and mental health centers. We combined the teaching of basic behavioral education principles with instruction in setting up and running parent groups, and the provision of on-site consultation when the professional trainees instituted their own training programs.

The trainee I worked with was a mental health professional with good behavioral skills and an eagerness to serve families with handicapped children. We worked as a team to develop her parent-training program. When she worked individually with her parent-trainees, she treated them as partners in the mutual effort to help their children. In our private consultation, her concerns were "How do I reach this family? Am I asking too much or not enough? Is my instruction clear?" My role was largely one of support and guidance, assurance that she was doing the right thing, and, on occasion, advising her that she was doing too much when the parents needed to do more. Here was another example of the parent-professional and the professional effectively teaming. I was the leader then, but when I was finally forced to place my son in the state school that year, she became the sympathetic mental health professional offering me, the parent, support and advice.

Dealing with a Double Status. This past year I ran a short training program outside the project. I introduced myself as a parent first, then added my credentials. I told them a little about Rob so that they would not by chance happen onto personal information that might cause them to question the value of the training model. I told them that my 25-year-old son had been recently institutionalized; that because of the skills I taught he was at the front of the institution, which was better than being in the back wards; that because of his skills, I had hopes of getting him back into the community; and that I had no cause to regret all of the effort, energy, and love that went into helping and teaching him. I told the parents that with the new skills they were about to acquire, their children would have better opportunities and make better use of the new services available. They accepted this information, and then we got down to the business of acquiring skills and developing good home programs.

By now, I think my special contribution to parent training has been thoroughly assimilated by my colleagues in our project and that we may be more productive trainers because we respect and support parents. After 5 years as a parent trainer, I feel that I have earned my professional status and contributed to the field by applying my special understanding and experiences as a parent.

This account of my career as a parent and a professional reviews many experiences that parents still undergo. I have been allowed to incorporate the lessons learned as a parent into a training program for parents and professionals. It should be eminently clear that this trainer progressed because of the support of some accomplished professionals, only a few of whom are mentioned here, who were interested more in a person's competencies than in her circumstances.

ISSUES IN THE DEVELOPMENT OF PARENTS AS PROFESSIONAL TRAINERS

Few parents of autistic children aspire to be human service professionals. Some have established careers in other fields; others lack the interest because they want and need something totally divorced from autism. Others, however, who have the potential skills and interest to become effective trainers may hesitate because they anticipate that the professional community may fail to receive them as equals and/or deny the special value of the parent perspective.

Issues of Acceptance

With the erosion of the psychogenic hypothesis of autism, parents can develop more productive relationships with professionals. However, working as client and professional implies a hierarchical rather than an equal relationship, and professionals can and do assert varying degrees of authority. When problems confound the expert, resorting to old attitudes about parental emotionalism and inability to teach (Cutler, 1981) may spare the professional the problem of testing his or her own assiduously acquired expertise. Many professionals will at least question their own theories and methods, but some will continue to rely on their old rules and maintain the myths.

Professional Acceptance. Parents who wish to become professionals need to be supported and legitimized by professionals who are not parents of handicapped children. Professionals who want to let colleagues and clients know that they believe parents to be reasonable and competent people can best deliver this message by enlisting a parent-professional as a respected partner. Assurances are never so strong as the action of openly collaborating with the "otherwise qualified" parent, i.e., hiring and/or training parents as professionals, paraprofessionals, and ancillary staff. Partial acceptance, on the other hand, not only weakens the status of the parent-professional but sooner or later undermines the whole enterprise; everyone suffers, including professionals, clients, and especially the children, who are denied the effects of better programming through collaboration.

Self-Acceptance. Parents must openly accept the status and experience of being the parent of a handicapped person, understanding that they can never be "above reproach," because of the fact their children are handicapped. In this small world of clients and services it is better to be up-front rather than silent about one's parent status. Eventually someone will discover the undisclosed status and see in the parent's silence a denial that will raise the very suspicion of credibility that the parent sought to avoid.

Aspiring or practicing parent-professionals will define the parent status as an asset for understanding the daily problems of the handicapped family and use their special expertise to assist them in evaluating family difficulties. Knowing that it would be arrogance to insist that only parents can understand other parents, they avoid assuming the role of omniscient spokesperson for all affected families. They see their special parent knowledge as a contribution to, not a usurpation of, the field of parent training and do not deny the competence of other trainers. Of course, parent-professionals should not be so invested in the appearance of professional "excellence" that they forget the status that gives a special edge to their credentials.

By continually striving to increase their professional competence, by being prepared to deal with the potential bias they may encounter in their professional training and practice, and by recognizing the unique value of their personal experiences, parent-professionals can become confident and effective trainers.

Acceptance by Other Parents. This is largely determined by the parent-professional's competence and self-confidence and by the professional community's full acceptance of that role. Problems arise when the acceptance is limited. Like other minorities, parents of handicapped children are sensitive to tokenism. If they see that the image of inept, pathetic parents still clings to all of them, regardless of qualifications, they realize that the partnership is a sham with little hope of the genuine collaboration that leads to the greatest benefit for their children.

Two groups of clients respond strongly to the parent-professional. One group includes parents so stigmatized by their children's disabilities and so intimidated by earlier professional experiences that they reject the help of any parent. They are best assigned to a staff member who is not a parent. The other set of parents are those who have been so traumatized by their dealings with professionals that they have trouble trusting a professional trainer. These benefit from working with the parent staff member, with whom they can identify. During the program, as they are exposed to instances of productive teaming between staff members including the "otherwise qualified" parent member, both sets of parent-clients can learn that all staff respect parents and merit their trust. As clients experience full acceptance of the parent staff member, their own self-image can be strengthened and their capacity for beneficial change improved.

Special Contributions

The parent-professional's perspective, presence, and participation provides the training team with opportunities for framing new questions and revising assumptions and attitudes that may otherwise limit the team's effectiveness in helping parents.

A training team committed to instructing parents in coping and teaching skills has already taken steps to dispel the myths of parental incompetence and emotionaliam discussed earlier. Still, there are times when parents' failure, resistance, or lack of motivation can stonewall the trainer, who may respond in frustration by blaming parents. A common parental response is to ask, "Where did I go wrong?" Professionals who experience failure or trouble with their clients can take a lesson from parents and ask first. "Where did *I* go wrong?" then move to examine their own expectations and performance before assigning blame to someone else.

If parents are being resistant, that resistance may be appropriate from their perspective. Are we asking them to do things that seem meaningless or offensive? Have we clarified the training issues and methods to their satisfaction? Have we tried to accommodate *their* goals? Are *we* in fact resistant when they want to put their efforts into communication rather than good sitting or toothbrushing? If parents differ from us, how hard are we willing to work to resolve those differences?

A parent-professional can help colleagues to understand a range of parent perspectives, e.g., time. Although some parents tend to overprotect or baby their children, most parents feel that time is running out for their children. Can we help them to see that there is still time to make a significant difference in their lives and the lives of their children? By respecting their concerns, we can help them to reshape their views and redefine their goals so that progress is possible (Cutler, 1982).

A parent's presence on the professional team can have a unique impact on language, i.e., to constrain deprecating remarks and reduce the expressions of unsubstantiated assumptions by staff. Since language tends to shape thought, this constraint may over time aid professionals in improving their perception of parents.

The parent–professional team can become the iconoclasts of those cherished professional myths that have negatively affected the development of parental competence and independence. They can replace those beliefs with guidelines for new assumptions that are less dangerous, e.g., that most parents will tend to cooperate in any venture they believe will be helpful to their children. This kind of assumption puts the burden of help and conviction squarely on the shoulders of the professionals.

These are the ways that the parent–professional team can improve training programs to the benefit of their clients, both parent and professional. Still, the most significant contribution the parent–professional team can make is to work together, equally and publicly. Their joint efforts are an affirmation of the professional commitment to serve families of handicapped children.

REFERENCE NOTES

1. Schopler, E. *Parents of psychotic children as scapegoats.* Paper presented at the Symposium of the American Psychological Association, Washington, D.C., 1969.
2. Neufeld, R. Keynote address. AMIC-McLean Conference on the Emotionally Disturbed Child., Belmont, Mass. 1971.

REFERENCES

Abeson, A., Bolick, N., and Hass, J. Due process of law: Background and intent. In F. J. Weintraub, A. Abeson, J. Ballard, and M. L. Lavor (Eds.), *Public policy and the education of exceptional children*. Reston, Va.: Council for Exceptional Children, 1976.

Akerley, M. False gods and angry prophets. In A. P. Turnbull and H. R. Turnbull (Eds.), *Parents speak out*. Columbia, O.: Charles E. Merrill, 1978.

Bettelheim, B. *The empty fortress*. New York: Free Press, 1967.

Biklen, D. *Let our children go*. Syracuse: Human Policy Press, 1974.

Cutler, B. *Unraveling the special education maze*. Champaign, Ill.: Research Press, 1981.

Cutler, B. Education for parents. In D. Park (Ed.), *The proceedings of the 1981 International Conference on Autism*. Washington, D.C.: National Society for Children and Adults with Autism, 1982.

Des Jardins, C. *Your rights as parent of a handicapped child*. Chicago: Coordinating Council for Handicapped Children, 1969.

Des Jardins, C. *How to organize an effective parent group and move bureaucracies*. Chicago: Coordinating Council for Handicapped Children, 1971.

Kanner, L. Autistic disturbance of affective contact. *Nervous Child*, 1943, *2*, 217–250.

Kozloff, M. *Reaching the autistic child*. Champaign, Ill.: Research Press, 1973.

Kozloff, M. *Educating children with learning and behavior problems*. New York: Wiley, 1974.

Kozloff, M. *A program for families of children with learning and behavior problems*. New York: Wiley, 1979.

Kyne, J. The evolving parent–professional relationship. In B. Wilcox and A. Thompson (Eds.), *Educating autistic children and youth*. Washington, D.C.: U.S. Department of Education, 1980.

Martin, R. *Educating handicapped children: The legal mandate*. Champaign, Ill.: Research Press, 1979.

Park, C. *The siege*. Boston: Little, Brown, 1967.

Rimland, B. *Early infantile autism*. New York: Appleton-Century-Crofts, 1964.

Risley, T. R., and Wolf, M. M. Experimental manipulation of autistic behavior and generalization into the home. In R. Ulrich, T. Stachnik, and J. Mabry (Eds.), *Control of human behavior*. Glenview, Ill.: Scott, Foresman, 1966.

Rutter, M. The description and classification of infantile autism. In D. Churchill, G. Alpern, and M. DeMyer (Eds.), *Infantile autism*. Springfield, Ill.: Charles C. Thomas, 1971.

Schopler, E., and Reichler, R. Parents as cotherapists in the treatment of psychotic children. *Journal of Autism and Childhood Schizophrenia*, 1971, *1*, 87–102.

Walder, L. *Teaching parents and others principles of behavior control for modifying the behavior of children*. Final Report. Silver Springs, Md.: Institute for Behavioral Research, 1968.

Warren, F. A society that is going to kill your children. In A. P. Turnbull and H. R. Turnbull (Eds.), *Parents speak out*. Columbus, O.: Charles E. Merrill, 1978.

Wing, J. K. *Early childhood autism*. Oxford: Pergamon Press, 1966.

Wing, L. *Autistic children: A guide for parents*. London: Constable, 1975.

Wolfensberger, W. *The principle of normalization in human services*. Toronto: National Institute on Mental Retardation, 1972.

VI

Emotional Support and Siblings

16

Explaining Mental Retardation and Autism to Parents

VICTORIA SHEA

INTRODUCTION

To be told that his or her child has a serious disability is one of the most painful experiences in a parent's life. Numerous articles by parents eloquently describe the feelings of despair, anger, shock, or fear that the news of the child's diagnosis precipitated (Massie and Massie, 1976; Murray and Murray, 1975; Shigley, 1980; Turnbull and Turnbull, 1978; Wolfensberger and Kurtz, 1969). Some of the distress that learning their child has a serious disability causes parents is unavoidable. Parents must grieve the loss of the hoped-for normal child, and the normal grief process is often lengthy and painful. Some pain is unnecessary, however; this is the pain caused by thoughtless or unskilled professionals. Unfortunately, many parents have described experiences of being told abruptly, coldly, or superficially about their child's disabilities and future potential.

The lack of skill on the part of many professionals in explaining developmental handicaps to families is a serious, but not surprising problem, given the limited training that most professionals receive in this area. Research and professional literature on this topic is also limited (Doernberg, 1982; Matheny and Vernick, 1969; Miller, 1979; Morgan, 1973; Rockowitz and Davidson, 1979;

VICTORIA SHEA • Division for Disorders of Development and Learning, University of North Carolina, Chapel Hill, North Carolina 27514.

Schnell, 1982; Shea and Saur, 1981; Knobeloch, Note 1). The purpose of this chapter is to provide a guide for professionals in interpreting developmental handicaps in general, and mental retardation and autism in particular, to parents.

An interpretive session with parents (sometimes called an informing interview) should serve as a bridge between assessment and treatment. Thus, the interpretive session should accomplish three goals: (1) answering parents' questions and providing diagnostic information about their child's developmental status; (2) helping parents begin to cope emotionally with the knowledge of their child's handicap; (3) assisting parents in making plans to carry out recommendations. Parents must have a clear understanding of their child's developmental status and needs if they are to function effectively as caretakers and as advocates for their child in society. In addition to information, parents generally need emotional support to deal with the pain of learning about a serious developmental handicap. This is not to say that a goal of the interpretive is for parents to "accept" the child's handicap. The process of coping emotionally with having a handicapped child continues throughout a parent's life; there is no magic moment of "acceptance," in the interpretive session or at any other time. So the second goal of the interpretive is simply to support the parents as they begin to cope in their own ways with the diagnostic information. The third goal of facilitating treatment is based on the premise that evaluating and labeling a child, at great expense and sometimes pain, is pointless unless the diagnostic information leads to some kind of intervention that makes the child's or the family's life better. Parents are almost always responsible for implementing these interventions (e.g., agreeing to special class placement, carrying out a behavior management plan, teaching a self-help skill, applying for SSI), and they often need help in understanding and following through with the suggestions.

Many interpretives are unsuccessful because one or more of these goals is not met. For example, sometimes test results are presented, but parents are not given the opportunity to ask questions or to express their feelings. In other cases, parents are encouraged to grieve, but no concrete help is given. In these situations, the interpretive must be considered incomplete or unsuccessful.

What can professionals do to increase the likelihood that all the interpretive goals will be met? This chapter will focus on five elements that can be arranged to contribute to a successful interpretive.* These elements are the *assessment* of parents' ideas and feelings, the focus of the *staff conference,* the *structure* of the interpretive session (e.g., who is present, how long it lasts), the *content* of information conveyed to parents, and the interpretive *process,* which refers to the techniques of communication used with the parents.

*This work was supported in part by U.S. Public Health Service, Maternal and Child Health Project, No. 916 and Grant HD-03110.

ARRANGING SUCCESSFUL INTERPRETIVES

Assessment of Parents' Concerns

Traditionally, assessment of the parents of children with developmental problems focused on obtaining information about developmental milestones and/or identifying parental psychopathology. These approaches frequently did not result in useful information for designing and facilitating treatment. A complete discussion of the assessment of family functioning and developmental disabilities is beyond the scope of this chapter. There are, however, two topics that should be included in preinterpretive discussions with parents, specifically in order to achieve the interpretive goals delineated here. These topics are the parents' information about the child's skills and behavior, and their ideas and questions about the child's problems.

Many parents are good observers of their children's behavior, although they may not understand the implications of certain behaviors or developmental lags. Questioning the parents about the child's typical daily routine, favorite activities, special skills, and areas of developmental or behavioral difficulty often yields valuable information. Similarly, Schopler and Reichler (1972) found that many parents' estimates of their child's current developmental levels were strikingly similar to test results, although parents' predictions of the child's future potential were somewhat less realistic. Thus, it is generally good practice to ask parents if they think their child acts like other children his or her age, or if not, what age the child most resembles. In addition to providing information about the child's skills and/or the parents' perceptions, these questions are useful in laying the groundwork for the interpretive session. When parents and professionals can begin an interpretive discussion in general agreement about the child's behavior and skills, the diagnostic findings are less likely to produce anger or shocked disbelief on the part of parents. Conversely, when parents do not feel that their ideas and observations have been included in the professionals' formulation of the child's disability, they are more likely to be skeptical and defensive, or to feel unprepared for the diagnostic labels they hear.

In addition to exploring parents' observations, professionals should learn from the parents what diagnoses they suspect, what their understanding is of these diagnoses, and how they feel about them. Such discussions can be initiated by asking parents what they think their child's problems are, or what labels other professionals have used for their child. If parents mention a specific handicap by name, the professional can then go on to ask what the term means to them, and how they feel about having that label applied to their child. If parents do not bring up a disability by name, it is appropriate to ask them directly if they have considered the possibility of a diagnosis of mental retardation, since this is usually the handicap parents have worried about. For example, the professional could ask, "Have you ever thought that Johnny might be mentally retarded?" If a parent agrees that mental retardation has been a concern, the professional could ask, "What do those words mean to you?" or "What did hearing 'mental retardation" make you think of?" If parents indicate that they have never considered the possibility of mental retardation, the professional can point out that the child's assessment is still in progress, and that the question is being asked only because mental retardation is a common developmental problem that many parents worry about. Some basic information about mental retardation and/or suspected handicaps can be given at this time, but it is obviously not appropriate to confirm the diagnosis of a specific disability before the child's assessment has been completed and the staff conference held.

Another topic that should be explored at this time is the issue of etiology. Almost all parents have questions or hypotheses about causes for the child's problems, although their ideas are frequently unexpressed, even to their spouses. Some parents relate the child's problems to a specific cause, such as the mother's emotional distress during pregnancy, a minor health problem or accident, or perceived medical mismanagement. Others parents have more global fears about having been negligent or incompetent as parents, or being "punished" by having a handicapped child. During the assessment phase, professionals should ask parents if they have had any ideas or worries about why the child has developmental problems. Later, in the interpretive, it will be important to return to this issue and discuss what is and is not known about the causes of the child's problems.

Discussing possible diagnoses and causes during the assessment phase allows parents time to prepare themselves emotionally for the information that may be presented in the interpretive. Additionally, professionals who understand the parents' perceptions can focus the staff conference on the parents' primary concerns and anticipate their reactions during the interpretive.

Focus of Staff Conference

The apportionment of time in a typical staff conference bears little logical relationship to the purpose of the assessment, which is to develop effective interventions for the developmentally handicapped child. Frequently, the major part of the staff conference time is used in describing test results, a brief period is spent integrating and formulating findings, recommendations are implied or quickly listed (often with no plan for implementation), then the interpretive is planned hastily and superficially in the final moments of the conference. When this pattern is followed, the staff conference can become a stage for displaying narrow diagnostic acumen, rather than a forum for integrating information and developing appropriate recommendations. The interpretive becomes an after-thought, rather than a vital link between professional knowledge and parental understanding. By losing sight of parents' perspectives and instead seeing the assessment as belonging to themselves, professionals severely reduce the like-lihood of a successful interpretive.

The leader of a staff conference should make sure that time is spent ra-tionally, with sufficient time allowed for planning recommendations and the interpretive. Sometimes this means urging the professionals to keep their presen-tations of test results brief and pointed; at other times the leader must point out that the allotted conference time is not sufficient and must be extended. If the professionals are committed to providing good service to families, they will respond to this leadership.

There are two additional guidelines for professionals to remember during staff conferences: Listen to each other, and keep the parents' questions in mind.

A frequent problem in staff conferences is that some professionals seem to be simply waiting for their turn to speak, rather than listening to each other's information. This pattern is particularly a problem in multidisciplinary settings in which roles are rigidly defined and staff don't recognize the limits of their own knowledge and the value of other professionals' perceptions. The interests of a child with a pervasive developmental disability are much better served by a team in which members rely on others to complement their information about one aspect of the child or family with additional information from another perspec-tive (e.g., physical examination, psychoeducational testing, family interview).

During staff conferences, professionals must make a special effort to keep parents' questions in mind, because these usually do not relate directly to test results. Instead, parents' questions tend to require integration of information from a variety of sources. For example, parents are much more likely to ask, "Will he learn to talk?" or "How can I toilet train her?" than they are to wonder, "What age level are his visual-perceptual skills?" or "How retarded is her adaptive behavior?" In a staff conference that focuses mainly on the results of individual evaluations, it is unlikely that answers to the parents' complex questions will be developed. Since the parents are likely to ask the questions again during the interpretive, the professionals will be in the position of having to respond spontaneously, when they could have taken the time during the staff conference to gather information and opinions and prepare complete responses.

Structure of the Interpretive Session

Choosing Participants

Information about the child's developmental status and needs should be given to all of the child's primary caretakers. When the child lives with both parents, every effort should be made to hold the interpretive session with them simultaneously. This structure both allows the parents to support each other when hearing distressing news and avoids placing or perpetuating one parent in the role of caretaker and liaison with professionals and the other parent in a less involved role.

If parents are separated or divorced, individual interpretives with each parent usually should be arranged. Specific plans depend both on the parents' degrees of involvement with the child and each other and on individual state laws regarding release of information to the noncustodial parent. Similarly, when there are other relatives (e.g., grandparents) or agencies (e.g., Department of Social Services) involved, decisions about interpretive participants must be made carefully, taking into account both clinical and legal considerations.

Thought should also be given to which professional(s) should participate in the interpretive. The general principle is that these should be the professionals who *from the parents' perspective* are the most authoritative and trustworthy. The parents' interests should take precedence over clinic routine or professionals' schedules. Thus, if there are indications that parents will place more trust in an interpreter of a particular sex, race, or age, these preferences should be respected. Similarly, for many parents the professional status of the interpreter is an important factor in their acceptance of the diagnostic findings, so it is often wise to include an M.D. or a Ph.D. in the interpretive session. This is particularly true for highly educated parents, who are generally interested in the details of the assessment procedures and have many questions about medical findings and theories. For parents who are relatively uneducated or who are retarded themselves, however, the presence of several highly educated professionals in the interpretive can be overwhelming. With these parents, the session is usually best conducted by only one interpreter; occasionally it is helpful to include a community worker, such as the Head Start health/handicap coordinator or a Department of Social Services homemaker who has a good relationship with the family.

Planning the Number of Sessions

In many diagnostic clinics only one interpretive session, lasting approximately 1½ hours, is held with a family. Although with careful preparation this is generally sufficient for completing the basic interpretive tasks, having only one session increases the pressure on both professionals and parents to accomplish all their business in a short period of time. In clinic settings with an "extended diagnostic," "follow-up," or "treatment" component, there is more opportunity to reexplain complicated concepts, work through emotional reactions, and provide support for following recommendations. In all settings, professionals should offer as many sessions as are necessary to accomplish the interpretive goals.

Arranging the Environment

The physical setting of the interpretive session can either contribute to an atmosphere that allows the goals to be met or interfere significantly with this. Interpretive sessions should be private and uninterrupted. Participants should have comfortable chairs that are at appropriate angles and distances for conversation. Seating should be arranged so that parents can choose to sit together or apart, and professionals should make sure that facial tissues and ashtrays are available. All of this should be set up before the session beings. The essence of these prescriptions is that everything possible should be done to ensure that parents feel comfortable and supported.

Content of the Interpretive Session

Presenting Basic Concepts

The theme underlying the presentation of diagnostic and developmental information should be ''We have seen and worked with children like yours before, and we can help your child.'' This message, which is helpful in interpreting many medical and developmental problems, can be especially reassuring to parents of children with autism. Often these parents are confused or frightened by their child's behavior and have never encountered other children like theirs. To be told that their child's pattern of development has a name, can be understood, and can be helped is often a great relief to parents, and can be the beginning of a solid working relationship between parents and professionals.

Parents have the right, by the end of the interpretive session(s), to have a clear understanding of the name, nature, cause, severity, and future course of their child's developmental handicaps, to the extent that these can be known. This means that terms like *mental retardation* or *autism* must be used honestly and explained fully. (Of course, it does not mean that these terms should be brought up abruptly or used without acknowledging their emotional as well as their technical meanings.)

In explaining test results and implications, professionals should use simple language and should present information in small conceptual steps, waiting for parents' indications of understanding before moving on. This sounds easier than it actually is, because there is usually a large amount of test data and interpretation to present. Most professionals need to think through the diagnostic material carefully and organize their notes before the interpretive session begins.

Explaining Mental Retardation

The following material forms an outline that could be followed in explaining mental retardation and autism to parents. The ideas are presented in a logical sequence, which is suggested as a good general pattern. The specific pace and language used would have to be modified according to the parents' needs.

1. *Restate the parents' questions and concerns related to the child's development.* For example, the professional could say, "When we began Billy's evaluation, there were several areas you wanted help with. You asked why Billy seems to understand what you say to him, but doesn't talk. You were also wondering how to discipline him when he has temper tantrums, and what to do when he gets upset in the grocery store and at church. Were those the main things you wanted help with? Have you thought of other questions that you would like us to try to answer today?"

Beginning in this way has several effects. First, it establishes that the parents' questions are a legitimate focus of the interpretive session, and that the session is intended to be a discussion rather than a lecture. Second, beginning with the parents' questions gives them an opportunity to discuss issues that may have arisen during the diagnostic process. It often happens that observing diagnostic testing or answering questions about their child's development has changed parents' perceptions of their child, either by preparing them for the seriousness of the child's problems or by raising questions that had not previously occurred to them. Finally, beginning in this way indicates that there is a logical relationship between the parents' questions and the diagnostic information that will be presented. This is highly preferable to the professional's launching into test results that bear no apparent relationship to the family's daily life and concerns.

2. *Explain that the child's development was assessed using standardized tests.* The professional might begin by saying, "As you know, we did several tests to help us understand Billy better, so that we could answer your questions." Describing test procedures and results is significantly simpler if parents have observed at least part of the child's testing. During this observation or the interpretive session, it is appropriate to mention the name(s) of the test(s) used, if parents indicate an interest. It is usually helpful to explain that the tests have been administered in exactly the same way to many youngsters (thousands throughout the country, in the case of most intelligence tests) so that the child's performance could be compared to that of normally developing children of different ages.

3. *State that the assessment indicated that the child's development was delayed in some or all areas.* An example of this step in the interpretive is a

simple statement like "On all the tests Billy came out behind his age level. In other words, the tests showed that he is not doing all the things that other children his age can do."

At this point it is helpful to refer back to the parents' observations and estimates of the child's development, if these paralleled test results. For example, "So what we found was similar to what you thought: Billy is behind in his development and does a lot of things like a younger child." A statement like this supports the parents' judgment and competence as parents, which can be therapeutic at this time when their anxiety about their child is growing.

4. *Follow this general information with specific test results.* At this time the child's developmental age equivalents in different areas (e.g., fine and gross motor, receptive and expressive language) should be explained. An example of this type of explanation is "Billy can understand words and sentences like a 2½-year-old. This is what we call receptive language: his ability to understand what you say to him. But his expressive language, or his ability to use words to tell you things, is even more delayed. His expressive language is around the 18-month level." Most parents automatically make the comparison between the child's developmental level(s) and chronological age. For those who do not, this should now be made explicit.

5. *Compare the child's chronological age and developmental level(s) and explain that the child's rate of development has been slower than average.* For example, the professional could say, "Now, when we think about the fact that Billy is 6 years old, but most of his skills are like those of a 2- or 3-year-old, we can see that he has been developing at a slower rate than most children. He has learned a lot of things, but it has taken him more time to learn them."

It is extremely helpful to introduce the idea of the "rate" or "speed" of development early in the presentation of information. This is particularly true in the interpretives with parents of young or mildly retarded children, for whom the absolute value of the developmental delay may appear small. For example, if parents are told that their 4-year-old is functioning like a 3-year-old, they may assume that when the child is 14, he or she will have the skills of a 13-year-old, which does not seem like a significant problem. This type of misconception can usually be avoided if an early part of the explanation includes the idea that the child's rate of development is slower than average. This lays the groundwork for a discussion later in the session of the implications of the child's current developmental delays.

6. *Reassure the parents that the child will continue to learn and develop, although his or her rate of development in the future will be slower than average.* Many people have the misconception that a child's mind can stop growing at an early age, and that the child then retains that mental age throughout life. This idea is often unspoken, but professionals should anticipate and counteract it by reassuring parents that the child's developmental progress will continue. The

professional could say something like "We know that Billy is going to keep on learning and developing. He's not going to stay at the same level he is now. But his rate of development is probably going to be slower than average in the future, just the way it has been slower than average up until now."

The prediction of future development based on a single assessment is controversial. (This is another reason that obtaining information from parents about the child's skills at home is a valuable adjunct to testing.) There are certainly circumstances in which test results cannot be considered reliable indicators of future potential. These circumstances include (1) the presence of sensory or motor handicaps or severe behavior problems that interfered with test performance; (2) a history of extreme environmental deprivation (including prolonged hospitalization), which can be assumed to have affected the child's development in the past but may not in the future; and (3) extremely young age. (Some professionals are unwilling to diagnose mental retardation before children are 2 years old, although in many cases of severe neurological damage this reluctance seems unreasonable.)

When any of these factors is present to a substantial degree, then current developmental delays may not be reliable predictors of future developmental potential. However, some professionals tend to "excuse" all developmental delays on the basis of these or other, milder factors (e.g., the child had a cold or was hungry, sleepy, or irritable during testing). This tendency seems to stem from the professionals' own distress at the idea of mental retardation. Unless there is clear evidence that current behavior and test results are not representative of the child's true abilities, it is most likely that a slow rate of development in the past indicates a slow rate in the future. This is particularly true for children functioning at the moderately retarded range or below (Lockyer and Rutter, 1969; Robinson and Robinson, 1976).

7. *Introduce the term* mental retardation *as a synonym for slow development.* The point at which mental retardation is mentioned is usually the most difficult moment of the interpretive session. The diagnosis of mental retardation is painful for almost every parent to hear. Even parents who have previously heard the term applied to their child often become sad at having this finding confirmed. When the diagnosis is new for parents, their emotional distress is much greater.

There are numerous factors that contribute to parents' reactions to the diagnosis of mental retardation. These include realistic concerns about the child's welfare and the family's ability to find the extra time, energy, and money the child's care will require. The diagnosis of mental retardation confirms the parents' fears that the child has a chronic problem that will not go away. Additionally, there are common societal attitudes and misconceptions about mental retardation that may influence parents. Mentally retarded people are among the most stigmatized and devalued members of our society; parents may share these

feelings about mental retardation and be distressed that the disability has occurred in their family. In addition, many people confuse "mental retardation"
and "mental illness," so that the diagnosis may connote insanity and all its
manifestations. Still other people think of mental retardation as synonymous with
physical stigmata or handicaps, institutionalization, or complete lack of self-care
skills. These common ideas or others unique to individual parents can contribute
to their distress at the diagnosis of mental retardation.

Discussion during the assessment phase of the possibility of a diagnosis of
mental retardation is helpful in dispelling some misconceptions and preparing
parents for what they may be told in the interpretive. Even with preparation,
however, the pain that parents experience at hearing that their child is mentally
retarded cannot be completely avoided. Parents' grief, fear, and tension in the
interpretive room are almost tangible at this time.

Another factor that may contribute to the tension of this part of the interpretive session is that many professionals have difficulty discussing mental retardation in a straightforward manner. These professionals are usually extremely
sensitive to the social stigma associated with mental retardation and/or to the
parents' distress, and are therefore reluctant to use the words *mentally retarded*.
Usually this phenomenon is seen among young professionals, but occasionally
even experienced professionals have identified so closely with the parents that to
cause them pain is extremely difficult. When professionals are uncomfortable
with mental retardation, they have been observed to ramble around the topic and
"forget" that the term has not been used, to become dysfluent and almost
incoherent as they approach the use of the term, or to report that they had to
"force" themselves to say it. Unfortunately, these reactions on the part of the
professionals usually increase the stress and tension felt by the parents.

The term *mental retardation* should be introduced calmly and directly. For
example, the professional could say, "Another way of saying that Billy's rate of
learning is slower than average is that he is mentally retarded." Parents should
then be given time to react before the professional moves on to the next point in
the outline. (Techniques for eliciting parents' reactions are discussed in detail
under Process).

8. *Explain that there are different degrees of mental retardation that correspond to different rates of development.* Many parents are not aware that mental
retardation ranges in severity. Even those who have the concept of a continuum
are generally unfamiliar with the terms *mild, moderate, severe,* and *profound.* A
concrete way of presenting this information is to compare slow rates of development to a "normal" rate of 12 months' progress in a year. Although the following figures are oversimplified to some extent, mild retardation can be described
as representing 7–8 months' progress per year, moderate retardation as 5–6
months' progress, severe retardation as 3–4, and profound retardation as 1–2
months' progress in a year. (These figures correspond roughly to ratio IQs of 67,

50, 33, and below 25, respectively.) This explanation is both accurate and simple enough for almost all parents to understand.

A decision about how much to explain to a family about the degrees of mental retardation should be based on the family's situation and the child's handicap. Parents of mildly and moderately retarded children often benefit from having the professional describe more severe retardation and state explicitly that their child is not in that category. This is particularly helpful when parents are struggling to understand and accept the diagnosis because their only image of mental retardation is that of a profoundly retarded institutionalized person. In addition, explaining the whole spectrum of mental retardation is helpful with parents of young mildly and moderately retarded children, because it is often difficult to predict whether these children will continue to function in the same range, speed up in development with appropriate stimulation, or fall relatively further behind as developmental tasks become more abstract and language-based. Their parents should be prepared for all these possibilities, if they have the cognitive abilities and emotional energy to handle the information. (This does not necessarily have to be done during the initial interpretive session if there will be follow-up contacts.) It is generally not necessary or helpful to describe mild retardation to parents of severely or profoundly retarded children, since there is very little chance that these children will ever develop at a mildly retarded rate.

An issue that must be considered when informing parents of mental retardation is using the child's IQ score. In almost all diagnostic settings (i.e., medical facilities and schools) parents are entitled to review the child's records. Therefore, if the family is likely to request the records or if it is clinic policy to report the IQ to parents, it should be discussed at this time. The intelligence test scores associated with different levels of mental retardation could be mentioned when the ranges are first described, but before the individual child's IQ is reported. This procedure is recommended in order to prepare parents gradually for their child's score. Professionals who are accustomed to dealing with IQs in the mentally retarded range should be careful not to underestimate the devastating impact the IQ number may have on a family. Possibly because of the American grading system, in which a score below 70 is "failing," an IQ in the 40s, 50s, or 60s can be extremely distressing for parents. As one parent said, compared to an average IQ of 100, she felt as though a child with an IQ of 50 was "half a person."

9. *State that the child is unlikely to catch up in development.* Even at this point in the interpretive, many parents retain the hope that the child's problems are temporary. This hope is probably based on both cognitive and emotional factors. Parents may have been told by other professionals that their child had a "developmental delay"; this term can foster unrealistic hopes, since "delay" does not imply permanency, and in fact suggests that the child will catch up eventually. Additionally, many parents do not understand that intelligence stops

growing at the end of childhood. Thus, parents who understand the explanation that the child is developing at half the average rate might still expect that when the child is 40 he or she will have the skills of a 20-year-old. The professional must explain that childhood is a unique time of development and growth, which comes to an end during adolescence. It is often helpful to compare intelligence and height, saying something like "Just as our bodies stop growing in height and we don't get any taller, in the same way everyone's intelligence stops growing during the teenage years, and we don't get any 'smarter.' We can still learn new facts and skills as adults, but our basic intelligence remains pretty much the same."

Even parents who understand all the facts about development and the child's test results may hope that the child will become normal. It is neither necessary nor appropriate to attempt to take this hope away, as long as it does not interfere with decisions about the child's treatment. When parents respond to the professionals' information with expressions of hope and faith, the most helpful response is a simple statement like "I hope you're right" or "I wish you could prove us wrong."

Explaining Autism

The interpretation of autism should parallel the interpretation of mental retardation in explaining the diagnostic label in a way that helps parents understand the child's current behavioral patterns and predict the child's future developmental course. Thus, a technical definition of all aspects of the syndrome is often not as helpful as a simpler explanation tailored to the individual child's characteristics.

10. *State that in addition to mental retardation the child has another developmental handicap called autism.* The diagnosis of autism is generally less upsetting to parents than mental retardation, probably because autism is less familiar to the lay public and thus has fewer negative connotations. In fact, the ideas that people do have about autism may contribute to its relatively benign image, since these include the misconceptions that autism can be cured by psychiatric treatment, and that autistic children can have above-average intelligence. Thus, it is sometimes necessary to impress on parents the idea that autism is an additional handicap that complicates the global developmental delays already discussed. (Of course, sometimes a child with autism is not mentally retarded, in which case the issue of overlapping handicaps does not arise.) As with mental retardation, decisions about what information to convey about autism should be based on the parents' knowledge and attitudes as these were determined during the child's assessment.

11. *Explain that children with autism have in common difficulties in two areas of development: organizing and understanding information from their*

senses, and understanding communication with other people. This segment of the interpretive focuses on a description of the child's unique pattern of sensory interests and communication skills. Frequently this kind of information is the most difficult for parents to understand and conceptualize. Most people are unaccustomed to thinking about individual senses (e.g., vision, hearing, smell, touch, movement in space) and are even less familiar with the concept of perceptual organization of sensory stimulation. Thus, the idea that there are recognizable patterns of sensory interests and perceptual abilities is foreign to many parents. Similarly, most parents have not given much thought to the various skills that underlie communication (e.g., understanding gestures and facial expressions, discriminating sounds, attaching symbolic labels to concrete objects and events, organizing the information required to produce a word).

Clearly, there is a great deal of information that could be presented at this time. However, when parents are cognitively or emotionally overwhelmed by the information they have already received, it is reasonable to postpone discussion of the details of the child's perceptual and communication skills to a follow-up session (ideally in the context of treatment). During this first interpretive session a simple explanation of the fact that the child has difficulty learning through certain senses, and/or does not understand all the steps involved in communication with people, is often sufficient. Again, it should be stressed that these are characteristic problems of children with autism.

12. *Describe how the child's pattern of perceptual organization and communication skills makes his or her behavior more understandable.* It is likely that the child's behaviors that are the most confusing or distressing for parents are related to the child's autism. Most often these are behaviors like understanding some language but speaking very little, echolalia, fascinations with certain toys or ways of playing (e.g., lining up objects), stereotyped behaviors, lack of interest in cuddling or playing with the parents, or seemingly irrational fears or temper tantrums. It is usually possible to explain at least some of these behaviors in terms of the perceptual and cognitive deficits that have previously been described. For example, the professional might say, "One of the things Billy's autism means is that he doesn't pay attention to sounds in the same way that other children do. Sometimes he doesn't seem to be listening to anything at all, then at other times he pays as much attention to the fan or the traffic outside as he does to the words we say to him. On the other hand, he always pays very close attention to the things he sees. He likes to look at toys from different angles, and he likes to see things spinning or falling through the air. Since he prefers vision to sound so strongly, it makes sense that he would rather play by himself with toys that he can watch, rather than play with people who are talking to him in words he doesn't understand. Also, lots of loud or sudden noise in places like church or a shopping center might be very confusing for him. He doesn't understand where the noises come from or what they mean, and sometimes he is probably overwhelmed by them and gets upset or has a temper tantrum."

Clearly, there are many other points about mental retardation and autism that could be made, depending on the individual child's behavior and skills and the parents' concerns. One issue that should always be addressed, whether or not parents raise it, is the question of what caused the child's handicaps.

Discussing Etiology

Professionals should be sensitive to the fact that most parents feel some guilt or responsibility for their child's handicap. (This is especially true in the case of autism, because of the influence of early psychiatric theories on current popular literature.) This is the reason it is helpful to have explored during the assessment process the parents' ideas and fears about possible causes of the child's problems, so that these ideas can be addressed during the interpretive session. If, after medical studies, the cause of the child's problems is known or strongly suspected (e.g., inherited syndrome, maternal viral infection during pregnancy, oxygen loss at birth), this information should be given to the parents, along with whatever is known about the chance of recurrence. Although it is painful for parents to think about the time at which damage to their child's nervous system probably occurred, most parents say that they take some comfort in knowing exactly what went wrong and why. It is usually more stressful for parents to be told that the cause of the child's handicap will probably never be known, because the parents' fears and guilt remain unresolved. For most developmental disabilities, unfortunately, an exact cause cannot be found (although many factors suspected by parents can be ruled out). It is therefore most important to include in interpretives the reassurance that the child's disabilities are not the parents' fault. Parents need to hear that nothing they did caused the child's problems, and that there was nothing they could have done to prevent them. With time and the opportunity to discuss their ideas and fears, most parents can accept the idea that the disability is a sad reality that "just happened."

Answering Parents' Questions

There are certain questions that are asked in many interpretives and that professionals should be prepared to answer. There can be no standard replies to these questions, because the answers depend on an individual child's skills and needs. There are some general guidelines, however, for understanding the questions and formulating answers.

1. *Will our child talk?* The answer to this question depends on the child's age, level of retardation, and degree of autism, as well as the presence of other sensory or motor handicaps that might affect the development of speech. If the child has normal hearing and oral-motor mechanisms and is only mildly-moderately retarded and autistic, it is extremely likely that he or she will develop speech. Most severely retarded people also develop some speech, although they

might use only single words or short phrases rather than longer sentences to express their meaning; this is particularly true of severely retarded people who are also autistic. Some profoundly retarded people and individuals with severe autism never master all of the cognitive prerequisites for speech (Mount and Shea, 1982).

2. *Does our child need speech therapy?* Parents who ask this question often have the idea that the child is "trying to talk" but is unable to form intelligible sounds. They reason that speech therapy would help the child learn correct speech production and thus enable him or her to talk. However, most speech and language delays associated with mental retardation and autism can be attributed to the child's cognitive level. It should be explained to parents that language development depends on a combination of developmental readiness and exposure to words that represent meaningful objects, people, and activities. Thus, speech therapy sessions are often not as helpful as a more general program of language stimulation throughout the day. This program might or might not be planned by a speech/language clinician.

3. *Should our child go to private school?* Because most private schools are expensive and exclusive, parents tend to think of them as generally "better" schools, without reference to the issue of the child's handicaps. Certainly there are some excellent private schools for children with mental retardation and/or autism. In most communities, however, the private schools are not equipped to work with handicapped children. Especially since the implementation of Public Law 94-142 (Education of All Handicapped Children Act), most public school systems are better prepared than most private schools to educate handicapped youngsters. However, if there are private schools available in a particular family's community, professionals have an obligation to evaluate them before offering an opinion about their appropriateness for the child.

4. *Should our child have an EEG or a CAT scan?* The answer to this question is ultimately a medical decision. If a physician has not been involved in the child's evaluation, and the parents describe any behaviors that suggest illness, seizures, or developmental regression, medical consultation should be arranged. In the absence of those concerns, however, parents sometimes wonder in vague terms about a "brain test" that would pinpoint the child's problem; the implied hope is that the problem could then be cured. If there are no focal neurological signs by history or examination, however, physicians say it is unlikely that an EEG or CAT scan would contribute to an understanding of the child's problem, and even less likely that they would suggest a treatment.

5. *How much should we push our child?* This question is asked in many interpretives, but it seems to mean something different to each parent who asks it. It is wise to clarify parents' meaning before beginning to answer. Some parents mean, "Should we make him obey rules (e.g., pick up his toys, sleep in his own bed) or should he always have his own way?" Other parents are really

asking, "How many hours a day should we work with her?" In other cases parents explain, "Our neighbors and relatives tell us that if we were stricter he wouldn't act the way he does, but we don't want to spank him all the time, so what should we do?" Once the initial question has been translated into behavioral terms, the professional can either answer it on the basis of what is already known about the child or, if necessary, defer an answer until a later session when more time and information are available. An excellent reference for practical suggestions is found in the book by Schopler, Reichler, and Lansing (1980).

6. *What will our child be like in the future?* Rather than bombarding parents with detailed predictions, many of which would at best be educated guesses, the professional should provide general information about the usual developmental course and/or adult outcome of the child's handicap(s), then attempt to clarify parents' specific concerns. When parents of preschool-age children ask this question, they are rarely asking about the child's adulthood; instead, they are usually wondering whether the child will master self-help skills, go to school, and make friends. Some parents also wonder about the child's life expectancy, even when this issue does not occur to professionals. As children get older, parents usually begin to think about specific goals for adulthood, such as holding a job, managing money, and marrying.

As a general rule, mildly retarded adults without autism can live independently, marry, and work in competitive employment, usually at unskilled or semiskilled jobs. Moderately and severely retarded adults without autism usually master basic self-help skills and function well in supervised living situations and sheltered workshops (Baroff, 1974; Robinson and Robinson, 1976). Profoundly retarded individuals will always need assistance with daily living tasks; they too can be served in community-based residential facilities (group homes), although the number of these that currently exist is quite small. The outcome for children with autism at any intelligence level is generally less favorable than for children at the same intelligence level without autism (DeMyer, 1979). However, some individuals with autism are able to live independently, and others are served well within residential and vocational programs for the mentally retarded. (Often they are less retarded than the other clients but need equivalent amounts of supervision and structure.) For individuals whose handicaps include autism, moderate-severe mental retardation, and serious behavior problems, specialized and intensive programs will probably always be needed.

Making Recommendations

The recommendations that should be included in an interpretive depend on the type of setting in which the evaluation was done. In a diagnostic clinic with little or no treatment component, the interpretive session (and possibly a follow-up letter or set of reports) is the only mechanism for meeting the goals of providing concrete help to the parents. In these settings, therefore, it would be important to include the following kinds of recommendations:

1. Names, addresses, and telephone numbers of appropriate community agencies and/or personnel, such as the Coordinator for Exceptional Children in the school system, the director of an early intervention team, the contact person for parents' organizations, such as the National Society for Children and Adults with Autism, or the Association for Retarded Citizens.
2. Authors and titles of books related to the child's disability, such as *Is My Baby All Right?: A Guide to Birth Defects,* V. Apgar and J. Beck (New York: Simon & Schuster, 1972); *Your and Your Retarded Child: A Manual for Parents of Retarded Children,* S. Kirk and S. Kirk (Palo Alto: Pacific Books, 1968); *Autistic Children: A Guide for Parents and Professionals,* L. Wing (New York: Brunner/Mazel, 1972).
3. Specific suggestions derived from the child's evaluation, such as language stimulation ideas, gross motor activities, materials to develop fine-motor skills.
4. A specific plan for trials of medication or a behavior management program, including plans for follow-up contact.

When the diagnostic and the interpretive are the first stages of an ongoing treatment program, there is less need to include all possible information and recommendations in the interpretive session. However, even in these settings, parents should leave the first interpretive session with a clear understanding of what the follow-up procedure will be, including who will call whom for the next appointment, exchange of telephone numbers, and similar details.

Process of the Interpretive Session

The communication techniques that professionals use with parents are extremely important in ensuring that the interpretive goals are met. Suggested techniques for beginning the session, organizing the content, dealing with parents' feelings, and ending the session will be described in this section.

Beginning the Session

As the interpretive begins, many parents are quite tense, because the session is the culmination of a lengthy and anxiety-arousing diagnostic procedure that probably began months before, when the child was referred for evaluation. Professionals, also, can be anxious about going into an interpretive, knowing that they will soon be presenting parents with upsetting information. Because of these factors, the first few minutes of the interpretive session are sometimes characterized by seemingly endless forced small talk, followed by an uncomfortable silence.

Although informal conversation is normal and appropriate for transition times such as walking with parents to the interpretive room, it is a professional's responsibility to finish the small talk and begin the interpretive as soon as all the participants are present. If several professionals are involved, the interpretive leader should reintroduce them and remind the parents of what roles the different professionals played in the child's evaluation. The interpretive leader should also explain the structure of the session to the parents, by communicating the following ideas: We will give you all the test results, we will make recommendations, we want to answer all your questions and make sure you understand us, and we can take as much time as you need. (If there is a time limit on the session because of parents' or professionals' schedules, this should be acknowledged at the beginning of the session, along with the option of scheduling additional sessions.)

Organizing the Information

Although the outline of ideas presented in the content section works well for most families, the sequence in which information is presented must be individualized on the basis of each child's unique pattern of test results and each family's pattern of current understanding and readiness to hear new information. As described earlier, it is important to move in a logical sequence from describing test behavior to interpreting it. This logical procession, however, must be balanced by sensitivity to the parents' major concerns. Thus, for example, if parents ask a global question such as "Will he talk?" the professional must be willing to leave the prepared sequence of content and respond to the question. At times, of course, this response must be "I want to answer your question, but I need to give you some background information so that my answer will make sense."

Dealing with Parents' Feelings

While presenting logical, factual content, professionals should remain aware of the fact that the diagnosis of a developmental disability is an emotional shock for almost all parents. For some, the degree of shock approaches the level of an emotional crisis, in which the individual's normal coping skills are temporarily overwhelmed by the immediate problem (Schmitt, 1980). Emotional crises are usually precipitated by sudden, unexpected events that involve a loss of some kind (Parad and Caplan, 1965). Hearing that their child has a serious developmental disability has been conceptualized (Menolascino, 1965) as implying such a loss (e.g., the loss of a "normal" child or the loss of aspirations of the child's future). When parents experience acute emotional reactions, techniques of crisis intervention (Parad and Caplan, 1965) can be adapted for use in the interpretive session. Crisis intervention follows a progression of four steps: building a relationship, facilitating expression of feelings, focusing on a problem, and problem solving. The reasoning behind these steps is that a trusting relationship is necessary before individuals in crisis feel safe to express feelings, and that feelings must be ventilated before rational thinking can resume.

Planning for interpretives should include this sequence when it is known beforehand that the diagnostic information will be extremely upsetting to parents. In addition, professionals should be prepared in any interpretive session to respond to parents' expressions of grief, anger, or other emotions by encouraging further expression of feelings. Information-giving and treatment planning should be resumed only after the intensity of emotions has decreased.

The specific applications of modified crisis intervention techniques in interpretives are discussed below.

Building the Relationship

Developing a relationship with a family obviously begins long before the interpretive session, at the first contact between the family and the agency. Professionals form positive relationships with families by respecting their ideas, responding directly to their questions, and demonstrating an interest in their feelings. Within the interpretive session, these practices should continue. Professionals should maintain good eye contact with each family member and should communicate concern for each as an individual. This is sometimes difficult when one parent is more active and verbal than the other, but it is extremely important to include both parents in the discussion. On occasion this requires asking one parent to wait while the concerns of the other parent are addressed.

Facilitating Expressions of Feeling

It should be make clear in all interpretives that feelings will be accepted as a normal part of the interpretive discussion. This can be done by making statements like the following:

> "It can be confusing for parents when children are good at some skills but have great difficulties in other areas."
> "You must have been very frightened when the doctors told you that."
> "So you've been worried about Laura since she was a young child."
> "I'm sure it was frustrating for you to know that something was wrong but not be able to convince anyone that Billy needed help."

Unfortunately, some professionals become uncomfortable when parents express strong feelings. For example, when parents begin crying, inexperienced or unskilled interpreters occasionally either ignore the tears or rush to reassure parents that the child is "cute" or "happy." When parents disagree with diagnostic findings, some interpreters enter into an intellectual discussion of the validity and reliability of the tests used, rather than acknowledging to parents that it is difficult and painful to hear diagnostic labels given to their child.

To be skilled interpreters, professionals must first accept the assumption that it is normal and safe for parents to express strong feelings in interpretives. Even among professionals who believe this, however, many still have difficulty knowing how to go about encouraging and handling parental expressions of feeling. Identification of three styles of parental communication may be useful.

Sometimes parents are direct and vivid in the emotional response. For example:

"I know Bobby wouldn't have these problems if his pediatrician had listened to me sooner."

"I just don't want to believe it." (begins crying)

In these situations, the professional can simply accept the feelings and reflect them in a gentle, supportive way (Rogers, 1951). For example:

"It makes you angry to think about all of this."

"This is sad news we're giving you, and it's hard to believe it's true."

It is also helpful to state that the parents' feelings are very understandable, because the diagnostic information about the child would be distressing to any parent.

A second common pattern of parental response is seen when parents don't state their feelings explicitly but the feelings are clearly close to the surface. Often such feelings are expressed in nonverbal behavior, when parents become tearful or sit in a position that says they want to leave the interpretive room. At other times, parents' feelings might be obvious because of the nature of their comments, such as asking many questions about the mother's pregnancy, or explaining why the child did not perform well on a number of test items. In such situations, the professionals can bring feelings into the open through asking leading questions, such as:

"How do you feel about what we're saying?"

"Are you thinking that something about your pregnancy led to Mary's problem?"

"Do you think we're wrong about Andy?"

If parents and professionals have developed a trusting relationship, parents will generally respond to these questions with expressions of their fears and feelings.

A third pattern of parental response is occasionally seen in which parents give no indication of what their reactions are. Interpretives with these parents are the most difficult and often the shortest: The professional presents diagnostic information and recommendations, the parents do not respond, so the professional reluctantly ends the session. Experienced professionals have found, however, that it is often possible to overcome the parents' barrier of silence by inquiring directly about their reactions. while implicitly communicating that any number of responses would be understandable. For example, the professional might say, "I'd like to talk a little about what you're thinking about the things we've told you. Some parents have a hard time learning that their child has mental retardation and autism. It's hard for them to believe that it could happen to their child, or it makes them feel sad, or scared about the future. It is hard for you to hear?"

Usually it will take parents some time to decide whether or how to respond to these questions. It is therefore very important that the professional allow enough time and silence for the parents to organize their thoughts. Although periods of silence can be extremely uncomfortable for inexperienced professionals, they can be very important for parents who are trying to cope with complicated and distressing information.

Sometimes when parents are fairly noncommunicative, the professional has a hunch about how the parents are feeling or what they are worried about. At these times it is appropriate to follow the hunch and ask direct questions. Examples might be:

> "Are you wondering how you're going to explain this to his grandparents?"
> "Does it sound as though we're saying that she can't learn?"
> "Are you thinking about who will take care of her when she is older?

Obviously it is inappropriate to insist that parents discuss their feelings if they do not wish to. One or two direct questions is the maximum amount of probing appropriate for parents who do not express reactions to the diagnostic information.

Moving to Recommendations

Parents, rather than professionals, should determine when the discussion shifts from the parents' reactions to treatment recommendations. Rational treatment-planning cannot be done while parents are emotionally overwhelmed by the diagnostic information. The usual indication that they are ready to discuss treatment plans is that their expressions of sadness or fear have diminished, and they have begun to ask questions about the future. For example:

> "What should we do next?"
> "Can anything be done to help him?"
> "Can autism be cured?"

Some parents will ask these questions as soon as the diagnostic information is presented. These tend to be parents who cope with painful feelings by being well-controlled, rational, and efficient. Their style should be respected, and their questions about treatment should be answered right away. However, bearing the goal of emotional adjustment in mind, the professional should at some point gently probe for the feelings that have not yet been expressed.

Ending the Session

The interpretive should be brought to a close by the professional when the parents' behavior or statements indicate that the interpretive goals have been met—that is, when all the diagnostic information has been discussed, feelings expressed, and concrete plans made. If possible, the professional should end the interpretive on a note of reassurance and hope. It can almost always be said that the child will continue to learn and develop, and the child's strengths and appealing qualities can be reviewed. Parents who have had difficulty dealing with the diagnostic findings can be reassured that they showed courage in seeking help for the child, particularly since the evaluation process was painful for them personally. Finally, it is often helpful to remind parents that although they may have new labels for their child's problems, the child waiting at home hasn't changed from the unique being they know and love.

CONCLUSION

Although the interpretive session is often a painful and sad time for parents, it can also be the beginning of increased understanding of their child's needs and ways in which they can meet these needs. Professionals bear the responsibility for ensuring that parents receive complete information, emotional support, and concrete help from an interpretive. These goals are more likely to be achieved when professionals keep as an organizing principle during the assessment and staff conference the idea that parents' thoughts and feelings are as important as professionals' test results. With this background, the structure, content, and process of the interpretive session can then be individualized according to the family's needs and the child's characteristics. When all these elements converge, the interpretive session can be a significant professional contribution to the parents of handicapped children.

REFERENCE NOTE

1. Knobeloch, C. (Ed.). *Proceedings of the workshop on the interpretive conference, March 1–2, 1973.* Unpublished manuscript, University of North Carolina at Chapel Hill, 1973.

REFERENCES

Baroff, G. *Mental retardation: Nature, cause, and management.* Washington, D.C.: Hemisphere, 1974.

DeMyer, M. K. *Parents and children in autism.* Washington, D.C.: Winston, 1979.

Doernberg, N. Issues in communication between pediatricians and parents of young mentally retarded children. *Pediatric Annals,* 1982, *11,* 438–444.

Lockyer, L., and Rutter, M. A. Five- to fifteen-year follow-up study of infantile psychosis: III. Psychological aspects. *British Journal of Psychiatry,* 1969, *115,* 865–882.

Massie, R., and Massie, S. *Journey,* New York: Warner Books, 1976.

Matheny, A., and Vernick, J. Parents of the mentally retarded child: Emotionally overwhelmed or informationally deprived? *Journal of Pediatrics,* 1969, *74,* 953–959.

Menolascino, F. Psychiatric aspects of mental retardation in children under eight. *American Journal of Orthopsychiatry,* 1965, *35,* 852–861.

Miller, N. Parents of children with neurological disorders: Concerns and counseling. *Journal of Pediatric Psychology,* 1979, *4,* 297–306.

Morgan, S. Team interpretation of MR to parents. *Mental Retardation,* 1973, *11,* 10–13.

Mount, M., and Shea, V. *How to recognize and assess pre-language skills in the severely handicapped.* Lawrence, Kans.: H & H Enterprises, 1982.

Murray, J., and Murray, E. *And say what he is: The life of a special child.* Cambridge, Mass.: M.I.T. Press, 1975.

Parad, H., and Caplan, G. (Eds.). *Crisis intervention: Selected readings.* New York: Family Service Association of America, 1965.

Robinson, N., and Robinson, H. *The mentally retarded child; A psychological approach* (2nd ed.). New York: McGraw-Hill, 1976.

Rockowitz, R., and Davidson, P. Discussing diagnostic findings with parents. *Journal of Learning Disabilities,* 1979, *12,* 11–16.

Rogers, C. *Client-centered therapy: Its current practice, implications, and theory.* Boston: Houghton Mifflin, 1951.

Schmitt, R. Crisis theory and parent interpretive sessions. *North Carolina Journal of Mental Health,* 1980, *9,* 27–32.

Schnell, R. The psychologist's role in the parent conference. In G. Ulrey and S. Rogers (Eds.), *Psychological assessment of handicapped infants and young children.* Denver: LADOCA Publishing Foundation, 1982.

Schopler, E., and Reichler, R. How well do parents understand their own psychotic child? *Journal of Autism and Childhood Schizophrenia,* 1972, *2,* 387–400.

Schopler, E., Reichler, R., and Lansing, M. *Individualized assessment and treatment for autistic and developmentally disabled children, Vol. II: Teaching strategies for parents and professionals.* Baltimore: University Park Press, 1980.

Shea, V., and Saur, W. Interpreting developmental handicaps to parents: A guide for professionals. *JSAS Catalog of Selected Documents in Psychology,* 1981, *11,* 17.

Shigley, R. Parent and professional: Personal views from both perspectives. *Pointer,* 1980, *25,* 8–11.

Turnbull, A., and Turnbull, H. (Eds.). *Parents speak out: Views from the other side of the two-way mirror.* Columbus, O.: Charles E. Merrill, 1978.

Wolfensberger, W., and Kurtz, R. (Eds.). *Management of the family of the mentally retarded.* Chicago: Follett Education Corporation, 1969.

17

Family Resources and Successful Adaptation to Autistic Children

MARIE M. BRISTOL

The negative effects of autistic children on families have been poignantly documented by parents and, more recently, by clinicians and researchers (DeMyer and Goldberg, 1983; Holroyd and McArthur, 1976). Much less is known, however, about the characteristics of autistic children and the resources in their families and communities that enable some families to cope successfully in the face of such chronic stress. Mary Akerley (1975) spoke of "invulnerable" parents of autistic children, those parents who are able to persevere and even to grow in the presence of their autistic children. The purpose of this chapter is to focus on research on family resources and their role in facilitating such successful family adaptation to autistic and autistic-like children.

The information in this chapter is drawn from the research literature on family coping in general and the TEACCH program of research on families of autistic children. The TEACCH clinical program's ways of working with families are described in more detail in Chapter 4. The TEACCH family research program consists of a series of studies beginning with early research on parental cognitive functioning (Schopler and Loftin, 1969) and continuing with a series of collaborative studies of mothers, fathers, and siblings of autistic children. (Bristol, 1979; in press; Mates, 1982; Short, 1980; Bristol and Schopler, Note 1; McHale, Sloane, and Simeonsson, Note 2).

The data in this chapter are drawn from our ongoing research on stress and coping in mothers of autistic children, a collaborative effort between TEACCH and the Frank Porter Graham Child Development Center at the University of

MARIE M. BRISTOL • The Frank Porter Graham Child Development Center and Division TEACCH, University of North Carolina, Chapel Hill, North Carolina 27514.

North Carolina at Chapel Hill. The chapter will draw from an initial cross-sectional study of 40 mothers of autistic children aged 4–19 (Bristol, 1979), the pretreatment data from a short-term longitudinal study of 45 families of autistic and communication-handicapped children (Bristol, in press), and a study of sources of support reported by approximately 200 parents of autistic and autistic-like children (Bristol, Note 3).

The chapter will first review briefly some issues relevant to successful family adaptation in general, and some factors that place families of autistic children in particular at high risk for stress and family crisis. It will then discuss the contributions of selected family resources—family psychosocial environment, social support, and specific coping responses—to successful family adaptation. Finally, the implications of these findings for interventions with autistic children will be discussed.

GENERAL FAMILY ADAPTATION

Successful family adaptation to autistic children can be best understood in the context of successful family coping with any kind of stressful event. For more than 30 years, researchers have studied families under stress—families enduring hardships such as military separations, physical illness, or natural disasters such as tornadoes (Cohen and Lazarus, 1979; Hill, 1958; McCubbin, 1979). From their research and our own investigations, it is clear that no stressor or stressful event, including the care of an autistic child, invariably causes a family crisis. What is it then that enables some families to adapt successfully to having an autistic child while other families are overwhelmed by the stress?

Let us look first at what we know about successful family adaptation to any kind of stress. Hill (1949, 1958) proposed a classic ABCX model of family coping with stress. In his review of research on stressful events ranging from infidelity through military separation (1958), he stated that whether any stressful event (A) will result in a family crisis (X) depends on the event itself and its attendant hardships interacting with the family's crisis-meeting resources (B) and the definition the family makes of the event (C). The applicability of this total model to families of autistic children has been discussed at some length elsewhere (Bristol and Schopler, 1983) and has been supported empirically in research on families of autistic children (Bristol, in press). The focus of this discussion will be primarily on expanding our understanding of the contribution of one component of this ABCX model, the family's crisis-meeting resources (B), to successful family adaptation to autistic children.

Although all families need crisis-meeting resources, families of handicapped children, particularly parents of autistic children, are especially in need of such resources. Research on other types of stressors reveals a number of factors common to families of autistic children that increase the likelihood of family crisis and the consequent need for family resources. These include the ambiguity of the stressor and its severity, duration, and lack of congruence with community norms.

High Risk Factors

Ambiguity

As McCubbin and Patterson (1982) point out in their review of studies of war separations, a significant contributing factor to family crisis is ambiguity. In the case of families of prisoners of war, it was not clear within the family whether the father would return, or, within the community, what the appropriate family behavior should be in his absence. For these reasons, stress- and crisis-proneness were significantly increased. Because the autistic child appears physically normal and often extraordinarily attractive, whether or not the child is actually handicapped is ambiguous. Until the mother understands that the child's deviant behavior stems from an inborn disorder of behavior and communication, she may feel inadequate as a parent because the child is obviously not responding the way she imagined well-raised children should.

When such misplaced feelings of guilt are intentionally or unintentionally reinforced by professionals who imply either that there is no problem or that the problem is one of parental mismanagement, the ambiguity of the child's handicap significantly increases the risk of family crisis.

Recent research (Bristol, in press) suggests that, at least before formal diagnosis, more retarded autistic children have a less adverse effect on families, especially on the marital relationship, than children who have disordered behavior but are not recognized as handicapped. Similarly, in a study of how parents understand their own child (Schopler and Reichler, 1972), parents of mildly autistic children were worse estimators of the child's current developmental level than were parents of severely autistic children whose degree of handicap was quite clear. The ambiguity of the mildly impaired child's handicap makes it difficult for the parent to know what to realistically expect from the child. Apparently, such ambiguity leads to disagreements both within the family and in the larger community as to the nature and cause of the child's problem. Such disagreement reinforces parental feelings of uncertainty and increases stress and the risk of family crisis.

This ambiguity also complicates community acceptance and support of the child and the family. When a child who is obviously handicapped throws his milkshake on the floor at McDonald's, the majority of other diners are sympathetic, if not enthralled by the child's behavior. When an autistic child who appears to be prefectly normal does the same thing, the sympathetic understanding may turn to hostility and to unsolicited advice on child-rearing, heightening the naive mother's sense of inadequacy and contributing to potential family crisis.

Severity

Both the severity and the duration of any stressful event also affect the likelihood of family crisis (Hill and Hansen, 1962; McCubbin, Cauble, and Patterson, 1982). Autism is a severe, lifelong disability that affects not only the child's ability to learn and function in the "outside world" but also his ability to relate to other members of his own family. A mother tearfully explained that her daughter was 8 years old when she first came to the TEACCH program. Before that time, the child had never called her mother "Mama," nor did she appear to recognize her in a group of strangers. The severity of the autistic child's social and cognitive deficits makes families of these children particularly vulnerable to stress.

In comparisons of families of autistic children with families of children with different types of handicaps, parents of autistic children do report more stress than families of other groups, such as Down's syndrome or psychiatric outpatient children (Holroyd and McArthur, 1976). Both mothers of autistic children and mothers of the Down's syndrome children reported problems that may be related to a common retardation factor. Both of these groups of mothers reported similar problems of excessive time demands, poor health, depressed moods, pessimism about the child's future, and limits on educational or occupational opportunities for their families because of the child.

Examination of scale scores reported by Holroyd and McArthur reveals that mothers of autistic children reported more stress than mothers of Down's syndrome children in areas such as taking their children to public places, and more embarrassment and disappointment than the parents of the Down's syndrome children. The autistic children were also reported to have fewer activities that occupied them, fewer services, and poorer prospects for employment and independent living. Autistic children were more disruptive of family integration as measured by activities such as family mealtime, vacations, or outings. The autistic children were also reported to have more difficult personality characteristics.

Comparing Holroyd and McArthur's (1976) data on stress in families of autistic children in California with TEACCH data collected in North Carolina suggests that there may, in fact, be a characteristic pattern of stress associated with parenting an autistic child (Bristol and Schopler, 1983).

Duration

Although it has been clearly demonstrated that all autistic children, regardless of their functioning level, benefit from instruction (Rutter and Bartak, 1973), the majority of autistic children will never become fully "normal" and will require at least some assistance throughout their lives. One mother who was coping well with her 6-foot-tall autistic adolescent commented that she had resigned herself to always having a young child in the house. For other parents, the prospect of permanent dependency is overwhelming, especially when the community has made little provision for the child's care when the parent can no longer care for the child.

Lack of Congruence with Community Norms

McCubbin and Patterson (1982) point out that *the* major determinant of successful family adaptation to stress may well be the *fit* between the family and the community. McCubbin points out that family crisis may depend upon the efficacy and/or "adequacy of the solutions the culture, or community . . . provide. However, these community solutions may lag far behind the times and offer little to families struggling to manage a difficult situation." In the not-so-distant past, the community offered little understanding or support and few appropriate services for autistic children. The parent, then, far from feeling the support of the community, often felt rejected and isolated. This sense of social isolation has been documented for parents of retarded children as well (Farber, 1959). One mother of an autistic child commented that she knew what a leper must have felt like. As she walked down the street with her bizarre little child, both children and adults disappeared from sight as she approached. Such social rejection may become particularly acute as the child gets older and the community has less tolerance for deviant behavior in someone who appears to be a normal adult. Efforts of groups such as the National Society for Children and Adults with Autism have done much to educate the general public and bridge this ignorance gap. Our discussion below will highlight the importance of preventing such unnecessary feelings of isolation.

Given the special characteristics of autism that heighten the risk of problems in these families—the early ambiguity of the child's handicap, the severity and duration of this problem, and the frequent lack of community understanding and support—it is clear that these families need resources in order to prevent family crises.

FAMILY RESOURCES AND SUCCESSFUL ADAPTATION

What are resources, then, and how do they assist families in their long-term adaptation to having an autistic child? McCubbin and Patterson (1982) define resources for family adaptation as

> the psychological, social, interpersonal, and material characteristics of individual members, the family unit, and the community that may be brought into play in reducing tension, managing conflicts, and in general, meeting demands and needs. Individual resources include education, psychological stability, the capacity to be nurturing, the ability to manage the home, the ability to function independently, and

the ability to manipulate various resources to one's advantage. Family resources could include integration, cohesion, flexibility, organization, moral religious values, and expressiveness. Finally, environmental resources might include social support networks, medical and psychological counseling services, and social policies that enhance family functioning and protect families from financial disaster.

Although a number of personal resources such as ego-strength (Gallagher, Cross, and Scharfman, 1981), mastery, self-confidence (McCubbin, Joy, Cauble, Comeau, Patterson, and Needle, 1980), and intelligence and good health (Rabkin and Struening, 1976) are surely important in family adaptation (see a recent review by Gallagher, Beckman-Bell, and Cross, 1983), this section will deal primarily with what McCubbin terms family and environmental resources, including the role of family environment, informal social support, and specific coping responses in facilitating adaptation in families of autistic children. For a discussion of some other needed resources, see chapters 5 and 6 by Akerley and Warren.

Family Psychosocial Environment

A number of studies of families of nonhandicapped children have pointed out that there are certain family attributes or styles that make families more resistant to family crisis or more able to "regenerate" themselves after a crisis. The importance of family psychosocial environmental characteristics such as integration, cohesion, and organization, as well as adaptability, has been noted (Angell, 1936; McCubbin *et al.*, 1980; Hill, 1949; Hill and Hansen, 1962). In their study of families with spina bifida, Nevin and McCubbin (Note 4) found that family cohesion and an active recreational orientation, together with selected parental coping patterns and severity of the child's handicap, were related to levels of family stress. This study raises the question of whether particular characteristics of the family environments of autistic and autisticlike children would also be related to successful adaptation to the child.

To answer that question, a study was recently completed of 45 mothers recruited from consecutive referrals to Division TEACCH. Twenty-seven families had autistic children. The remainder ($N = 18$) had children who were not autistic but who had significant communication and/or behavioral problems. The children ranged in age from 2 to 10, with a mean age of 5. Seventy-six percent of the children were retarded. (See Bristol, in press, for a more complete description of selection criteria and sample characteristics.)

Data were collected through parental self-assessments, interviews, interviewer ratings, and direct assessment of the child. We assessed factors related to family adaptation to the child, marital adjustment, and decreased symptoms of depression, a problem frequently reported by mothers of handicapped children regardless of the type of handicap. Results of the larger study are reported in Bristol, in press.

One of the family resources assessed was the family home environment. Using the Moos Family Environment Scales (FES; Moos and Moos, 1981), we measured dimensions of family relationships (cohesion, expressiveness, and conflict), personal growth (independence, achievement orientation, intellectual-cultural orientation, active-recreational orientation, and moral-religious emphasis), and system maintenance (organization and control) and assessed the relationship between maternal reports of these environmental characteristics and successful family adaptation.

Successful Adaptation

Successful adaptation for the total group of families was most closely related to the degree of cohesion, expressiveness, and active recreational orientation of the families. Families with a higher degree of commitment, help, and support for one another (cohesion) were rated by interviewers as having significantly greater acceptance of and greater competence in family coping with the child. These mothers also reported marginally fewer depressive symptoms ($p = .07$) and marginally better marital adjustment ($p = .06$). The extent to which family members were encouraged to act openly and express their feelings directly (expressiveness) was significantly related to marital happiness, but not to family acceptance or coping with the child, or to depressive symptoms. Families with an active-recreational orientation—that is, those who participated in social and recreational activities outside the home or with persons outside the immediate family—were rated by interviewers as being more accepting of the child and having better family adaptation. Depressive symptoms were not related to such social and recreational activities, but families who did engage in these activities tended to report having happier marriages.

Although these data are merely correlational and do not prove any relationship between family environment and successful family adaptation, they tend to support the contention that particular family environments may make some families less vulnerable to the stress of having an autistic child. A close-knit, supportive home environment, being able to express feelings openly, and actively participating in activities outside the home appear to contribute to a more accepting and competent relationship with the child and with the spouse. It is important to note that although different families have different family environments or styles, some of these characteristics of the family environment can be changed through intervention (Koegel, Schreibman, Britten, Burke, and O'Neill, 1981).

Comparison with Norm Group

The families of both autistic and nonautistic handicapped children in our study were similar to the Moos and Moos norm group of well-adjusted families on 8 of the 10 scales. The most striking differences between the families of autistic children and the Moos and Moos norm group of families with nonhandicapped children were a markedly higher moral-religious emphasis and a lower reported level of participation in social and recreational activities for families with autistic children. On both of these scales, mean scores for families of autistic children were more than 1 standard deviation above or below the means for the "normal" sample. (Although mean scores for the nonautistic handicapped sample approached these limits, only the means for the families of autistic children went beyond plus or minus 1 *SD*.) Because the North Carolina samples and the national norm sample may differ in many important respects, such comparisons must be considered tentative, but they do suggest potentially important differences that merit further investigation.

Some aspects of moral-religious beliefs are discussed in more detail below under Specific Coping Responses. For many of these families of autistic children, belief in God (see below) and/or adherence to clear moral standards facilitates survival by giving greater meaning and purpose to the sacrifices the family is making for the care of the autistic child. Whether this greater moral-religious emphasis is characteristic of families of autistic children or is a function of the Bible Belt region from which our families come is uncertain. However, these North Carolina families of autistic children scored higher on this scale than did the contrast group of families of handicapped but nonautistic children from the same region.

The mothers of autistic children also reported less involvement with persons and activities outside the household than did the North Carolina contrast group of families of nonautistic handicapped children. It is not known, of course, whether this social isolation from community activities is freely chosen or whether it reflects the fact that the family is so overwhelmed by the demands of the handicapped child that there is neither time nor energy left for such pursuits. It is also true that many of the recreational activities in which the family might participate exclude the autistic child. As a result, the entire family stays home. Many parents also report that they lack trained baby-sitters or respite care services that make participation in adult recreational activities possible. The relationship described above between such active recreational orientation and family adaptation, however, suggests the importance of understanding and overcoming such lack of involvement in activities outside the home.

Social Support

Informal Support and Successful Adaptation

Another important resource that families draw upon either in preventing or recovering from family crisis is an informal social support network of immediate and extended family, friends, neighbors, and other parents of handicapped children. Cobb (1976) defines social support as information leading the person to believe that he is cared for and loved, valued and esteemed, and is important in a network of mutual obligation and communication. Cobb notes that the actual exchange of goods and services in such a relationship is less important than having the persons know that they are loved and valued and that they can count on help from others and are expected to provide assistance in return. We know that research has demonstrated a link between such social support and improved health outcomes for people in other types of stressful situations ranging from unemployment to the complications of pregnancy (Cassel, 1974, 1976; Cobb, 1976; Gore, 1978; Nuckolls, Cassel, and Kaplan, 1972). The importance of such social support in families of autistic children has been demonstrated in two consecutive studies at TEACCH.

In our earlier research (Bristol, 1979; Bristol and Schopler, Note 1), it was clear that high-stress families of autistic children aged 4–19 differed significantly from similar but low-stress families. Within a group of 40 mothers of autistic children, the highest stress group (top quartile) could be distinguished from the lowest stress group (bottom quartile) even though the two groups were comparable in terms of mother's age, socioeconomic class, number of children in the family, the children's average IQs, percent of firstborn children, and percent of children who were more severely autistic. In spite of these similarities, the groups were markedly different in terms of specific characteristics of the children and the resources that were available to the mothers. With an equal number of families of boys and girls participating in the study, only 30% of the children in the lowest stress group versus 70% of the children in the highest stress group were boys. The age difference between the children in both groups approached significance, with mothers of older autistic children reporting more stress than mothers of younger children. In addition, the low-stress group had children who were perceived by their mothers to have less difficult personality characteristics (including behavior management problems) and to be less socially obtrusive.

Mothers in the low-stress group also reported that their children had more activities and better occupational prospects as gauged by such things as the availability of services and the likelihood of independent living arrangements.

Perhaps even more striking than the child characteristics and formal services that separated the highest stress and lowest stress groups were the differences in the informal support networks of the mothers. Although the highest and lowest stress groups reported an almost identical degree of support from their own children, the lowest stress mothers reported greater perceived support on a measure that included support from spouse, immediate and extended family, friends, and other parents of handicapped children.

For the total group of mothers ($N = 40$), the most important sources of support related to lower stress were spouses, the wife's relatives, and other parents of handicapped children. This informal support network, then, appears to be an important family resource in successful adaptation to the autistic child.

Similar results were found in our most recent study of 45 mothers described earlier. First, the importance of informal social support to successful family adaptation was again clearly demonstrated. Although family adaptation to the child, as rated by an interviewer, was related to characteristics of the child, successful family adaptation was more closely related to the perceived adequacy of the mother's informal social supports, to the pattern of coping strategies used (see below), to maternal beliefs regarding the child's handicap, and to other stresses in the family. Once again, the strongest relationship was found between successful family adaptation and the amount of perceived support the mother received from her spouse. Mothers who felt this strong paternal support reported significantly fewer depressive symptoms and happier marriages, and were rated as being more accepting and having better family adaptation to the handicapped child. Support from both the wife's and husband's relatives was positively related to both acceptance and quality of parenting and marital adjustment.

Greater support from the husband's relatives was related to a significant reduction in depressive symptoms, a relationship that was marginally significant ($p = .10$) for support from the wife's relatives. Farber's work with families of retarded children (1959) suggested that frequent contact with in-laws may be a potential source of stress, not support. For these parents, however, when in-laws were perceived as supportive, the family adaptation to the child was rated more positively by interviewers.

For this group of mothers just coming for initial diagnosis, the support of other parents was not significantly related to family adaptation. Most (62%) of the parents interviewed stated that they didn't have contact with any other parents of handicapped children. Part of the TEACCH intervention program consists of encouraging parents to find support in other parents of autistic children. When they do, as in our first study of "experienced" TEACCH parents, they apparently experience less stress related to the child.

Formal Support and Successful Adaptation

It is clear that parents of autistic children need the ongoing informal support provided by spouse, friends, and their immediate and extended families. They also need the formal support provided through services that require a more formal organizational structure or the exchange of money. Successful family adaptation depends on adequate and appropriate educational, vocational, recreational, medical, and other services (see Chapter 4). The low-stress parents in the initial study described above (Bristol and Schopler, Note 1) differed not only in informal social support but also in availability of activities and services and prospects for independent living for their autistic children. In addition, a *post hoc* analysis revealed that the vast majority (80%) of the mothers in the low-stress group had children who were currently receiving TEACCH services. The majority (70%) of the children in the highest stress group were receiving services in "regular" local special education programs that generally do not provide parent support services.

There is convincing evidence that parent training is needed by these families since it has been shown to be superior to direct child intervention alone in maintaining and generalizing child skills (Koegel *et al.*, 1981). Studies of TEACCH parent training have also demonstrated that providing information and training parents to be cotherapists for their autistic children is effective in improving parent's teaching skills, reducing children's inappropriate behaviors, increasing functional skills, and preventing unnecessary institutionalization (Marcus, Lansing, Andrews, and Schopler, 1978; Schopler, Mesibov, DeVellis, and Short, 1981; Short, 1980). Clearly, then, both informal and formal support services are necessary for successful family adaptation to an autistic child.

Specific Coping Responses

General Coping Strategies

As we discuss the resources that families use to prevent or to recover from family crisis, it is somewhat tempting to think of the family or parent as a rather passive recipient. Although it is certainly true that parents and other family members receive emotional support, advice, or assistance, there is much that they themselves do to cope with having an autistic child.

Drawing upon previous research with families of nonhandicapped children, McCubbin (1982) defines coping as cognitive and behavioral efforts to master conditions of harm, threat, or challenge when a routine or automatic response is neither readily available nor a natural part of the individual's or family's repertoire. Anyone who has ever spent an extended period of time with an autistic child will recognize that something beyond routine or automatic response is necessary for survival. Parents, then, develop specific coping strategies or responses, some effective and some ineffective, in dealing with the stress of their autistic child.

In studying coping responses, Cohen and Lazarus (1979) speak of instrumental and palliative types of coping. Instrumental coping strategies actually change the stressful situation. Palliative coping responses do not directly affect the stressful situation but are designed to help the family tolerate, minimize, or ignore the stressful situation. Both types of coping strategies are necessary to cope with the chronic stress of having an autistic child. One mother of an autistic child says that she is often reminded of the old prayer "Dear Lord, give me the courage to change those things which must be changed, the patience to accept those things which cannot be changed, and the wisdom to know the difference.'' Both changing and accepting must be important parts of the parents' repertoire.

Before discussing the types of coping strategies actually used by parents of autistic children, it is well to consider two concepts related to coping—freedom from stress and the roller coaster effect.

Freedom from Stress. There is a fantasy indulged in by both parents and professionals alike that if the parents were only to use the ''correct'' coping strategies, their problems would be resolved and stress eliminated. First, it is not possible or even desirable to eliminate all stress. It is not possible to create a life that is completely without stress, particularly a life that includes an autistic child. Second, a certain level of stress is necessary before we are motivated to bring a child in for an evaluation, to carry out a home program that requires some effort, or to go to the school board to complain about our child's placement. Stress, then, can be a useful prod to accomplish great things. When the stress we experience exceeds the resources we have to deal with it, however, stress is counterproductive and a family can be on the way to the ''burnout'' phenomenon described by Lee Marcus in Chapter 18. Freedom from stress, however, is not possible. Coping, even effective coping, as McCubbin points out (1982), does not automatically resolve the problem of stress.

The Roller Coaster Effect. Hill (1958) has described the process of family coping with stress as illustrating a ''roller coaster'' effect. The advent of the stressor is first accompanied by a period of disorganization, then finally reorganization, and this is repeated over and over as elements of the stressful event or the family itself change. Families that are coping successfully with their autistic children are not families who never feel overwhelmed by the stress. They are families, just like all families of autistic children, who are sometimes discouraged, who sometimes feel like giving up. They are families that cry and families who may sometimes feel that their burden is insupportable. The critical difference between families who cope successfully, however, and those who do not is that somehow these ''invulnerable'' families spring back and do not give up. They have what Burr (1973) might call ''regenerative'' ability, the power to somehow knit themselves back together as a family just when it seemed as if the fabric of their lives was unraveling.

Perceived Helpfulness of Coping Responses

What do these families do to cope with having an autistic child? What are the specific coping responses they use and how effective are they?

In the study of 45 mothers described earlier, we gave mothers a list of 45 specific coping responses that parents might use in dealing with the stress of a handicapped or ill child. The list of coping responses (The Coping Health Inventory for Parents [CHIP]) was developed by McCubbin and his associates (McCubbin and Patterson, 1981) to measure the perceived helpfulness of three major types of coping patterns in dealing with the stress of a handicapped or chronically ill child. The first pattern of coping responses comprises coping strategies aimed at maintaining family integration, cooperation, and an optimistic definition of the situation. It includes items such as "Doing things with my children" and "Telling myself I have many things to be thankful for." The second factor or pattern of coping strategies involves those aimed at maintaining social support outside the family, and maintaining self-esteem and psychological stability. This pattern includes items such as "Engaging in relationships and friendships which help me to feel important and appreciated" and "Doing things with relatives." The third factor or pattern involves seeking information and services, and carrying out prescribed activities. It includes items such as "Talking with other persons in the same type of situation and learning about their experience" and "Learning more about how I can help my child improve."

We asked mothers to indicate whether or not they used each coping strategy and, if so, how helpful they felt that particular strategy was to them in overcoming stress related to their child. We wanted to assess which coping strategies parents used, which they themselves thought were most helpful, and, finally, whether any particular patterns of coping were related to a more objective measure of favorable adaptation to the autistic child.

First, we found that all 45 coping strategies were used by at least some of the parents, that each of the 45 were thought to be extremely helpful by at least one of the parents, and that 33 of the 45 coping strategies were thought to be "no help at all" by at least one parent. Preferences for using particular coping strategies were highly varied. Since these mothers were seen *before* their child was evaluated for autism and before they had regular services for their children, contact with professionals did not, of course, play a large part in their coping repertoire. The most commonly used coping strategy used by virtually all parents (44 of 45) was "Reading more about the special problems which concern me." Professional help was not yet a part of their support system. Up to this time they had had to rely on themselves to read and obtain information.

Since there was clearly a range regarding the frequency of use of the various coping strategies, we wanted to know which coping strategies the vast majority of these parents found both most and least helpful, at least at this point before they had received any formal training. Table I lists the 10 most helpful coping strategies that were used by at least two-thirds of the mothers. The coping strategies are ranked in decreasing order of mothers' perception of helpfulness in coping with stress regarding the child.

Helping the Child. The two top-ranked coping strategies involve direct services to the child. ("Learning how to help my child improve" and "Believing that my child's program has my family's best interests in mind"). The desire

Table I. Ten Most Helpful Coping Strategies

---

1. Believing that my child's program (TEACCH) has my family's best interest in mind.
2. Learning more about how I can help my child improve.
3. Believing in God.
4. Talking over personal feelings and concerns with my spouse.
5. Building a closer relationship with my spouse.
6. Trying to maintain family stability.
7. Developing myself as a person.
8. Telling myself that I have many things I should be thankful for.
9. Doing things with my children.
10. Believing that my child will get better.

---

to learn how to help their children improve probably impelled the family to seek TEACCH services in the first place. Data collected at Division TEACCH do indicate the importance (Marcus *et al.*, 1978; Schopler *et al.*, 1981; Short, 1980) to both child and parent outcomes of having the mother learn how to teach her child. The number 1 ranking given to the belief that the child's program has the family's best interest in mind also emphasizes the importance to parental coping of the belief that their children are receiving adequate and appropriate services.

Controlling the Meaning. Pearlin and Schooler (1978) emphasize the importance to coping of controlling the meaning of a stressful event. As both Lazarus (1966) and Pearlin and Schooler (1978) point out, stress is neither in the person nor in the stressful event, but rather in the person's perception of that event. The meaning attached to an event determines to a large extent the threat that experience presents to a family. The single most common form of individual coping in general is what Pearlin and Schooler call "cognitive neutralizing." In this form of coping, the ability of an event to precipitate a crisis is neutralized by beliefs that endow the event with a higher meaning (see Belief in God, below) or by a process such as "positive comparison" where people count the blessings that they do have and realize that they are better off than at least some other people who are significant to them.

As seen from Table I, 4 of the top 10 coping strategies rated most helpful by these mothers of autistic and autistic-like children were beliefs rather than actions. Some parents in this study, for example, believed they were better off than families that had a physically handicapped child. Another form of the positive comparison strategy involved comparing the present situation with either the past, which was worse, or the future, which they expect will be better. The mother whose autistic child finally sleeps through the night remembers her sleep-deprived days and is grateful for the child's nocturnal improvement even though his behavior leaves much to be desired. All parents of autistic children also cope to some extent by looking forward to their children's expected improvement.

A few of these mothers, however, may unrealistically expect complete cure rather than simply improvement. In this study, only families of children subsequently found to have a significant handicap were included. Before formal evaluation of the child, these mothers were asked if they thought their child was, in fact, handicapped. Twenty percent of the mothers did not believe that their child was handicapped. The remaining 80% acknowledged that the child was handicapped, but almost half of these parents expected that their child would outgrow the handicap and eventually be normal. Although some of these children may have such a fortunate outcome, the majority will not. The mothers' unrealistic hopes are not surprising considering the fact that at the time of the study, the children had been referred but had not yet been diagnosed as handicapped. This type of coping, which can be seen as a form of denial, is effective only when children are young. Marcus (1977) has pointed out that when children are young, parents can be optimistic that, with the proper training, the child will eventually be normal. As the child gets older, the permanency of the child's handicap is apparent, and the belief that the child will be cured, which was effective in dealing with stress when the child was younger, must be replaced with an alternative strategy. A particular coping response, then, is neither good nor bad. There is no such thing as the "best" coping response, but only a question of what is the best coping response for this parent with this child at this particular time.

Belief in God. The high rating given by mothers to the importance of belief in God is consistent with our previous interview findings. Parents frequently express the sentiment that knowing that this child is "part of God's plan" makes it easier to cope with the day-to-day difficulties. Other mothers express the thought that "God will give me the strength to carry on with my child," and, occasionally, parents have expressed the belief that they expect that God will "cure" their child.

From our studies, it appears that the strength of this religious support, however, seems to be more a function of a personal belief system than an endorsement of organized religion. In three separate studies (Bristol, Note 3), organized religion failed to place in the top third of the most helpful of 27 sources of social support. Although individual parents have spoken of the understanding and support they have received from a particular clergyman or a particular church, the majority have expressed sadness and even bitterness about the lack of such support. Many reported that churches or synagogues have either actively excluded their autistic children from the life of that group or have only grudgingly admitted them, but made it clear that they were intruders. One mother recounted that she had always taught Sunday school before her autistic son was born. When it was time for him to participate in Sunday school, however, the child was sent home as too disruptive. The family decided, as this mother expressed it, "If they don't want him, they don't get me." She gave up her

Sunday school teaching, a considerable loss to both her church and herself. Parents seem particularly hard-hit by such events. One mother, the wife of a minister, noted that she expected her autistic child to be misunderstood and even sometimes rejected in other settings, but not in church. Mothers have noted that most clergymen have had little training and less contact with handicapped children. Their avoidance or lack of understanding of autistic children stems more from ignorance than from malice, but it is still a painful reality with which families must often deal.

Seeking Spousal Support. In the discussion of social support above, the importance of the perceived receipt of support from the child's father is highlighted. In this instance, 2 of the top 10 extremely helpful coping strategies involve active involvement in enlisting that support ("Talking over personal concerns and feelings with my spouse" and "Building a closer relationship with my spouse"). The paternal support alluded to here is emotional support rather than direct assistance with the child, and the wife appears to play an active role in choosing to seek that support. (Surely some spouses are more receptive to such requests.)

It is also interesting to note that the coping strategy "Going out with my spouse on a regular basis," although not one of the top 10 for the total group, was seen as extremely helpful by 52% of those mothers who used it, but that almost a third of the mothers indicated that it was simply not possible for them to go out with their spouses regularly. (The single parents, of course, do not have this option available to them.) A rather vicious cycle can sometimes get set in motion in circumstances such as this. Burke and Weir (1982) and DeMyer (1979) point out that stress can have debilitating effects on the marital helping and sexual relationships. If the demands of caring for the child further erode the relationship by preventing the couple from spending time alone together, the relationship can further deteriorate, making it even more unlikely that parents will actively seek that time together. The importance of adequate child care and respite arrangements so that parents will have time to invest in their own relationship cannot be overestimated, both for the sake of the couple and, ultimately, for the long-term benefit of the child.

From our own research (Bristol, in press) we do know that single mothers without spousal support are rated by interviewers as providing less optimal family environments for autistic and autistic-like children than two-parent families. This greater stress in single-parent families of handicapped children has also been documented by Beckman-Bell (1980) and Holroyd (1974). There is also some evidence that single parents of handicapped children may be more apt to institutionalize their children (McAndrew, 1976), a finding that is not surprising, particularly as the handicapped child's size and strength begins to exceed his mother's.

Focusing on the Family. The coping strategies in Table I regarding the spouse, together with those of trying to maintain family stability, and doing things with the children, all contribute to increasing the integration and stability of the family, coping behaviors that McCubbin has found helpful to improved child and family adaptation in families of chronically ill children.

Self-Development. Finally, one important aspect of coping with the chronic stress of having an autistic child appears to be the necessity of having the mother develop herself as a person so that she has interests, activities, and especially reinforcements that do not depend solely on the child.

Least Helpful. Among the least helpful coping strategies used by at least two-thirds of the mothers were eating, allowing themselves to get angry, entertaining friends at home, and explaining their family situation to friends and neighbors. Mothers spoke of "feeding their frustration" by snacking and then having the added stress of worrying about being overweight. Regarding anger, mothers often stated that although getting angry helped them let off steam, they ended up feeling guilty about having gotten angry either at the child or about demands the child made. With many of these children, entertaining at home was a stress-provoking rather than a stress-releasing event, with the child rampaging through and upsetting all their careful preparations. Mothers sometimes resented explaining their child to people "when it was none of their business," or often felt inadequate in trying to explain autism to those they did care to have understand. Again, education of the general public so that such repeated explanations are unnecessary should reduce stress in these families.

Coping Responses and Family Adaptation

We were interested in knowing whether, in fact, some patterns or clusters of coping strategies were also related to a more objective evaluation of positive family adaptation to the child. McCubbin and Patterson (1981) have empirically grouped the coping strategies used in this study into the three factors discussed above, one focusing on maintaining family integration and an optimistic definition of the situation, one that includes maintaining self-esteem and reaching out for informal social support, and the final one involving contact with professionals and other experts in seeking information and services for the child. We found that higher scores on all three of these coping factors (i.e., more coping strategies and/or greater utility of various coping strategies) were significantly related to a more favorable interviewer rating of acceptance and quality of parenting. Mothers who relied on a coping pattern involving maintaining self-esteem and seeking informal social support also reported fewer depressive symptoms and marginally happier marriages. Particular patterns of coping strategies, then, do seem to be related to more positive family adaptation to the child.

Overall group scores on these coping patterns for mothers of autistic children did not differ significantly from scores for the mothers of nonautistic handicapped children in this study. Scores for mothers of autistic children were also comparable to scores found by Nevin and McCubbin (Note 4) for a group of families of children with cystic fibrosis and to scores for mothers of severely handicapped infants (Saur, 1980). Apparently, coping with the home care of handicapped children, regardless of the type of handicap, elicits similar coping responses from parents, at least prior to any specific family training or intervention.

SUMMARY AND IMPLICATIONS FOR INTERVENTION

This chapter reviewed some of the issues related to family resources and successful adaptation in families of autistic children. The risk of family crisis in families of autistic children may be increased because of a number of factors shown to affect family adjustment and adaptation in families of nonhandicapped children. The risk may be heightened because of the ambiguity of the child's handicap and the uncertainty regarding expectations the community has for autistic children and their families. It is reasonable to expect that this risk of family crisis could be substantially reduced if the ambiguity surrounding the child's handicap were dispelled through early diagnosis and parental education regarding the nature of autism. Akerley (1975) has also emphasized this need for a clear diagnosis in helping to make the family "invulnerable" to self-doubt and criticism. She also points out that parent-training programs attempting to change parental behavior should make clear that parent changes are required because of the child's organic deficiency and not because of any failing on the parent's part.

The amount of perceived support received by mothers from an informal network of spouse, extended family, friends, and other parents of handicapped children was found to be related to levels of perceived stress and to an interviewer rating of family adaptation. The role of the father was especially critical. Intervention programs are careful to provide a responsive and supportive environment for children by involving the mother in the treatment program. Many programs, however, fail to consider the need to go beyond the mother–child dyad and identify persons in the child's environment who can support the mother. Involving other family members or friends in understanding the child's diagnosis and treatment may be an important way to both reduce maternal stress and maintain the mother's newly acquired skills.

Although there is general agreement that fathers should be more involved, it is not clear whether they should be trained and encouraged to work directly with the autistic child or whether it may be more important for them to provide other task assistance to the mother or under what circumstances their emotional support is more important. There is much that we need to learn regarding the optimum role for fathers both in families of autistic children and in programs for handicapped children in general. Equally important, as the number of single parents increases, we need to learn more about alternative sources of support in these families, especially since findings reported here indicate greater problems in coping in these families. As part of a 5-year institute funded through the Special Education Program of the Department of Education, Dr. Eric Schopler, Dr. James Gallagher, and I will be investigating these issues and making recommendations for intervention.

The importance to successful family adaptation of cohesion and an active recreational orientation emphasizes the need for a family focus for intervention. One important objective of intervention should be encouraging a family-oriented rather than an autistic-child-centered home. Intervention programs should not make such excessive demands on parents that the parents need to focus all their time and energy on the autistic child to the detriment of other family needs and activities. Because of the extremely demanding nature of these children, and the often well-intentioned but narrow, child-centered focus of professionals, some parents make the autistic child the center of the family universe and withdraw from social and recreational activities to meet the child's needs. The findings in this chapter suggest that it may be the mutual support of *all* family members and the family's active engagement in outside activities that are critical for successful family adaptation to the child. Only by taking care of themselves and each other can parents hope to have the resources necessary to care for their child.

Before involvement in an intervention program, most of the mothers in our study did not even know any other parents of handicapped children from whom they might receive encouragement and support. Our research indicates the importance to both two-parent and single-parent families of linkages with other parents of handicapped children. Encouraging families to participate in support groups such as the National Society for Children and Adults with Autism provides them not only with contact with potential sources of support but also with an opportunity to join with other parents in gaining more control over their own lives and the lives of their children by shaping the future of services for autistic children and adults. Without adequate services, it is unlikely that any amount of psychosocial support can prevent family stress.

The importance of personal religious beliefs in coping with the stress of an autistic child was clearly revealed in our studies, although there was also disappointment with the lack of support from churches or synagogues. Since this is one source of support potentially available in virtually all communities, efforts should be made to sensitize both clergymen and church members to the special needs of families of autistic and other handicapped children.

It is not possible or desirable to remove all stress from life, but it is important to be able to keep it in manageable bounds, knowing that there will be recurrent periods of disorganization and reorganization as well as relative equilibrium. It is well to remember that successful adaptation or coping is a process and not an achievement. The "best" way to cope with having an autistic child depends on the individual child, the particular family, and the particular situation the family is dealing with. Successful adaptation to any child, however, depends upon a combination of intervening and changing the child to fit the family, and also helping the family adapt to fit the child and to find a positive purpose or meaning in having an autistic child in spite of the very real and chronic stress involved.

Mothers ranked as most helpful to them coping strategies that involved helping the child, controlling the meaning of having a handicapped child through the use of cognitive neutralizing, and using strategies such as positive comparisons. There appears to be an active role the mother plays in eliciting support from her spouse and in maintaining family integration. Investment in self-development by mothers was also perceived as helpful in reducing stress. Patterns of coping strategies that involve maintaining family integration and an optimistic definition of the child's handicap, maintaining self-esteem and seeking social support, and seeking information and professional advice and services were positively related to successful family adaptation.

Although all of the families involved in this research were experiencing the stress of having an autistic child and had a real need for services for their child, the vast majority of them were functioning well as families and had succeeded in adapting to their autistic child. Previous emphasis on pathology in families of autistic children has limited our study and knowledge of successful coping in families of autistic children. Research reported here suggests that we have much to learn from families who have adapted successfully to the awesome task of caring for their autistic children.

REFERENCE NOTES

1. Bristol, M. M., and Schopler, E. *Coping and stress in families of autistic children*. The Gatlinburg Conference on Mental Retardation and Developmental Disabilities, Gatlinburg, April 1982.
2. McHale, S., Sloane, J., and Simeonsson, R. *Sibling relationships of children with autistic, mentally retarded, and nonhandicapped children: A comparative study*. Paper presented at the Annual Conference of the National Society for Autistic Children, Omaha, July 1982.
3. Bristol, M. M. *Sources of help for parents of autistic children*. Paper presented at the International Conference of the Society for Autistic Children, Boston, July 1981.
4. Nevin, R. S., and McCubbin, H. I. *Parental coping with physical handicaps: Social policy implications*. Paper presented at the National Council of Family Relations annual meeting, Boston, August 16, 1979.

REFERENCES

Akerley, M. The invulnerable parent. *Journal of Autism and Childhood Schizophrenia*, 1975, 5, 275–281.

Angell, R. C. *The family encounters the depression*. New York: Scribner's, 1936.

Beckman-Bell, P. *Characteristics of handicapped infants: A study of the relationship between child characteristics and stress as reported by mothers.* Unpublished doctoral dissertation, University of North Carolina at Chapel Hill, 1980.

Bristol, M. M. *Maternal coping with autistic children: The effect of child characteristics and interpersonal support.* Unpublished doctoral dissertation, University of North Carolina at Chapel Hill, 1979.

Bristol, M. M. The home care of developmentally disabled children: Some empirical support for a conceptual model of successful coping with family stress. In S. Landesman-Dwyer and P. Vietze (Eds.), *Environments for developmentally disabled persons.* Baltimore: University Park Press, in press.

Bristol, M. M., and Schopler, E. Coping and stress in families of autistic adolescents. In E. Schopler and G. B. Mesibov (Eds.), *Autism in adolescents and adults.* New York: Plenum Press, 1983.

Burke, R. J., and Weir, T. Husband–wife helping relationships as moderators of experienced stress: The "mental hygiene" function in marriage. In H. I. McCubbin, A. E. Cauble, and J. M. Patterson (Eds.), *Family stress, coping and social support.* Springfield, Ill.: Charles C. Thomas, 1982.

Burr, W. R. *Theory construction and the sociology of the family.* New York: Wiley, 1973.

Cassel, J. C. Psychosocial processes and stresses: Theoretical formulation. *International Journal of Health Services,* 1974, *4,* 471–482.

Cassel, J. C. The contribution of the social environment to host resistance. *American Journal of Epidemiology,* 1976, *104*(2), 107–123.

Cobb, S. Social support as a moderator of life stress. *Psychosomatic Medicine,* 1976, *38,* 300–314.

Cohen, F., and Lazarus, R. Coping with the stresses of illness. In G. C. Stone, F. Cohen, and N. Adler and Associates (Eds.), *Health psychology—A handbook.* San Francisco: Jossey-Bass, 1979.

DeMyer, M. K. *Parents and children in autism.* Washington, D.C.: Winston, 1979.

DeMyer, M. K., and Goldberg, P. Family needs of the autistic adolescent. In E. Schopler and G. B. Mesibov (Eds.), *Autism in adolescents and adults.* New York: Plenum Press, 1983.

Farber, B. Effects of a severely mentally retarded child on family integration. *Monographs of the Society for Research in Child Development,* 1959, *24*(2, Serial No. 71).

Gallagher, J. J., Beckman, P., and Cross, A. H. Families of handicapped: Sources of stress and its amelioration. *Exceptional Children,* 1983, *50*(1), 10–19.

Gallagher, J. J., Cross, A., and Scharfman, W. Parental adaptation to a young handicapped child: The father's role. *Journal of the Division for Early Childhood,* 1981, *3,* 3–14.

Gore, S. Effect of social support in moderating the health consequences of unemployment. *Journal of Health and Social Behavior,* 1978, *19,* 157–169.

Hill, R. L. *Families under stress: Adjustment to the crises of war separation and reunion.* New York: Harper, 1949.

Hill, R. Sociology of marriage and family behavior, 1945–1956: A trend report and bibliography. *Current Sociology,* 1958, 7(May), 1098.

Hill, R., and Hansen, D. The family in disaster. In G. Baker and D. Chapman (Eds.), *Man and society in disaster.* New York: Basic Books, 1962.

Holroyd, J. The questionnaire on resources and stress: An instrument to measure family response to a handicapped member. *Journal of Community Psychology,* 1974, *2,* 92–94.

Holroyd, J., and McArthur, D. Mental retardation and stress on the parents: A contrast between Down's syndrome and childhood autism. *American Journal of Mental Deficiency,* 1976, *80,* 431–436.

Koegel, R. L., Schreibman, L., Britten, K. R., Burke, J. C., and O'Neill, R. E. A comparison of parent training to direct child treatment. In R. L. Koegel, A. Rincover, and A. L. Egel (Eds.), *Educating and understanding autistic children.* San Diego: College-Hill, 1981.

Lazarus, R. *Psychological stress and the coping process.* New York: McGraw-Hill, 1966.

Marcus, L. Patterns of coping in families of psychotic children. *American Journal of Orthopsychiatry,* 1977, *47*(3), 383–399.

Marcus, L., Lansing, M., Andrews, C., and Schopler, E. Improvement of teaching effectiveness in parents of autistic children. *Journal of the American Academy of Child Psychiatry,* 1978, *17,* 625–639.

Mates, T. *Siblings of autistic children: Performance at school and at home.* Unpublished doctoral dissertation, University of North Carolina at Chapel Hill, 1982.

McAndrew, I. Children with a handicap and their families. *Child Care, Health and Development,* 1976, *12,* 213–237.

McCubbin, H. Integrating coping behavior in family stress theory. *Journal of Marriage and the Family,* 1979, *41*(2), 237–244.

McCubbin, H. I. Introduction. In H. I. McCubbin, A. E. Cauble, and J. M. Patterson (Eds.), *Family stress, coping and social support.* Springfield, Ill.: Charles C Thomas, 1982.

McCubbin, H. I., Cauble, A. E., and Patterson, J. M. (Eds.). *Family stress, coping and social support.* Springfield, Ill.: Charles C Thomas, 1982.

McCubbin, H. I., Joy, C. B., Cauble, A. E., Comeau, J. K., Patterson, J. M., and Needle, R. H. Family stress and coping. A decade review. *Journal of Marriage and the Family,* 1980, *42*(4), 855–871.

McCubbin, H. I., and Patterson, J. M. *Systematic assessment of family stress, resources, and coping.* St. Paul, Minn.: Family Stress Project, University of Minnesota, 1981.

McCubbin, H. I., and Patterson, J. M. Family adaptation to crisis. In H. I. McCubbin, A. E. Cauble, and J. M. Patterson (Eds.), *Family stress, coping and social support.* Springfield, Ill.: Charles C Thomas, 1982.

Moos, R. J., and Moos, B. S. *Family Environment Scale manual.* Palo Alto: Consulting Psychologists Press, 1981.

Nuckolls, C., Cassel, J., and Kaplan, B. Psycho-social assets, life crises and prognosis of pregnancy. *American Journal of Epidemiology,* 1972, *95,* 431–441

Pearlin, L. I., and Schooler, C. The structure of coping. *Journal of Health and Social Behavior,* 1978, *19,* 2–21.

Rabkin, J. G., and Struening, E. L. Life events, stress, and illness. *Science,* 1976, *194*(3), 1013–1020.

Rutter, M., and Bartak, L. Special education treatment of autistic children: A comparative study. II. Follow-up findings and implications for services. *Journal of Child Psychology and Psychiatry,* 1973, *14,* 241–270.

Saur, W. G. *Social networks and family environments of mothers of severely handicapped infants.* (Doctoral dissertation, Florida State University, 1980).

Schopler, E., and Loftin, J. Thought disorders in parents of psychotic children: A function of test anxiety. *Archives of General Psychiatry,* 1969, *20,* 174–181.

Schopler, E., Mesibov, G., DeVellis, R., and Short, A. Treatment outcomes for autistic children and their families. In P. Mittler (Ed.), *Frontiers of knowledge in mental retardation* (Vol. 1). Baltimore: University Park Press, 1981.

Schopler, E., and Reichler, R. J. How well do parents understand their own psychotic child? *Journal of Autism and Childhood Schizophrenia,* 1972, *2,* 387–400.

Short, A. *Short-term treatment outcome using parents as co-therapists for their own children.* Unpublished doctoral dissertation, University of North Carolina at Chapel Hill, 1980.

18

Coping with Burnout

LEE M. MARCUS

During the past decade the topic of burnout has become increasingly popular among the helping professions as a way of describing and understanding work-related stresses (Edelwich and Brodsky, 1980; Freudenberger, 1974; Greenberg and Valletutti, 1980; Patrick, 1981; Pines, Aronson and Kafry, 1981; Welch, Medeiros, and Tate, 1982). Viewed as the end result of chronic stress, this phenomenon has generated the development of a literature that touches upon and attempts to integrate a range of psychological perspectives from Albert Ellis (Ellis and Harper, 1961) to transcendental meditation (Jaffe, 1980) to sports psychology (Nideffer, 1981). Although burnout has been observed in business executives, police officers, and lawyers (Welch *et al.*, 1982), its widest application has been to the helping professions such as nursing, teaching, and counseling (Patrick, 1981; Pines *et al.*, 1981; Welch *et al.*, 1982), in which the common denominator is the impact of providing constant care and meeting the multiple needs of clienteles, often without essential agency support.

Families of autistic individuals experience stresses that would appear comparable to those of the helping professionals, although there is relatively little written on burnout in this area (Sullivan, 1979). This chapter is intended to deal with this phenomenon as it pertains to these families by first reviewing some of the relevant literature, including a discussion of the definition and description of burnout, discussing factors that are faced by families, examining natural coping techniques families have utilized, and, finally, presenting a system or set of strategies for intervention.

LEE M. MARCUS • Division TEACCH, University of North Carolina, Chapel Hill, North Carolina 27514.

BURNOUT IN THE HELPING PROFESSIONS

Burnout has been defined as the physical and emotional depletion of resources (Sullivan, 1979); a progressive loss of idealism, energy, and purpose
experienced by people as a result of work conditions (Edelwich and Brodsky,
1980); the feeling of emotional exhaustion, negative attitude shift, and sense of
personal devaluation that occurs over time and in relation to high-stress work
environments (Patrick, 1981); a feeling of hopelessness, helplessness, and ineffectiveness (Pines *et al.*, 1981); and the effect on people who feel they give more
than they receive (e.g., those people who work with clients who are unmotivated
or are incapable of reciprocation, Pines *et al.*, 1981). These definitions are
usually given with the caution that exactness is elusive and burnout is more a
gradual process, a series of events rather than an overnight experience. There is
some disagreement about whether it should be viewed as the inevitable outcome
of prolonged stressful conditions that result in pathological apathy or resignation,
or as a potentially growth-producing set of experiential states that can be managed with varying degrees of effectiveness. Regardless of one's orientation,
awareness of burnout has inspired a diverse array of countermeasures that can
promote better understanding of the circumstances under which caretakers or
service providers carry out their responsibilities.

Although there are variations in the definition of burnout, its symptoms
have been well articulated. Symptoms include physical and somatic difficulties,
damage to interpersonal and family relationships, loss of interest, emotional
detachment, and resentment or anger. Patrick (1981) divides the symptoms into
objective and subjective categories. Objective signs include increased amount of
work, often frenzied, skipping of food and rest breaks, irritability, social withdrawal, and self-medication. Subjective reactions include weakened self-image,
feeling of being trapped, depression, sense of isolation, and low motivation.
Rubenstein (Note 1) describes the effects as the decrement in performance across
four dimensions: attentional skills, coordination, problem solving, and human
relations. Welch *et al.* (1982) examine the impact and symptomatology as it
involves five areas of human functioning: physical, intellectual, emotional, social, and spiritual.

Causation

The causes of burnout stem from a variety of factors. Patrick (1981) dis-
tinguishes between system-generated and self-generated causes. System-generated variables include work demands (e.g., intensity, specific clients, interactional nature of involvement), decision-making requirements, knowledge and
skill requirements, atmospheric elements (i.e., level of stress, pattern of stress,

methods of resolving conflict, and authority), nature of surroundings, how one's efforts are acknowledged, and amount of stimulation or challenge. Self-generated variables include role expectations, gaps in self-awareness, personal life pressures, existing coping strategies, internal or external belief systems, life-style habits (e.g., drinking, exercise, nutrition), and communication styles. Professionals deal with ongoing and multiple needs of their clientele in the face of inadequate fiscal resources, excessive and irregular hours, relatively low pay, and lack of participation in the decision-making process (Pines *et al.*, 1981).

An important factor is disillusionment, which ties into a comparable major source of pressure facing parents. The typical health service provider enters the field with high hopes and expectations for achieving success and having a significant impact on the lives of his or her clients. Although many of the expectations may be partially fulfilled, especially in the initial period of high enthusiasm, it becomes apparent to the worker that this idealistic fervor cannot be sustained in the face of reality—repetitive, intense, often one-sided relationships, job monotony, and inconsistent support.

Burnout factors are also referred to as stressors, the prolonged and unresolved effects of which lead to the loneliness, emptiness, frustration, and fatigue of the worker who finds him- or herself with few options. Stressor analysis (Rubenstein, Note 1) is a method that helps identify and specify potential causes for burnout. Stressors may be dichotomized into macrostressors (e.g., organizational roles or structures) and microstressors (e.g., threat to body or property). An understanding and awareness of these potentially etiological factors is the logical first step in managing the burnout syndrome.

Edelwich and Brodsky (1980) present a stage model of burnout. They describe five steps, each of which requires vigilance and lends itself to the development of coping strategies. The first is enthusiasm, characterized by high ideals and aspirations, but hazardous because of the potential of disillusionment and the impact of devastating failures. Second is stagnation, when the job continues to be carried out but with increasing doubts about its value and the sense of "dead end." Third is frustration, considered the core of burnout with the feeling of powerlessness and the presence of symptoms such as psychosomatic illness, unhealthy indulgence in food and drugs, and damage to personal and family relationships. Fourth is apathy, or boredom and resignation, in which one retreats from the commitment to help others and attempts only to survive, considered the hardest stage to bounce back from. Finally there is intervention, discussed as the implementation of inadequate or poor strategies such as legitimatized malingering or changing jobs without really effecting professional or personal change. These stages are viewed as cyclic and inevitable, but not in and of themselves harmful. Handled with awareness and sound action, they can be growth-producing; managed poorly or denied, burnout can be irreversible.

Assessment

The burnout literature emphasizes the importance of assessment as a critical step in the process of dealing with burnout (Maslach and Pines, 1977; Patrick, 1981; Pines *et al.*, 1981; Rubenstein, Note 1). Depending on the level at which the issues are being studied (e.g., organizational, interpersonal, personal), specific questions and methods of examining multiple variables can be delineated. Patrick (1981) describes a self-assessment guide consisting of 78 questions divided into five categories: personal responsibility (e.g., what are your life goals? when things do not go well, whom do you blame?); emotional resources (e.g., when were you last angry? dejected? anxious?); self-care (e.g., physical exams? junk food? cigarettes? recreation?); communication (e.g., communication style? assertive? passive? how do you communicate frustration or anger?); and job resources (e.g., what areas of your job are unsatisfying? very satisfying? what would you like to change about the environment in which you work?).

Maslach has developed a burnout inventory (Maslach and Pines, 1977), which measures four dimensions: emotional exhaustion, negative attitudes toward clients, negative self-evaluation as a helper, and emotional distance from clients. Rubenstein (Note 2) utilizes a variety of assessment tools to help individuals pinpoint the source and strength of potential burnout stressors. Some involve appraisal of life-style habits, including physical and nutritional evaluations; another involves a checklist covering identification of stressors (e.g., sources and types), perception (e.g., as things are vs. as I see things), stress cues (e.g., physical responses like flushed face or tight stomach muslces; feeling responses like fear, confusion, or discomfort; thinking responses such as Why me? or Making mistakes is terrible; attentional responses such as distractibility or thought confusion), performance deficits (physical coordination and timing off), danger signs (how often does heart pound? lack of concentration? persistently keyed up?), common physical symptoms of stress (e.g., excessive sneezing, alcoholism, overeating, frequent headaches), common psychological symptoms of stress (e.g., nightmare, overwhelming sadness), and diseases (e.g., cardiovascular, metabolic, peptic ulcers, addictions, general disorientation). The Schedule of Recent Experiences (Holmes and Masuda, 1974) is often used as one means of monitoring life events that have the potential of generating considerable stress, perhaps at a time when one is particularly vulnerable to a major negative reaction.

Intervention

What is becoming apparent in the field of burnout is the proliferation of techniques of examining numerous aspects of one's personal and work-related life to help anticipate and fend off possibly damaging events. As writers and workshop trainers endeavor to organize their thinking and methods, they draw upon concepts and strategies for practical application across diverse settings and groups of individuals. Examples of constructs include disillusionment, which will be linked later to the parental experience of grieving; internal versus external systems of beliefs or locus of control; overt versus covert strategies; reframing; Ellis's irrational beliefs (Ellis and Harper, 1961); Glasser's "small world" (Glasser, 1976), which refers to the encapsulated psychological environment in which the helping professional finds him or herself. These concepts can provide a cognitive map to guide the individual to constructive action, which remains the goal of burnout intervention.

Finally, the literature covers the need for intervention. Although practitioners in burnout intervention may approach the problem with somewhat different perspectives, all touch upon the importance of self-care as well as developing concrete strategies for dealing with the stressors or causes themselves. Also critical to most systems is the need for knowledge of the signs and nature of burnout, means of assessing them, the relevance of social support systems, and having an arsenal of techniques, activities, or "tricks" at one's disposal.

Patrick's model (1981) emphasizes knowledge as the starting point, which leads to assessment of the problem across contexts. The next step is to make a responsibility shift, in her view the key to prevention and management of burnout. Once the impact one can have on altering burnout is acknowledged, specific changes can be made and coping capacities can be expanded, resulting in the reduction or avoidance of burnout.

Edelwich and Brodsky (1980) link successful prevention of burnout to the understanding of the five stages of the process mentioned earlier. Thus, during the initial stage of enthusiasm, the worker needs to develop a realistic attitude and tone down high aspirations. Stagnation can be blunted by movement; that is, with further education and related actions a stalled career can be reenergized. The stage of frustration, considered pivotal, can be managed by channeling the energy of discontent into constructive action. Apathy, the most difficult stage to handle, is best helped by involvement, the need to somehow turn this negative state around.

Welch et al. (1982) have developed a specific set of strategies and activities for the five areas affected by burnout, geared to different professionals whose experiences and needs may vary from one another. Pines et al. (1981) utilize a model related to Lazarus's work in stress research (Lazarus, 1974). They describe a grid of coping strategies based on the dimensions of direct/indirect action and active/inactive level of intensity. The resultant four strategies, direct-active (changing and confronting the source of stress), direct-inactive (ignoring, avoiding, escaping), indirect-active (talking, redirecting, adapting), and indirect-inactive (unhealthy indulgences, collapsing) characterize the response styles of individuals; three out of the four can serve as choices, depending on the type of situation and problem faced.

Rubenstein's model of stress modification is a four-step approach involving stress awareness, stress analysis, context for change (determining what is changeable in the situation), and programming for change based on an examination of the previous information (Rubenstein, Note 1). The program involves restatement of the description of the stressor, stating what is stressful about it in what way, developing several change strategies (e.g., new skills, reframing, or life-style habits), examining the consequences of each, and contracting to test one of them.

Later in this chapter these intervention systems will serve as a basis for considering ways of helping families of autistic individuals deal with burnout.

BURNOUT FACTORS IN FAMILIES OF AUTISTIC INDIVIDUALS

Elsewhere in this book issues involving stress and the needs of families have been discussed (Kozloff, Chapter 10; Bristol, Chapter 17). Previous writings by professionals (Bristol and Schopler, 1983; DeMyer, 1979, 1983; Marcus, 1977) and parents (Akerley, 1975; Warren, 1978) have considered the multiplicity of demands on coping skills of parents of children and adolescents with autism. Relatively little has been written on the burnout phenomenon itself or on methods of dealing with it in a systematic way (Sullivan, 1979). To get a clearer perspective on those critical factors likely to lead to burnout, a review of this literature will select the major points repeatedly raised by both professionals and parents.

The *unrelieved care* of raising a chronically handicapped youngster appears foremost among stressors. This is related to the severity of the condition as well as the lack of available, appropriate resources (Sullivan, 1979). Autistic individuals who are relatively self-sufficient are better able to adjust to regular school and a respite/baby-sitting arrangement, allowing the parents more freedom and time to themselves. This "luxury," however, was not available to parents of younger autistic children prior to this decade and the advent of public awareness and federal and state education laws. Thus, parents of adults with autism, regardless of level of severity of handicap, have had to face constant caretaking demands.

Obtaining a proper diagnosis and appropriate, supportive services has been a typical source of stress for most families. Although this may be more prevalent during the early years of life, for many families, the search for an accurate appraisal may continue until adolescence and beyond. The strain this generates stems from the uncertainty of what is wrong, the self-doubts engendered by the puzzling condition, the misinterpretations and suspicions aimed at parents by professionals and the public, the frustrations of finding an understanding teacher or therapist, and the lack of an opportunity to deal honestly and completely with the essential nature of the disorder.

This latter point is worth elaborating because it is becoming increasingly clear that the best hope for families is early diagnosis and explanation, not just to get intervention started for the child and services for the parents, but to begin the process of enabling the parents to come to grips with the painful reality of having a handicapped child for life. Several writers and speakers have commented on the nature of the stages or states of parental reaction and grieving (Searl, 1978; Moses, Note 3). As discussed earlier, a potential cause of burnout in professionals is untempered and unrealistic enthusiasm. In a comparable way, parents have high hopes and aspirations for their offspring that have to be readjusted, drastically in most cases, for their autistic child. The longer this process is deferred, the harder this essential step becomes. Some lack of acceptance of one's handicap is often necessary to continue coping efforts, however. Interestingly, parents who have recently dealt with this topic claim that acceptance or resolution of this process never is fully achieved. Moses (Note 3) describes five grieving states he considers potentially growth-producing (and presumably preventive of burnout): denial, anxiety, anger, guilt, and depression. These states are not sequentially ordered; rather, parents move from one to another as they struggle with the reality of their child's condition, working toward acceptance or positive coping as the ultimate outcome. Searl (1978) describes the conflicting feelings he experienced over his severely retarded daughter, including the tension between a sincere commitment and dedication to her total care and a recognition of the toll it took upon the family dominated by the handicap; the awareness that her condition was as much a social as a medical problem and that society places little value on such individuals; and the slow and painful recognition of the need to abandon the "American myth of progress and success" (p. F28) in the face of minimal growth.

Hagamen (1979) reiterates the factor of unfulfilled expectations, the element of disappointment and disillusionment, which suggests the need for early awareness of what lies ahead and other strategies that will be discussed later in this chapter.

A third factor that increases the vulnerability of parents to burnout is the pervasive *loneliness and isolation* that results from rearing a child whose idiosyncratic needs and continual demands set the family apart from other families. Morton (1978) lists the following elements that contribute to this isolation: the relative infrequency of the situation of having a severely handicapped child and the limited knowledge of the outside world in responding to families; the confusion family and friends have in knowing what role to serve, often keeping their distance or helping to "cover up" or downplay the problem; the discomfort experienced by others; the irrelevance of "normal" social organizations such as PTA; and the special programs and arrangements (such as buses) that separate parents from the mainstream. Morton pleads for more practical help, time, and manpower from parents who are less burdened, a point that will be reemphasized in the section on intervention.

Inadequate supportive services is a major contributor to burnout (Sullivan, 1979). At the governmental level this includes the failure to provide necessary fiscal resources to carry out various legislative mandates. At the professional level it involves lack of interest and knowledge of the problems of autism, how it differs from other developmental disabilities (and in some traditional circles the fact that it is still viewed as an emotional disorder), and the significant burden carried by the family. From the developmental perspective, the frustration experienced by parents trying to obtain a clear diagnostic opinion when their child first shows problems (anywhere from the first few months to 2½ years) was mentioned before. Once such a diagnosis has been made, finding the proper preschool or primary school program without considerable searching is a priority, unfortunately all too often unmet. Even if the primary school years pass by relatively smoothly with adequate services, the adolescent period reawakens the problem of adequate services and, coupled with the emergence of more difficult behaviors and diminished energy of the parents, presents the family with yet another dimension of this chronic crisis of care (DeMyer, 1983). Still, most autistic adolescents can be served in the public schools to one extent or another because of the federal law. Once they are "graduated" or aged out of this system, the threat to families of no adequate day program, whether competitive employment or training centers, becomes a realistic concern. It is doubly unfortunate and somewhat ironic that at the point that most parents deserve permanent respite and are most vulnerable to the ravages of chronic stress, the target of their efforts and the source of their energy drain, the autistic child, may be ineligible for even the most basic service, perhaps finally destroying whatever hopes the parents entertained for salvaging a partially "normal" future.

Lastly, *neglect of personal, social, and medical needs* of parents contributes to the physical and emotional exhaustion characteristic of burnout. The constant vigilance often required of parents, particularly mothers, permits relatively little time and freedom to take care of oneself. The need for self-care, of course, is even more urgent for parents under this type and intensity of stress than for the typical family, yet the opportunities for engaging in the variety of physical and social activities to strengthen coping capacities are less available. The emphasis in the burnout literature on the crucial role of self-care strategies in combating the effects of chronic stress points to a generally neglected factor in considering some of the basic needs of families struggling with autism. Morton (1978) writes about "stripping life to the essentials" (p. 145), especially evident during the adolescent and adult years. Many families lack the necessary inner resources to handle the fatigue, yet for most, few satisfactory alternatives remain.

NATURAL COPING STRATEGIES

Before discussing systematic approaches to preventing or reducing the effects of burnout, it is useful to consider some of the ways families have developed their own coping mechanisms, particularly those that enable many to adapt successfully. It should be noted that although there is a tendency to highlight the grave stresses facing parents—and professionals, for that matter—who are struggling with autistic individuals (DeMyer, 1979, 1983), there are many examples in the literature of positive outcomes, growth in families, and enriched lives (Akerley, 1975).

Actually, one coping technique is writing about one's personal experiences, whether successful (Kaufman, 1976; Park, 1972) or overwhelmingly negative (Greenfeld, 1978). Welch *et al.* (1982) suggest keeping a journal or diary in whatever loose or tight form is helpful as a way for teachers and other health professionals to channel the emotional stresses of their work. Not only does writing about one's experiences serve as an outlet for these feelings, it can enable a parent to make some sense out of the variety of events that may initially appear bewildering and add a meaning or dimension that is otherwise lacking. It counteracts the loneliness and isolation so often described. Some parents keep an ongoing log, which may be intended at some future date to become a book; others may expect it to be shared only within the family or with close friends; others may write letters to extended family or friends to help explain their personal experiences or their perception of the nature of their child's problems. In the TEACCH program in North Carolina (Schopler, Mesibov, Shigley, and Bashford, Chapter 4), prior to the initial evaluation, parents fill out a narrative questionnaire covering their major concerns, what a typical day is like, and their goals from the program. The great majority of parents write at length, honestly, movingly, and trustingly, lending the impression that this has been the first opportunity for them to express in a direct way what their lives are like, what their concerns and hopes are.

These parent-authors have also made insightful contributions regarding the basic problems of autism, including possible causes, methods of managing and teaching their children at home, the appropriate role of the professional, and advocacy.

Becoming involved in parent advocacy or social action on behalf of autistic persons provides a channel for constructive action. For some parents who have difficulty in the day-to-day management of their child, participating in or organizing activities that might ultimately lead to improved services enhances feelings of self-worth and control over their personal predicament. One family that was totally at a loss in caring for their child worked tirelessly to establish a group home to serve others with autism, expressing the recognition that their "failure" to cope in one situation was matched by their competence in a different area. The mutual support and spirit of collaboration that evolves from such organized efforts works for only a minority of parents, a perennial source of frustration for those who remain active. There is thus an inherent risk of burnout itself in advocacy and social action if expectations are unrealistic.

"Dropping out" or finding ways of not centering their lives around their handicapped child becomes a focus for parents, many of whom have worked diligently on behalf of their child's needs, whether as a teacher at home or as a social advocate. This psychological separation is not so much an abandonment of their perceived parental obligations as an increasing awareness of the importance of personal needs. Some parents create opportunities for a vacation, something they have rarely, if ever, done before. Others may rely on older siblings to provide more caretaking. Decreasing or dropping altogether their involvement in parent organizational work is another indication of shifting the centrality of the role of the autistic child. This change in personal focus often has the positive effect of enhancing the parent's own identity and permits the development of meeting personal needs.

Parents whose youngsters make extremely slow progress, especially in communication and social skills, often successfully cope by magnifying the smallest accomplishment and recognizing its value given the severity of their child's handicap. Rather than dwelling on the deficits, parents build on more potentially achievable goals such as self-help. Others cope, perhaps less successfully, by "shopping around" for the latest fad or miracle cure. This search helps maintain a certain level of enthusiasm and goal-directedness, although usually at the cost of repeated disappointments and a failure to come to grips with the fundamental irreversibility of the disorder. Some parents, however, have been able to be sensibly selective about different treatment approaches and have not lost objectivity while keeping their expectations high.

Negative coping techniques, which are indices of possible burnout, include heavily sarcastic humor (as opposed to a beneficial flippant or teasing type of humor), chronic complaining, loss of interest in finding a solution, depression, distortion of facts to give an impression of satisfactory adjustment, and emotional distancing from the child. These signs reflect the feelings of hopelessness, helplessness, and ineffectiveness that characterize the experience of burnout (Pines *et al.*, 1981), more typical of the adolescent period and in families with chronically dependent, severely affected children (Bristol and Schopler, 1983).

STRATEGIES FOR INTERVENTION

Broadly speaking, there are two methods by which families with autistic individuals can be helped to manage burnout: first, through the help provided by professionals; second, by the help parents can provide for themselves. The former has been written about extensively, including chapters in this volume (Schopler, Mesibov, Shigley, and Bashford, Chapter 4; Kozloff, Chapter 10; Schreibman, Koegel, Mills, and Burke, Chapter 11). A few of the key points will be reiterated as they relate to the phenomenon of burnout. The latter has not been well-covered with respect to parents, although professionals in the field have been the target of burnout intervention.

Professionals can help families cope more effectively with the stressors that lead to burnout in several ways. They can provide honest, accurate diagnostic information to enable parents to establish realistic expectations. They can directly provide or help parents locate or obtain appropriate preschool, school, and related day services for their children, and home teaching and behavior management counseling for themselves. They can recognize the need for regular, low-cost respite care, either in-home or center-based, including summer residential camp programs. They should acknowledge the necessity of continuity of services across ages and settings, working with relevant agencies to develop adolescent and adult programs where they are lacking. They should not become judgmental about the parents' needs at some point to find permanent residential placement, even if the setting falls far short of a homelike environment (LaVigna, 1979). They should engage parents in a constant, collaborative, and equal relationship, which combines the expertise of the clinician in technical areas and knowledge of resources with the motivation and unique insights and skills the parents possess regarding their child (Marcus, Schopler, Lansing, and Logie, Note 4). They should be sensitive to the individuality of each family system, respect the family's values and style, and understand the limits to which the family can be pushed both by the stress created by having a handicapped child and by the pressures of living with that child in an often unsympathetic and uncaring social environment (Morton, 1978; Searl, 1978). The professional also helps families cope by supporting, within reason, the hope and optimism necessary to function well.

Parents can help themselves cope by using strategies developed within the helping professions (Adams, 1980; Patrick, 1981; Welch et al., 1982; Rubenstein, Note 1, Note 2; Marcus, Rubenstein, and Schopler, Note 5). The system proposed is a four-step process: (1) helping parents identify and assess stressors in their environment—*stress analysis;* (2) helping parents become aware of their reactions to those stressors—*stress awareness;* (3) considering whether or not a particular stressor is changeable and, if so, how or where—*context for change;* (4) developing intervention strategies to reduce stress and the potential for burnout and thus better utilizing themselves in responding to their children—*stress modification* (Rubenstein, Note 1). An underlying theme is that one major impact of stress is its interference with the proper utilization of existing skills and competencies. Methods that reduce the effects of stressors not only minimize the possibility of burnout but allow parents to maximize the effectiveness of their inner resources and the knowledge gained from working with professionals.

Step 1: Stress Analysis

Stress analysis involves the description of the stressful event (e.g., repeated aggressive outbursts at unpredictable times, lack of rudimentary communication skills, unresponsiveness of local school system), focusing on both the specific environmental condition that caused the stress and the internal stimulus within the parent that elicited a stress response. Thus, the event from an objective standpoint may not appear to be inherently stress-producing (e.g., hand flapping), but the internal reaction it stimulates (e.g., shame over their child's weird-looking behavior) produces stress. A second aspect of analysis is to determine the nature of the stressor, such as emergency or nonemergency (e.g., threat of bodily harm), personal loss, conflict, uncertainty, or expectations. A third aspect is frequency of occurrence, chronic or episodic, and, finally, the severity in terms of impact on parental effectiveness. Parents can list those stressful events, including those that can be referred to as macrostressors, environmental conditions involving broad-based elements (e.g., organizational roles or structures, awareness of the lifelong nature of the problem, loss of confidence in parenting skills), or microstressors, specifiable, discrete events that are analyzable and more controllable than the large-scale stressors (e.g., specific behavioral irritations, financial strain of obtaining a service), and assess their quality along the dimensions noted above. This process increases parental understanding of the specifiable components of what may initially appear to be undifferentiated or vaguely identifiable sources of tension and begin to give them a clearer sense of how they can better control these events. It ties in with the essential first step of self-knowledge recommended in the burnout literature (Edelwich and Brodsky, 1980; Patrick, 1981).

Step 2: Stress Awareness

Stress awareness involves the parents' describing and learning to understand how they react to particular stress situations. It includes a general description of the stress reaction in terms of emotional, physical, and cognitive cues, examples of which were given earlier in the chapter; the perception of causality, whether the stressor and its reaction are seen as under the control of the parent or under the control of external events; a focused description of the dimensions of physical cues, affective responses, cognitive responses or self-statements, and attentional responses; and the impact of the stress response on performance and well-being in the areas of problem solving, interpersonal skills, teaching and management skills, and long-term health effects. The coping styles described by Pines *et al.* (1981) can help parents become aware of their typical approach to stressor events: For example, when their child engages repeatedly in noncompliant behaviors, does the parent take a direct-active approach by confrontation or an indirect-inactive one by withdrawing, becoming overwhelmed by feelings of helplessness?

Step 3: Context for Change

Context for change, determining what is changeable in the stressful situation, is an important mediating step before implementing an intervention that may not be necessary. Certain stressors may not be changeable as perceived by the parent. An example might be the child's ability to live independently upon reaching adulthood. If the parent focuses on the child's lack of competencies as the stressor, rather than on their own worries of being responsible for lifelong care, there will be wasted energy placed on trying to teach unrealistically high skills, instead of changing the parental perception of what is attainable (e.g., group home and sheltered work situation).

There are four aspects in examining the context for change regarding the mutability of the stressful situation: eliminating the stressor, avoiding the stressor, accepting the stressor, and changing oneself (changing the perceptions or expectations or developing new skills). In addition, the hopefulness of being able to effect change and some estimation of the impact on the family of no change occurring along with the costs to the family of implementing change strategies need consideration.

Step 4: Stress Modification

Stress modification or intervention is regarded as the preventive measure against burning out. It involves restating the description of the stressor and what part of the stressor is generating the debilitating reactions in the parent. It should also be recognized that intervention is an evolutionary process, based on developing an individualized set of strategies derived from the assessment of one's own situation and adjusted according to changing circumstances. The situation for a family with a newly diagnosed autistic child is obviously far different from a family whose autistic child has reached adolescence. The same family goes through cycles—their life circumstances may be altered for financial or other sociological reasons and their coping capacities may vary from time to time. Once a clear description of the stressor has been made, various change strategies can be considered along the general dimensions noted above.

Usually, doing nothing, or no-change-strategy, should not be seriously considered, although there may be instances in the past where particular stressful behaviors were transient and inexplicably disappeared; a comparable behavior arising at another time may also be "treated" in this way, i.e., assumed to resolve itself.

More likely, the first choice will involve changing the stressor; such techniques as elimination, avoidance, distraction, and various behavioral methods fall into this category. Parent-training programs are built around these techniques, examples of which are discussed elsewhere in this book.

Changing one's perception should also be considered as a strategy. Acquiring new information by reading or speaking with a professional may alter one's expectations about what is realistically achievable with the child, which can reduce pressure and self-generated stress. One specific technique called reframing involves relabeling the stressor into something positive or useful (e.g., going through the painful experiences will strengthen the family for the future; autism is a challenge to be overcome). The impact of negative messages or self-statements has been well documented by Ellis (Ellis and Harper, 1961), among others. Reversing the content of many of these statements, particularly those that involve irrational beliefs such as "I must be a perfect parent," can enable the stressed parent to deal more realistically with the problems encountered.

A final strategy to be discussed of promoting change involves changing oneself. A number of books and articles focus on activities and methods of taking better care of oneself (Leatz, 1981; Mason, 1980; McGuigan, 1981; Patrick, 1981; Welch et al., 1982). Relaxation techniques, exercise and nutritional programs, life planning, and time management are easily accessible to individuals who are interested. Parents of autistic children are particularly vulnerable to neglecting personal needs and falling into nonproductive life-styles because of the time-consuming nature of the stress they face at home. Yet, in the long run, establishing a healthy life-style and giving oneself permission to take care of oneself may be more effective in preventing or diminishing the effects of burnout than other direct stress management procedures. In this regard it is essential that parents support one another's needs for personal care by sharing responsibilities around the child.

Other ways of changing oneself include knowledge and skill building through reading and attendance at conferences as well as specialized training programs or courses, assertiveness training (Kelley, 1979), interpersonal skills training (Gerrard, Boniface, and Love, 1980; Patrick, 1981), participation in stress management workshops, and involvement in social support groups (Pines et al., 1981).

Obviously, there is no one particular intervention or set of techniques that would meet the needs of all families. Perhaps, as several writers have pointed out, it may be sufficient just to have the awareness from the beginning that all parents face the pressures and problems that make the possibility of burnout very real, if not inevitable, but that its impact can be forestalled and diminished by taking constructive action and anticipating the events that lead up to it. Here, as in nearly every other area involving helping families in which there is autism, the more professionals and parents are informed and mutually cooperative, the less likely burnout will become a reality.

REFERENCE NOTES

1. Rubenstein, G. *A micro-analysis of self-care strategies for parents of disturbed children: A stress awareness/intervention program.* Unpublished manuscript, 1981.
2. Rubenstein, G. *Stress modification.* Workshop presented at the Piedmont TEACCH Center, University of North Carolina School of Medicine, Chapel Hill, December 1981.
3. Moses, K. L. *Parenting an autistic child: A manual for emotional survival.* Workshop presented at the Annual Conference of NSAC: The National Society for Children and Adults with Autism, Omaha, July 1982.
4. Marcus, L. M., Schopler, E., Lansing, M. D., and Logie, C. *Collaborating with parents of autistic children to enhance coping strategies.* Paper presented at the Annual Meeting of the American Orthopsychiatric Association, Washington, D.C., April 1979.
5. Marcus, L. M., Rubenstein, G., and Schopler, E. *Helping parents of psychotic children through skills training and stress reduction.* Paper presented at the Annual Meeting of the American Orthopsychiatric Association, New York, April 1981.

REFERENCES

Adams, J. D. Guidelines for stress management and life style changes. In J. D. Adams (Ed.), *Understanding and managing stress.* San Diego: University Associates, 1980.

Akerley, M. The invulnerable parent. *Journal of Autism and Childhood Schizophrenia,* 1975, *5,* 275–281.

Bristol, M. M., and Schopler, E. Stress and coping in families of autistic adolescents. In E. Schopler and G. B. Mesibov (Eds.), *Autism in adolescents and adults.* New York: Plenum, 1983.

DeMyer, M. K. *Parents and children in autism.* Washington, D.C.: Winston, 1979.

DeMyer, M. K. Family needs of the autistic adolescent. In E. Schopler and G. B. Mesibov (Eds.), *Autism in adolescents and adults.* New York: Plenum, 1983.

Edelwich, J., and Brodsky, A. *Burn-out: Stages of disillusionment in the helping professions.* New York: Human Sciences Press, 1980.

Ellis, A., and Harper, R. A. *A new guide to rational living.* Englewood Cliffs, N.J.: Prentice-Hall, 1961.

Freudenberger, H. J. Staff burnout. *Journal of Social Issues,* 1974, *30,* 159–165.

Gerrard, B. A., Boniface, W. J., and Love, B. H. *Interpersonal skills for health professionals.* Reston, Va.: Reston Publishing, 1980.

Glasser, W. *Positive addiction.* New York: Harper & Row, 1976.

Greenberg, S. F., and Valletutti, P. J. *Stress and the helping professions*. Baltimore: Paul H. Brookes, 1980.

Greenfeld, J. *A place for Noah*. New York: Holt, Rinehart & Winston, 1978.

Hagamen, M. B. Parents speak: The burn-out syndrome. *Journal of Autism and Developmental Disorders*, 1979, *9*, 120–122.

Holmes, T. H., and Masuda, M. Life change and illness susceptibility. In B. S. Dohrenwend and B. P. Dohrenwend (Eds.), *Stressful life events*. New York: Wiley, 1974.

Jaffe, D. T. *Healing from within*. New York: Knopf, 1980.

Kaufman, B. *Son-rise*. New York: Warner Books, 1976.

Kelley, C. *Assertion training*. San Diego, Calif.: University Associates, 1979.

LaVigna, G. W. Parents speak: The burn-out syndrome. *Journal of Autism and Developmental Disorders*, 1979, *9*, 124–126.

Lazarus, R. S. Psychological stress and coping in adaptation to illness, *International Journal of Psychiatry in Medicine*, 1974, *5*, 321–332.

Leatz, C. *Unwinding*. Englewood Cliffs, N.J.: Prentice-Hall, 1981.

Marcus, L. M. Patterns of coping in families of psychotic children. *American Journal of Orthopsychiatry*, 1977, *47*, 383–399.

Maslach, C., and Pines, A. The burn-out syndrome in the day care setting. *Child Care Quarterly*, 1977, *6*, 100–113.

Mason, L. *Guide to stress reduction*. Culver City, Calif.: Peace Press, 1980.

McGuigan, F. J. *Calm down: A guide for stress and tension control*. Englewood Cliffs, N.J.: Prentice-Hall, 1981.

Morton, K. Identifying the enemy—A parent's complaint. In A. P. Turnbull and H. R. Turnbull III (Eds.), *Parents speak out: Views from the other side of the two-way mirror*. Columbus, O.: Charles E. Merrill, 1978.

Nideffer, R. M. *The ethics and practice of applied sport psychology*. Ann Arbor, Mich.: McNaughton Gunn, 1981.

Park, C. *The siege*. Boston: Atlantic-Little, Brown, 1972.

Patrick, P. K. S. *Health care worker burnout: What it is, what to do about it*. Chicago: Blue Cross Association, 1981.

Pines, A. M., Aronson, E., and Kafry, D. *Burnout: From tedium to personal growth*. New York: Free Press, Macmillan, 1981.

Searl, S. J., Jr. Stages of parent reaction. *Exceptional Parent*, 1978, *April*, F27–F29.

Sullivan, R. C. Parents speak: The burn-out syndrome. *Journal of Autism and Developmental Disorders*, 1979, *9*, 111–117.

Warren, F. A society that is going to kill your children. In A. P. Turnbull and H. R. Turnbull III (Eds.), *Parents speak out: Views from the other side of the two-way mirror*. Columbus, O.: Charles E. Merrill, 1978.

Welch, I. D., Medeiros, D. C., and Tate, G. A. *Beyond burnout*. Englewood Cliffs, N.J.: Prentice-Hall, 1982.

19

Children with Handicapped Brothers and Sisters

SUSAN M. McHALE, RUNE J. SIMEONSSON, and
JERRY L. SLOAN

Helping children get along with their brothers and sisters has always been a major concern for parents. The importance that mothers and fathers place on sibling relationships is evident in the literature that instructs parents on how to understand and to change their children's behavior toward and feelings for one another. Writings on sibling relationships, for instance, offer descriptions about how parents can prepare older children for the arrival of a new brother or sister and about how they can cope with the jealousy and rivalry that will (inevitably, it seems) appear at some point in their children's lives (e.g., Calladine and Calladine, 1979; Ginott, 1965; Levy, 1934, 1937; Sewall, 1930; Spock, 1973). Parents seem to be particularly concerned about finding ways of minimizing physical aggression and arguments (overt conflicts) between their children and about providing their children with fair and equal treatment so as to reduce the possibility of jealousy and anger (internal conflict) between brothers and sisters. When one child in the family is handicapped, parents may experience these as well as other worries about their children's relationships with one another.

Given this level of popular interest, the paucity of empirical research on sibling relationships is surprising. Even though a variety of aspects of sibling relationships have been examined (e.g., the correlates of birth order, the nature of siblings' social interactions), a comprehensive set of baseline data on normal sibling relationships is not yet available. In addition, the field lacks a model that

SUSAN M. McHALE • College of Human Development, Pennsylvania State University, State College, Pennsylvania 16802. RUNE J. SIMEONSSON • Frank Porter Graham Child Development Center, University of North Carolina, Chapel Hill, North Carolina 27514. JERRY L. SLOAN • Southeastern TEACCH Center, Wilmington, North Carolina 28401.

would tie together disparate research efforts and illuminate the significance of each. Because our notions about normal sibling relationships are limited in these ways, it is often difficult to evaluate the implications of research on relationships between handicapped children and their siblings—a primary goal of this chapter.* Consequently, to ground our present review in some valid notions of why sibling relationships are important and what about them is important, we will move away from the research literature momentarily and focus on sibling relationships from the point of view of parents.

THE PARENTS' PERSPECTIVE

When we consider why most parents worry about their children's relationships with one another, several reasons come to mind. First, parents no doubt would like their children's daily activities together to be harmonious. When children can play together and work out their problems without arguments and fights, for example, parents will not be annoyed by their children's bickering or called upon to mediate their children's conflicts.

Parents may also want their children to get along with one another because they have a sense that the quality of sibling relationships has consequences for children's personal adjustment. A child who gets away with being bossy or domineering in his or her sibling relationships, for example, may begin to act that way outside of the family (with a peer group, for instance). A child who always gives in to the demands of his or her siblings, or whose needs and activities are given relatively little attention, could grow up with a lesser sense of self-worth.

The feelings of rivalry that may arise among siblings are an indication that the way brothers and sisters get along with one another may be, in part, a reflection of the functioning of the family as a whole. That is, relationships between brothers and sisters both influence and are influenced by the larger constellation of relationships among family members. Most parents are well aware that a child's feelings of jealousy and animosity toward a brother or sister may arise because that child sees his or her sibling as the more favored child— that is, as the recipient of more of the family's resources and more of the parents' time and attention.

From the parents' point of view, then, the important factors about sibling relationships have to do with the ways their children treat each another, the effects siblings have on each other's behavioral and emotional adjustment, and the way sibling relationships affect and are affected by the larger network of family relationships. Investigators who have studied sibling relationships of non-

---

*The authors wish to thank Dr. Ted Huston for his comments on early drafts of this chapter.

handicapped children have addressed each of these issues, sometimes obliquely and sometimes in a more straightforward fashion. Research in the area, for instance, includes observational studies of sibling interaction (Abramovitch, Corter, and Lando, 1979; Samuels, 1980), studies of the way children's personality and intellectual development are affected by their ordinal position in the family (Zajonc, Markus, and Markus, 1975), and studies of what child characteristics may affect sibling relationships. One child characteristic that researchers as well as parents have been concerned about is the existence of a handicapping condition in one sibling in the family. In the following sections of this chapter we will examine the research literature on relationships among handicapped and nonhandicapped siblings in terms of (1) the consequences of having a handicapped sibling for nonhandicapped children's adjustment, (2) the way these sibling relationships are affected by the larger constellation of family relationships, and (3) the nature of these sibling relationships—that is, the attitudes and behavior children display toward their handicapped brothers and sisters.

PERSONAL ADJUSTMENT OF NONHANDICAPPED SIBLINGS

When investigators began to study the families of handicapped children in the 1950s and 1960s, their interest in sibling relationships was focused on parents' (that is, mothers') concerns about how handicapped children affected their brothers' and sisters' personality development and on the way in which the presence of a handicapped sibling influenced the organization of the family as a whole, thereby affecting the development of the nonhandicapped children. One purpose of this early research was to determine whether the nonhandicapped children in the family would be better off if their handicapped sibling was institutionalized (e.g., Caldwell and Guze, 1960; Farber, 1959). The data on this question, however, remain equivocal. Although investigators have been concerned with the possible effects of having a handicapped sibling, findings across studies are inconsistent, probably because subject populations (e.g., the cohort, the nature of the handicapped sibling's disorder), methodologies (e.g., the use of data-collection procedures like behavior rating scales, behavior observation scales, standardized tests, interviews, or retrospective accounts), and outcome measures (e.g., personality measures, IQ, or general social attitudes) are so variable. In this section we will begin to examine some of the effects of having a handicapped sibling while noting the conditions under which different kinds of outcomes may occur.

As we mentioned, investigators have focused on a variety of problems in adjustment that may be exhibited by children with handicapped siblings. Several investigators, for instance, have discussed problems that children experience in establishing their self-identity (Cleveland and Miller, 1977; Grossman, 1972;

Kaplan 1969; San Martino and Newman, 1974). Young children know that they are, at least in some sense, similar to their handicapped siblings: They share the same home, the same parents, perhaps the same color of hair and eyes. The question for each of these children therefore becomes: How many of the handicapped sibling's characteristics do I share? That is, these children may come to think of themselves as somehow defective. When children mature, these doubts and questions may result in their developing a fear of giving birth to a handicapped child because of the genetic or biological makeup that is shared with the handicapped sibling. On the basis of information obtained in discussion groups of adolescents with mentally retarded siblings, Grossman (1972) defines this problem as one in which teenagers overidentify with their retarded brother or sister. She goes on to stress the importance of making children understand that they can be "normal" even though they have a retarded sibling.

This view of identity problems is based only on anecdotal accounts, but professionals who are concerned about the psychological well-being of children and young adults would do well to provide them with accurate information (including genetic counseling) about the causes of their handicapped sibling's condition. In addition, the incidence of this problem calls for more systematic investigation of how these identity problems may be related to parent behavior, to experiences children have with their handicapped siblings, or to experiences they have outside the home. In our own research, for instance, some children have reported that their peers tease them about their handicapped sibling by calling the nonhandicapped children names like "retard." Thus, the view that nonhandicapped siblings might share the salient characteristics of their handicapped brother or sister is not confined to the siblings themselves. Discussion groups for siblings of handicapped children may provide an effective mechanism for getting across this information and for demonstrating that other persons have faced similar questions and doubts.

In contrast to these descriptions of children's psychological problems, some empirical work provides evidence that children with handicapped siblings do not display extraordinary problems in psychological adjustment. For example, Mates (Note 1) studied the adjustment of 32 siblings of autistic children and found that these siblings as a group display higher than average levels of self-concept. In addition, studies of children's behavioral adjustment have found no unusual problems in this group as a whole. For instance, investigations have revealed very low rates of disordered behavior (Lonsdale, 1978; Schipper, 1959), disturbed peer relationships (Caldwell and Guze, 1960; Gralicker, Fishler, and Koch, 1962; Lonsdale, 1978), problems in sociobehavioral adaptation (Lauterbach, 1974), academic problems (Lloyd Bostock, 1976; Schipper, 1959), and anxiety (Caldwell and Guze, 1960) in children with handicapped siblings. In one of the few studies that actually compared the behavior of children with handicapped and nonhandicapped brothers and sisters (i.e., that provided a control group) Gath (1972) found no differences between these groups on parents' and teachers' ratings of children's disordered behavior.

Although these studies have shown that children with handicapped siblings as a whole do not have more problems in adjustment than do other children, additional, more detailed analyses have revealed that a number of factors may influence how a particular child adjusts to having a handicapped sibling. For example, when children are placed in a position where the responsibility for their handicapped sibling lies heavily on their shoulders, they may show more problems in adjustment. These responsibilities may involve caretaking for the handicapped child, household chores, or other tasks that a child must perform because the handicapped sibling requires much more time and attention than a "normal" brother or sister. The sibling of a handicapped child may experience "role tension" when "regardless of his birth order in the family, the severely handicapped child essentially becomes the youngest child socially" and other siblings are expected to care for him and subordinate their needs to him (Farber and Ryckman, 1965, p. 4). Relevant to this analysis, Farber (1959) found that siblings were adversely affected by the degree of dependence of their handicapped brother or sister because of these caretaking responsibilities. Thus, children with more severely handicapped siblings tend to have the greatest problems in adjustment. Along these lines, Mates (Note 1) interpreted his findings of decreases in school achievement scores of older brothers and sisters as being due to their increased caretaking role with the handicapped sibling.

Further supporting this notion are results from several studies indicating that the child who is most affected by the presence of a handicapped sibling is the oldest girl in the family. Again, an explanation for this finding is that the oldest female is the child who is most likely to assume responsibilities that fall to the mother in most families—like caring for the handicapped sibling or being in charge of household tasks or other children in the family while her mother is caring for the handicapped child (Cleveland and Miller, 1977; Farber, 1959; Gath, 1974). Both children (e.g., Caldwell and Guze, 1960; Cleveland and Miller, 1977) and their mothers (e.g., Holt, 1958; Lloyd-Bostock, 1976; Lonsdale, 1978; Schipper, 1959) have said that the care and supervision by one sibling of a handicapped brother or sister is time-consuming, and, in some cases, siblings may become resentful toward the handicapped child. This situation may become a problem especially when parents come to expect a great deal of help from their nonhandicapped children while at the same time being unable to give these children as much a share of their time, attention, and financial resources as the handicapped child receives. Professionals who are concerned about the welfare of children with handicapped siblings should note the potential importance of making available to these families community services like respite care or big brother and sister programs. Use of these services may save nonhandicapped children from becoming overwhelmed or resentful about the care and attention given to the handicapped sibling and may also allow for parents and other children in the family to spend time together without the distraction of having to deal with the handicapped sibling's needs.

Another factor that affects how children respond to having a handicapped brother or sister is how much parents expect from nonhandicapped children in the way of achievement. In some cases, for example, nonhandicapped children in the family may feel the need to make up for the limitations of the handicapped sibling by getting high grades in school or excelling in athletic skills (Taylor, 1974). One study found that this pressure seems to be the greatest when there is only one nonhandicapped child in the family (Cleveland and Miller, 1977).

Although one might expect that achievement pressure may have a detrimental affect on children's adjustment, some work shows that negative effects may be overcome by more positive forces that arise when children have handicapped siblings. Children who have the greatest responsibility for their handicapped siblings, for example, often display more idealism and humanitarian concern in their life goals (Farber, 1963). In interviews conducted with teenagers Farber found that boys and girls who interact frequently with their retarded brother or sister rank making a contribution to mankind and devoting their lives to worthwhile causes as their most important life goals. Teenagers who do not interact often with their handicapped sibling, on the other hand, rank having many friends, focusing life around marriage and family, and being respected in the community as more important life goals. Farber interprets these findings as indicating an internalization of social welfare norms by youngsters who are more involved with their handicapped sibling. Along these same lines, the extent to which having a handicapped sibling affects the career choices of adults was measured by Cleveland and Miller (1977). These investigators found that oldest females in the family (the group reported to have the heaviest caretaking responsibilities for the handicapped sibling) are the most likely to pursue the helping professions—to put into practice their social welfare norms.

Evidence that having a handicapped brother or sister can have a positive impact on a child in terms of their attitudes and their life goals comes from several additional sources. Schreiber and Feeley (1965) concluded that many children with handicapped siblings are characterized by greater maturity and are more responsible than their age-mates. Caldwell and Guze (1960) interviewed young adolescents with mentally retarded siblings and found that these youngsters show an increased understanding of retarded persons and, in general, are more empathic toward persons with problems. Almost half of a group of college-age students interviewed by Grossman (1972) were judged to have benefited from having a handicapped sibling in terms of their level of altruism and idealism, their tolerance toward others, and their orientation toward humanistic concerns. These findings are in accord with anecdotes from a number of other investigators (e.g., Farber, 1963; Holt, 1958; Lloyd-Bostock, 1976; O'Neill, 1965).

FAMILY FUNCTIONING

The presence of a handicapped sibling may directly influence nonhandicapped children's development, but more often these effects are mediated by the way the family as a whole operates. Consequently, a number of investigators have studied the ways in which handicapped children's effects on their brothers and sisters will vary, depending on characteristics of individual family members as well as the family as a whole. The age and gender of the nonhandicapped children are important, as are factors such as the family's socioeconomic status, size, and religious background. In addition, certain characteristics of the handicapped children themselves (like the nature and extent of their cognitive and physical disorders) are associated with the way in which children adapt to the presence of a handicapped sibling in their family. Simeonsson and McHale (1981) have reviewed research on such family and child variables, and a summary of their analysis is provided in Table I.

In addition to searching for factors that are related to nonhandicapped children's adjustment, some investigators have tried to explain just how these characteristics of children and families may contribute to their positive or negative effects. Isolating the processes through which these effects take place, however, is a much more difficult endeavor than simply identifying what factors have an effect, and consequently, descriptions of these processes are speculative as yet.

In trying to understand the influence of these processes, however, several investigators have looked at family functioning as a whole or the nature of the relationships among other family members. The goal of this work is to define the indirect effects of the handicapped child on other children in the family. A growing literature, for example, is addressed to the question of how handicapped children affect their mothers or the relationship between their mothers and fathers and, in turn, influence the nonhandicapped children in the family. Ricci (1970), for instance, examined the child-rearing attitudes of mothers who had mentally retarded children and found that these mothers' parenting attitudes were, on the whole, characterized by more rejection and punitiveness toward children in general than were the attitudes of mothers of nonhandicapped children. No direct measures of the siblings' adjustment were taken, but a large body of literature documents the potentially disruptive effects of this (i.e., punitive and rejecting) maternal style (e.g., Steinmetz, 1979).

In addition to child-rearing attitudes that may generalize to nonhandicapped children, a number of investigators have assessed the impact of a handicapped

Table I. Correlates of Adjustment in Children with Handicapped Siblings

Family characteristics	
1. Size	Children from large families are better adjusted, provided their families have sufficient financial resources.
2. Socioeconomic status	Families of low socioeconomic status have the problem of limited financial resources. Families of middle and upper socioeconomic status must adjust their high expectations for the handicapped child's accomplishments.
3. Parental acceptance	When parents are more accepting of the handicapped child's condition their other children are better adjusted.
4. Marital relationship	With a positive marital relationship, both parents and children adjust better to having a handicapped child in the family.
Child characteristics	
1. Birth order	Older children tend to be better adjusted, particularly when there is a span of ≥ 10 years between the nonhandicapped and handicapped siblings.
2. Gender	Oldest girls in the family are most adversely affected.
Handicapped sibling's characteristics	
1. Age	As the handicapped sibling grows older, other children in the family experience more problems.
2. Gender	Children of the same gender as the handicapped sibling experience more problems, except for the oldest female, who usually experiences the most difficulties.
3. Type of handicap	When the sibling's handicap is ambiguous or undefined, children tend to be more poorly adjusted, especially in higher SES families.
4. Severity of handicap	When the sibling's condition is severe (and the child requires a lot of care), children experience more problems, especially in low SES families.

child on mothers' and fathers' emotional well-being (e.g., Drotar, Baskiewicz, Irvin, Kennell, and Klaus, 1975; Olshansky, 1962; Parks, 1977). Drotar *et al.* (1975), for example, have delineated the stages of grief and acceptance through which parents pass in coming to grips with an understanding of their handicapped child's limitations. One or both parents in any given family may never achieve a realistic and accepting attitude toward the handicapped child, and some evidence indicates that the degree to which parents resolve their feelings about the handicapped child will affect the nonhandicapped children's acceptance of the situation (Grossman, 1972). In addition, studies by Caldwell and Guze (1960) and Gralicker *et al.* (1962) indicate that children's attitudes about their handicapped siblings' institutionalization are consistent with those of their parents. For example, when parents want their handicapped children at home and feel that home is the best place for the child, the other children in the family tend to see the situation in the same way. On the other hand, when parents want their children to be institutionalized, the other children in the family also tend to feel it best for the handicapped child to be out of the home (Caldwell and Guze, 1960).

The handicapped child may have an effect on his or her siblings by affecting the family as a whole, but findings regarding the nature of this effect are inconsistent. In several studies, the functioning of families with handicapped children has been measured, with many families showing relatively high rates of cohesiveness and adjustment (Caldwell and Guze, 1960; O'Conner and Stachowiak, 1971; Schipper, 1959). On the other hand, families of handicapped children may also be characterized by low marital integration, disturbed family roles, and poor family functioning (Fotheringham and Creel, 1974).

The family's level of functioning prior to the handicapped child's birth seems to be an extremely important factor in the ultimate level of adjustment: It may not be the handicapped child but the fact that one additional stress has been added to an already stressful situation that sets the stage for disturbances in the family, in general, and affects the well-being of the nonhandicapped children, in particular (Gath, 1974; Schipper, 1959).

SIBLING RELATIONSHIPS

We have discussed two of the concerns raised at the outset of this chapter: the ways in which handicapped siblings may affect children's development and the ways in which family relationships as a whole may mediate those effects. Our review has uncovered data that address each of these issues. Surprisingly, however, much less attention has been paid in the research literature to the issue of how nonhandicapped children and their handicapped brothers and sisters get along on a day-to-day basis.

In several of the studies described earlier, the quality of the sibling relationship was measured by assessing children's attitudes toward their handicapped brothers and sisters. These studies are consistent in their reports of positive attitudes of these children as a group. Parents, for instance describe the relationship between their handicapped and nonhandicapped children as basically positive, with any difficulties being temporary and remediable (Holt, 1958; Lloyd-Bostock, 1976). One estimate suggests that only about 13% of children have disturbed relationships with their handicapped siblings, and that most parents believe the problems between their children are not greater than would be seen in pairs of nonhandicapped brothers and sisters (Lonsdale, 1978).

Children themselves also report positive feelings about their handicapped siblings. When young adolescents were asked about their relationships with a handicapped brother or sister, for example, they demonstrated a general acceptance and tolerance toward the child (Gralicker et al., 1962) and reported that the child had brought pleasure to their own and their families' lives (Caldwell and Guze, 1960). Adults who looked back on their family life and on growing up with a handicapped sibling also said that they had had generally good relationships with that child (Cleveland and Miller, 1977).

The present authors recently completed a study comparing the sibling relationships of mentally retarded, autistic, and nonhandicapped children (McHale, Sloan, and Simeonsson, Note 2). In all, 90 children between the ages of 6 and 15 years were questioned in an open-ended interview (a modification of the interview developed by Grossman, 1972, for use with college students). Questions focused on (1) the children's feelings toward their handicapped (or nonhandicapped control) sibling (the Sibling Relationship Scale); (2) the ways in which the sibling affected their families' relationships (the Family Relationship Scale); (3) the ways in which their siblings affected the youngsters' own peer relationships (the Peer Relationship Scale); and (4) for the two groups with handicapped siblings, how well the youngsters understood their siblings' handicapping condition.

Comparisons of the youngsters' scores on the first three interview scales revealed minimal differences among the three groups. The interview questions were scored on a 6-point scale (1 = problematic to 6 = most adaptive responses), and the mean scores on each scale for all three groups fell in the moderately positive range (4.0–5.0). The only statistically significant difference found was on the scale dealing with family relationships as a whole, with children who had nonhandicapped siblings saying, for example, that their families spend more time together (i.e., with all members present) and that their families are the same as other families (see Table II).

As part of this study, mothers were also asked to rate the youngsters' behavior toward their handicapped (or nonhandicapped control) siblings using a 24-item rating scale developed by Schaeffer and Edgerton (Note 3). Factor analyses of this scale revealed four dimensions of behavior—the degree of accep-

Table II. Mean Scores[a] of Subject Groups (Children with Autistic, Mentally Retarded, and Nonhandicapped Siblings) on Interview Scales

Interview scales	Autistic siblings	Mentally retarded siblings	Nonhandicapped siblings
Sibling relationship	4.2	4.2	4.1
Family relationship	4.2	4.2	5.0[b]
Peer relationships	4.0	4.2	4.1
Understanding of handicapping condition	3.2	3.3	—

[a]Scores range from 1 to 6.
[b]$p < .00001$.

Table III. Group Means on Mother's Ratings of Children's Behavior toward their Siblings Using the Schaeffer and Edgerton Rating Scale[a]

Schaeffer and Edgerton rating scale score	Autistic siblings	Mentally retarded siblings	Nonhandicapped siblings
Acceptance	3.9	3.8	3.2[b]
Hostility	3.7	3.7	3.2[b]
Support	3.4	3.7	3.1[b]
Embarrassment	4.5	4.6	4.1
Overall mean	3.8	3.9	3.4[b]

[a]Scores range from 1 to 5; for all factors, higher scores represent more positive ratings.
[b]$p < .01$.

tance, hostility, support, and embarrassment that were displayed toward siblings. Behaviors constituting each of these dimensions were rated by mothers on a 5-point scale (1 = negative characteristics to 5 = positive characteristics of the sibling relationship). Comparisons of the three subject groups revealed that mothers tended to rate relationships between children and their *handicapped* siblings more positively than relationships between children and their nonhandicapped siblings. As before, however, the mean scores on all dimensions for each group were moderately positive (3.2–4.6 on the 5-point scale, see Table III), and statistically significant differences among groups may not reflect meaningful differences in the groups of children as a whole. Nonetheless, mothers' positive ratings of sibling relationships—the fact that handicapped and nonhandicapped brothers and sisters, on the whole, get along as well as pairs of nonhandicapped children do—is an encouraging finding and is consistent with findings from earlier investigations.

A closer look at the data from this study, specificially, at the range of responses within the three subject groups (rather than at overall group differences), provides a somewhat different picture of the situation. Far from providing *only* socially acceptable reports of their relationships with their siblings, children with handicapped siblings showed a wide range of responses to the interview questions. Children with nonhandicapped siblings, in contrast, clustered around the mean on each interview scale item. What happened, it seems, is that some of the children with handicapped siblings gave fairly negative reports about their sibling relationship and the other half of the children in these groups gave very positive reports. Averaged together, the group of children with handicapped siblings looks very similar to the comparison group—whose members all rated their sibling relationships within much more narrow bounds. In actuality, however, the sibling relationships of children with handicapped brothers and sisters seem to vary considerably—much more so than sibling relationships between nonhandicapped children. The next step in this line of research is to assess the conditions under which children establish good relationships with their handicapped brothers and sisters.

So far, we have concentrated on how well children can adapt to having a handicapped sibling, but we do not mean to imply that children will always have an easy time, even in the best of circumstances. For instance, the personal accounts offered by young adults who have grown up living with an autistic sibling reflect not only the warmth and concern that these individuals feel for their brothers and sisters but also the difficulties that they often face (Sullivan, 1979). DeMyer (1979) clearly describes the dilemma of siblings and other family members in terms of these questions: "(1) How much time and effort can I give to the autistic person without giving myself away? (2) Am I handling my grief and anger [feelings that must necessarily arise on occasion] in such a way that I can do my best not only for the autistic [child] but for other family members?" (p. 297).

A number of reports in the literature offer means of helping children deal with such issues and of improving upon the relationships of children and their handicapped brothers and sisters. Kaplan (1969) and Schreiber and Feeley (1965), for instance, held discussion groups with adolescents, the purposes of which were to help these boys and girls cope with any negative consequences of the handicapped siblings' presence (e.g., feelings of resentment, identity problems). These investigators also led conversations that focused on the ways in which the youngsters could learn to manage and to understand their siblings' behavior. The effects of these groups were not evaluated formally but were described by the authors of each report as beneficial experiences for the siblings.

In an even more ambitious effort, Weinrott (1974) established a special summer camp for handicapped children and their siblings. In this program, 10- to 18-year-old siblings of handicapped children learned basic principles of behavior therapy, and they observed the application of operant techniques by camp counselors. The children were then given the opportunity to use these techniques both with their own handicapped brother or sister and with other handicapped children. Follow-up assessments indicated that older children, in particular, were able to demonstrate their understanding of behavior modification principles on a multiple-choice test. Moreover, ratings by parents indicated that they were happy about the outcomes of the program for children of all ages. By the end of the camp program the quality of children's interactions with handicapped siblings had also changed—most markedly in two respects: (1) Children began to focus on adaptive behaviors exhibited by the handicapped siblings and to reinforce those behaviors rather than focusing on deviant behavior, and (2) children's interactions with their handicapped siblings began to involve teaching rather than the custodial care they had previously centered on.

Several other investigators have trained children with handicapped siblings in behavior modification procedures—but for the purpose of improving the handicapped siblings' behavior rather than promoting the quality of the sibling relationship itself. Miller and Miller (1976), for instance, used a procedure involving demonstration and practice of prompting and reinforcement (praise) techniques to increase compliance of mildly retarded preschool girls. Each of the childrens' older sisters showed increases in their use of commands and praise as a function of training. The handicapped child's level of compliance also showed a slight increase.

The older siblings of a physically handicapped, developmentally delayed child and a mentally retarded child were trained in behavior modification techniques and were also found to be effective behavior change agents for fostering their siblings' language development and independence and for reducing the incidence of siblings' disruptive behaviors (Miller and Cantwell, 1976). A side effect of this training program was to increase the rate of positive interactions between the handicapped and nonhandicapped siblings. Lavigueur (1976) also reported positive side effects on sibling relationships in two families in which children were trained to modify their handicapped brothers' or sisters' behavior.

In discussing the effectiveness of siblings as behavior change agents, investigators have noted that trained siblings provide for a more consistent environment for the handicapped child and that the training reduces the possibility that siblings may be inadvertently fostering undesirable behavior in the handicapped child. On an anecdotal level, parents report that siblings are often more effective in working with their handicapped brothers and sisters at home than are the parents themselves (DeMyer, 1979). Siblings may be more open and unprejudiced about the handicapped child's capabilities or may interact with the child more spontaneously in a playful context (Holt, 1958). Thus, siblings may be "more enthusiastic, committed, and, in the end successful" (Weinrott, 1974, p. 365) in working with their handicapped brothers and sisters. These studies document the significance of nonhandicapped children as resources for fostering their handicapped siblings' adaptive behavior. The ways in which and extent to which sibling training programs improve the quality of the sibling relationships by changing the children's behavior toward (e.g., Miller and Miller, 1976) and activities with (e.g., Weinrott, 1974) one another, however, should be explored in future research.

SUMMARY AND CONCLUSIONS

We have examined the literature relevant to three issues about children's relationships with their handicapped siblings: how handicapped children affect their siblings' development, how they influence family functioning, and how they and their brothers and sisters get along in everyday encounters. Our examination of the research findings has shown that the consequences of having a handicapped sibling are neither unequivocally positive nor negative. Rather, children's reactions to this experience seem to be mediated by other circumstances that prevail in their families.

The research literature offers some hints about what conditions might be particularly important for how children and families adjust to the presence of a handicapped child and for the quality of relationships that get established with that child. Factors like what kinds of responsibilities children have in regard to their handicapped siblings, how well parents, particularly mothers, have accepted the handicapped child's condition, and how well children are able to control the behavior of their handicapped brother or sister all seem to make a difference. The literature on which this analysis is based, however, is often outdated and, in addition, is beset by methodological difficulties (see Simeonsson and McHale, 1981, for a review of some of these limitations). In any case, many of these propositions have not yet been tested directly. As ever, definitive conclusions await future research.

Another topic that awaits systematic investigation is the study of how sibling relations affect the handicapped child. The focus of this chapter was almost exclusively on the consequences of the sibling relationship for the nonhandicapped children in the family simply because so little information is available about the effects of the sibling relationship on handicapped children. In fact, data about effects on handicapped children are confined to studies of how nonhandicapped siblings can modify their handicapped brothers' and sisters' behavior using reinforcement techniques. Especially given the move toward normalization, handicapped children's interactions with their siblings may have important developmental consequences for these children. Their first extensive social experiences with other children, for instance, are likely to be with their nonhandicapped siblings. Because these interactions are likely to precede encounters with children outside the home, sibling interaction may serve as a bridge between family relationships and peer relationships. Thus, previous activities with a sibling may influence how well a handicapped child adjusts to a mainstreamed school classroom, for example. In sum, the questions we have raised here in regard to nonhandicapped children also need to be studied from the perspective of the handicapped child's development.

REFERENCE NOTES

1. Mates, T. E. *Which siblings of autistic children are at greatest risk for the development* of *school and/or personality difficulties?* Paper presented at the annual meeting of the National Society for Autistic Children, Omaha, July 6–10, 1982.
2. McHale, S. M., Sloan, J., and Simeonsson, R. J. *Sibling relationships of children with autistic,*

mentally retarded and nonhandicapped children: A comparative study. Paper presented at the annual meeting of the National Society for Autistic Children. Omaha, July 6–10, 1982.

Schaeffer, E., and Edgerton, M. *Sibling behavior to handicapped or younger child.* Unpublished manuscript, University of North Carolina at Chapel Hill, 1979.

REFERENCES

Abramovitch, R., Corter, C., and Lando, B. Sibling interaction in the home. *Child Development,* 1979, *50,* 997–1003.

Caldwell, B. M., and Guze, S. B. A study of the adjustment of parents and siblings of institutionalized and non-institutionalized retarded children. *American Journal of Mental Deficiency,* 1960, *64,* 845–861.

Calladine, C., and Calladine, A. *Raising siblings.* New York: Delacorte Press, 1979.

Cleveland, D., and Miller, N. Attitudes and life commitments of older siblings of mentally retarded adults: An exploratory study. *Mental Retardation,* 1977, *3,* 38–41.

DeMyer, M. K. Comments on "Siblings of autistic children." *Journal of Autism and Developmental Disorders,* 1979, *9,* 296–298.

Drotar, D., Baskiewicz, A., Irvin, N., Kennell, J., and Klaus, M. The adaptation of parents to the birth of an infant with a congenital malformation: A hypothetical model. *Pediatrics,* 1975, *56,* 710–717.

Farber, B. Effects of a severely mentally retarded child on family integration. *Monographs of the Society for Research in Child Development,* 1959, *24*(2, Serial No. 71).

Farber, B. Interaction with retarded siblings and life goals of children. *Marriage and Family Living,* 1963, *25,* 96–98.

Farber, B., and Ryckman, D. B. Effects of severely mentally retarded children on family relationships. *Mental Retardation Abstracts,* 1965, *2,* 1–17.

Fotheringham, J. B., and Creel, D. Handicapped children and handicapped families. *International Review of Education,* 1974, *20,* 355–373.

Gath, A. The mental health of siblings of congenitally abnormal children. *Journal of Child Psychology and Psychiatry,* 1972, *13,* 211–218.

Gath, A. Sibling reactions to mental handicap: A comparison of the brothers and sisters of mongol children. *Journal of Child Psychology and Psychiatry,* 1974, *15,* 187–198.

Ginott, H. G. *Between parent and child.* New York: Macmillan, 1965.

Gralicker, B., Fishler, K., and Koch, R. Teenage reactions to a mentally retarded sibling. *American Journal of Mental Deficiency,* 1962, *66,* 838–843.

Grossman, F. K. *Brothers and sisters of retarded children.* Syracuse: Syracuse University Press, 1972.

Holt, K. S. The home care of severely retarded children. *Pediatrics,* 1958, *22,* 744–755.

Kaplan, F. Siblings of the retarded. In S. Sarason and J. Doris (Eds.), *Psychological problems in mental deficiency.* New York: Harper & Row, 1969.

Lauterbach, C. G. *Socio-behavioral adaptation of siblings of the mentally handicapped child.* Scranton, Pa.: The Print Shop, 1974.

Lavigueur, H. The use of siblings as an adjunct to the behavioral treatment of children in the home with parents as therapists. *Behavior Therapy,* 1976, *7*(5), 602–613.

Levy, D. M. Rivalry between children in the same family. *Child Study,* 1934, *11,* 233–261.

Levy, D. M. Studies in sibling rivalry. *American Orthopsychiatry Research Monograph,* 1937, No. 2.

Lloyd-Bostock, S. Parents' experiences of official help and guidance in caring for a mentally handicapped child. *Child Health, Care, and Development*, 1976, *2*, 325–338.

Lonsdale, G. Family life with a handicapped child: The parents speak. *Child Health, Care, and Development*, 1978, *4*, 99–120.

Miller, N. B., and Cantwell, D. P. Siblings as therapists: A behavioral approach. *American Journal of Psychiatry*, 1976, *133*, 447–450.

Miller, N. B., and Miller, W. H. Siblings as behavior change agents. In J. D. Krumboltz and C. E. Thoreson (Eds.), *Counseling methods*. New York: Holt Rinehart & Winston, 1976.

O'Connor, W., and Stachowiak, J. Patterns of interaction in families with low adjusted, high adjusted, and mentally retarded family members. *Family Process*, 1971, *10*, 229–241.

Olshansky, S. Chronic sorrow: A response to having a mentally defective child. *Social Casework*, 1962, *43*, 190–193.

O'Neill, J. Siblings of the retarded: Individual counseling. *Children*, 1965, *12*, 226–229.

Parks, R. M. Handicapped children. *Health and Social Work*, 1977, *2*, 52–66.

Ricci, C. Analyses of child rearing attitudes of mothers of retarded, emotionally disturbed, and normal children. *American Journal of Mental Deficiency*, 1970, *74*, 756–761.

Samuels, H. R. The effect of an older sibling on infant locomotor exploration of a new environment. *Child Development*, 1980, *51*, 607–609.

San Martino, M., and Newman, M. B. Siblings of the retarded: A population at risk. *Child Psychiatry and Human Development*, 1974, *4*, 168–177.

Schipper, M. T. The child with mongolism in the home. *Pediatrics*, 1959, *24*, 132–144.

Schreiber, M., and Feeley, M. Siblings of the retarded: A guided group experience. *Children*, 1965, *12*, 221–225. ·

Sewall, M. Some causes of jealousy in young children. *Smith College Studies in Social Work*, 1930, *1*, 6–22.

Simeonsson, R. J., and McHale, S. M. Sibling relations of handicapped children. *Child Health, Care, and Development*, 1981, *7*, 153–171.

Spock, B. *Baby and child care*. New York: Simon & Schuster, 1973.

Steinmetz, S. Disciplinary techniques and their relationship to aggressiveness, dependency, and conscience. In W. R. Burr, R. Hill, F. I. Nye, and I. L. Reiss (Eds.), *Contemporary theories about the family: Research based theories*. New York: Free Press, 1979.

Sullivan, R. C. (Ed.). Siblings of autistic children. *Journal of Autism and Developmental Disorders*, 1979, *9*, 287–298.

Taylor, L. S. *Communication between mothers and normal siblings of retarded children: Nature and modification*. Unpublished doctoral dissertation, University of North Carolina at Chapel Hill, 1974.

Weinrott, M. R. A training program in behavioral modification for siblings of the retarded. *American Journal of Orthopsychiatry*, 1974, *44*, 362–375.

Zajonc, R. B., Markus, H., and Markus, G. B. The birth order puzzle. *Journal of Personality and Social Psychology*, 1975, *37*, 1324–1341.

20

The Sibling's Changing Roles

ROBERT FROMBERG

My brother Steve is 19 years old—3 years younger than I. He is of average height, slim, and quite good-looking. Steve doesn't often talk unless urged; then he speaks in a monotone, or mimics the words or tone of the person he is talking to. Steve has many interests: traffic signs, elevators, apartments, interstate highways, big cities, music, and drawing. His knowledge in these areas, though limited, is acute, and he speaks most freely when the subject is, say, the new school crossing signs on Lakeshore Drive. Steve's artwork reflects his other interests. He draws amazingly accurate freehand road maps, signs, and floor plans of every one of our apartments.

Steve is considered moderately autistic. He was a passive baby and didn't begin to speak until he was almost 6. As a child he was hyperactive. He ran, never walked, and often had tantrums consisting of growling noises, shouting, and running out of the house. As he reached his late teens, Steve began to calm down, and many of his bad habits dropped off. Now, while he still has periods of frustration, Steve is generally a pleasant, but very reserved, young man.

THE DIFFICULTIES

My memories of Steve begin when he was just learning to speak and often had tantrums. One situation, when I was 12 and Steve was 9, remains vivid. Our family took a trip from Peoria, Illinois, where Steve and I grew up, to San Francisco, where we stayed with a family we knew. One night the adults went out, leaving the kids home alone, and, as usually happened, I was in charge of Steve. At one point that evening, as everyone sat around the television watching

ROBERT FROMBERG • 5411 Tralee Place, Raleigh, North Carolina 27609.

"All in the Family," Steve started to show signs of discontent. He grunted and growled, becoming increasingly upset. I watched closely and finally realized what was bothering him: he was annoyed every time one of us laughed, or any time the program's laugh track came on. I wasn't sure why that should bother him (I guessed he wanted nothing to interrupt the continuity of the show), but uppermost in my mind was how to keep Steve quiet, or if not that, how to keep him from getting more out of hand. I tried to get Steve to leave the room with me, but he wouldn't go. I couldn't very well ask everyone to stop laughing; even if I could, that wouldn't stop the laugh track on the program. I knew from experience that if I tried, orally or physically, to force Steve to be quiet, he would only get worse.

It occurred to me that the Ritalin Steve had recently started to take might help. As I looked through our luggage for the bottle, I thought about the situation. I didn't know when Steve had taken his last pill; I didn't know how strong the drug was; I didn't know what effect one pill too many might have.

I took the chance. I found the bottle, gave Steve one pill, and it did the trick. He calmed down in a short while and stayed that way for the rest of the evening. Despite the fact that everything turned out well, I remember thinking that it was a thorny situation for a 12-year-old to have to deal with.

Being Steve's brother meant I was a part-time parent—but without the maturity or experience of our real parents. Our mom and dad didn't go out often, but when they did, Steve was usually my responsibility, and his troubles weren't always solved as easily as in the episode above.

In dealing with Steve at his most difficult, I was always faced with several choices: talk to him, shout at him, spank him, give in to his demands, or wait for him eventually to calm down. I made my decisions on the spur of the moment, usually by impulse more than logic. Talking rarely helped. Shouting made things worse. And I didn't have the wits or patience to wait for Steve's yelling and running to stop. Spanking seemed to do some good, both moderating Steve's aggression and getting out some of my frustration. Occasionally I would give in to whatever was troubling Steve. For instance, one afternoon he decided to watch "Sesame Street" on the neighbors' color television. They weren't home at the time. When I tried to explain, and to keep Steve inside, he screamed, slammed doors, and ran out of the house and up the street. When he came back inside, I locked the doors, but that made Steve more furious. Finally, I scoured the house for change and took Steve on the bus to a department store where color televisions were on display. Unfortunately, the channel showing "Sesame Street" didn't come in very well, and another tantrum almost started. I don't remember how I got him out of the store and back home.

What I obviously needed was training. I needed someone to tell me not to get angry at Steve, to let him run around the house, to wait out his tantrums. I don't blame my parents for not giving me this kind of advice. I'm sure that when they came home and asked how we were, I said, "Just fine." At the time I don't think I realized how much difficulty I was having. I thought I was handling these situations as well as anyone could, and after they were over I tried to forget them as soon as possible. Mom and Dad, only seeing Steve and me interact in their presence, thought I got along with him very well, as I did most of the time. But when the difficulties started, some simple, practical advice would have helped immeasurably.

Though caring for Steve was often trying, it was not the most painful experience associated with him. There was a kind of constant pressure in our family regarding Steve. Whenever we went out, we monitored his behavior constantly, trying both to avoid major problems and to smooth out less troublesome actions—thumb-sucking, for instance. Sometimes keeping Steve in tow was as much trouble for the family as a whole as it was for me alone. Once, on a trip to New York, we spent hours driving to every grocery store we could find looking for Carl Buddig brand pressed and sliced corned beef, at the time the only lunch or dinner food Steve would eat.

A more difficult kind of pressure was also present in our household—one that I can only describe as the pressure of sadness. This came primarily from my mom's difficulties. She was a very talented, successful artist and teacher, with numerous shows around the country and works in such collections as the Library of Congress. When Steve was born, and she and Dad realized his problem, Mom painted much less and almost stopped her career as an artist.

More important than Mom's artistic output was her mood. As far back as I can remember, I sensed a great sadness about her, and the few times the subject came up, she attributed her frustration to the pressures of dealing with Steve and running a household. Mom took the setbacks in finding proper placements for Steve badly. When Steve was 12, the public schools told my parents that they could no longer serve him. I can clearly remember how this crushed Mom, though with my dad's help, she fought to have a program for the autistic set up in the schools.

Through my childhood I wished Mom could have borne up better under the strain. I wished that she didn't have to give so much of her time, give up so many of her pleasures. The sense of my mom's frustration and sadness—not intense, but constant—was the greatest hardship of being a brother to Steve.

CHANGING ROLES

While I was in my early teens, I tried to be a brother to Steve as well as a part-time parent. My efforts went largely unrewarded. I would occasionally knock on Steve's door when he was alone in his room; often his answer was a growl. Inside, Steve would stop whatever he was doing—playing records, drawing—and I would try to persuade him to let me hear the record, or to tell me about his drawing. I tried to be as casual as possible, keeping my voice conversational, hoping he would pick up that tone. And I tried to show my genuine interest in whatever he was doing. Steve usually tolerated me for a few minutes but made it obvious when I was overstaying my welcome. Despite his lukewarm receptions, I was always happy to spend those few minutes of comparable calm with Steve.

When I was 17, I left home, moved to New York City, and started a series of menial jobs. I was there for a year and a half, and during that time I had very little contact with Steve. I was told that I was no longer included in his family drawings. My stay in New York ended when my dad died suddenly of a heart attack.

Mom had a very difficult 2½ years between Dad's death and her own from hepatitis. One large problem was dealing with Steve's constant and varied needs. She tried to find proper vocational training for him; she worked with his teacher to help him at school; she attended to the endless small demands, from lunch money to new tennis shoes. Toward the end of this period, these demands were too many and too great, and Mom was less and less able to care for Steve. By that time I had moved out of the house into an apartment nearby, with my future wife. Several days before she died, Mom asked me to keep Steve for one night; the next day she became noticeably ill and had to enter the hospital.

For almost 2 years, from the time I was 20, Steve lived with my wife and me, and I became, in a much more accurate sense than before, his parent. Assuming that role gave me a great deal of sympathy for my parents, and an appreciation of all the time and effort they spent on Steve. Now I had to make sure he had lunch money, new tennis shoes, and help with his homework, that he caught the bus on time, and got to basketball class every Tuesday and Thursday. The small tasks involved with Steve's school and other activities seemed endless, and kept my wife and me very busy. Taking care of Steve made me sympathize in particular with my mom. Steve was hard enough for two people; I had no idea how she'd handled him alone.

I should note here that, though we were continually doing battle with Social Security, money was not much of a problem. I had inherited enough to keep my wife and me in school and to give us more than adequate food and shelter. Also fortunate was the fact that Mom had disinherited Steve in her will (over her lawyer's objections) and named me his legal guardian, allowing me to use the money to his best advantage and keeping it out of the hands of the state. In addition, Steve's and my Social Security benefits were a considerable help.

My legal guardianship over Steve was in effect only until he turned 18, several months after Mom's death. (In fact, I was too young by 1 year to be Steve's guardian, but our lawyer said not to worry, and no problems arose.) Since then Steve has not had a legal guardian, only because no situation has come up requiring one; the school system, Social Security, and others have been willing to work through me as though I were Steve's legal guardian. If at any time it becomes necessary, I can get partial guardianship of Steve, making me legally able to manage his affairs, but not responsible for him financially.

Steve, my wife, Becky, and I all changed as a result of Mom's death and having Steve with us. Though Becky and I were often busy with Steve, as well as ourselves, there was a strangely dull and monotonous quality to our lives. We adopted odd habits, like watching a certain weatherman every night on the 10 o'clock news, and going to the record store every day for no reason. Our new immersion in ritual was unsettling. It was as if my wife and I were becoming autistic too.

However, Steve's changes were more heartening. His hyperactivity, which had diminished greatly in the 2 or 3 years before, was less evident than ever. He seemed more socially aware, seemed to want friends his own age. Sometimes I would see him staring out the window at children playing outside. He didn't spend nearly as much time alone in his room. Instead, whenever Becky and I sat in the living room watching television or talking, Steve would join us. His teachers said that his work and behavior in school were also improving. As well, Steve easily picked up several skills I taught him: getting up in the morning with an alarm, showering and choosing his own clothes, and going outside to wait for his bus at the right time. Simply, Steve was becoming more mature and more self-sufficient.

I can't be certain, but the new environment was very likely responsible for many of Steve's changes. He seemed, for a time at least, to respond better to me than he had to Mom. I believe that was part of his growing social awareness: I was closer to his age, so more of a friend than a parent. I tried to keep our relationship like that of two friends, and usually Steve responded well. However, there were still times when scenes from our past were replayed. I would correct Steve too harshly; he would get mad. We would both shout, and he would run out of the apartment. But these blowups were more rare, and though Steve and I had our conflicts, his behavior was improving steadily, and I was getting better at dealing with him.

Along with Steve's day-to-day needs, I spent a great deal of time looking for proper vocational and residential placements for him. The prospects in both areas seemed bleak. Steve had once worked at the community workshop for the handicapped, but they had asked him not to return. Soon after he moved in with us, Steve started to work afternoons at Goodwill Industries, but that was no better. Nobody there had experience with the mentally handicapped, and eventually I went there several afternoons a week to train Steve myself. When it was obvious that Steve was only going to sweep the floor for hours at a time, I had him leave. I spent the rest of that year looking, without success, for vocational training for Steve.

An appropriate residential placement was just as hard to find. The Illinois Department of Mental Health, after 6 months of silence, said they had forgotten about Steve. After they resumed their efforts, they found one facility that I felt was inappropriate. I began to call them off and on with names of residential facilities I'd discovered in and out of the state, and each time they claimed not to have known, or not to be able to deal with, the place. They always promised to investigate, but I never heard of any progress. At one point Steve was accepted at a good vocational and residential community for the mildly retarded near Chicago, and we thought we'd finally succeeded. We were told the waiting list was approximately 1 year, and settled back to wait. Several months later, I called to check our place on the list and found out the waiting period was closer to 5 years than 1. We were frustrated, to say the least, and I felt I was getting an even better idea of what my parents had gone through.

After a year of letters, phone calls, and interviews, we were pretty much where we'd started in terms of a permanent residence for Steve. No matter how much everyone wanted to help, they finally said there was nothing they could do.

Next, I wrote to the National Society for Autistic Children and asked for a list of residential facilities for the autistic around the country. On this list, Division TEACCH was mentioned as a program that provided additional services. Since they were located in North Carolina, where I knew of an excellent graduate program in creative writing that I could attend, and where Becky could continue school, I wrote to their office in Chapel Hill. I soon received a letter outlining TEACCH's functions and what they might provide Steve. I called with a few more questions, visited twice in the next several months, and finally, a year and a half after Mom had died, the three of us moved to Chapel Hill.

What TEACCH offered was a set of reasonable options concerning every aspect of Steve's care and education. Though we had no guarantees when we moved, it was obvious that a suitable set of programs could be found in the area. From the minute we got to Chapel Hill, TEACCH took the initiative in finding the best settings for Steve, and in working to have him placed there. This drastic change in outlook took a huge weight from my shoulders. That we were finally moving forward in finding a place for Steve gave the whole family renewed optimism.

Steve began the year in a public school class for the trainable developmentally disabled. The class emphasized both academics and vocational training, and Steve was happy there. Steve also saw his TEACCH counselor once a week. In November, TEACCH phoned to say that a new group home was being built, and that I should call the agency in charge and have Steve apply. I did, and to make a short story shorter, Steve was accepted. In late January, Steve moved into the new group home. We'd moved to Chapel Hill just 6 months before.

Since that time my role in relationship to Steve has changed again. I now feel less like a parent, less like an autistic person myself, and in some ways less like a brother. I believe I am now more of a friend to Steve. Every Friday evening he calls, and we make plans to get together the next day. On Saturday we usually go to lunch at McDonald's, then drive wherever we want—to neighboring towns or shopping malls. With a little encouragement, Steve tells me about his week, about any problems he's had, or any good things he's done. As we drive, we try to work out his problems, and he talks about things he enjoys, like New York, elevators, or the state fair. Our weekend outings are fun for both of us, and we are as much like two friends getting together as anything else.

Even when, once a month or so, Steve calls me from the group home saying he's fed up and ready to move out, I still don't feel much like a parent. Usually I just sympathize with him and talk for a while until he calms down. Having Steve out of the house has given me a little breathing room and a little perspective. Now when Steve is upset, I can see that as something other than the end of the world.

My life apart from my relationship with Steve has changed as well. I feel younger, and my wife and I are able to relax and get out of the aparment more often. Along with this I have the comfort of knowing that Steve is being well cared for. At the group home he is cooking, cleaning, and becoming more self-sufficient than ever. He is getting along better with people, and we have high, but realistic, hopes for his future. Above all, I'm happy knowing Steve is happy.

THE PLEASURES

Though having Steve for a brother has been difficult, the pleasures have outweighed the troubles. Not only do I like Steve and enjoy his company, but I believe he has taught me as much as, or more than, I've taught him.

One of the most enjoyable aspects of spending time with Steve is being constantly amazed at what he does or says. His drawings for example, are marvelous. One of my favorites has a house and garage with windows that look like an odd face. Standing in front of the house is a crudely drawn family. Next to the family is a dog that is larger than the people, even larger than the house. And floating in the sky are various complete and half-complete Interstate 74 signs. It's an amazing work, and no one but Steve could have done it.

Also amazing are Steve's powers of observation and imitation. He can precisely mimic the sneezes of almost everyone he knows. At one time Steve had over a hundred diagrams of school buses, showing the most subtle differences among them. Steve knows more about road signs, streets, and interstate highways than anyone I could imagine. He knew Chapel Hill inside out before I could do much more than find my way downtown. This kind of knowledge that Steve has is a constant source of pleasure.

I also enjoy seeing Steve's language and personality develop. In the past year he's become much more casual, much more at ease. Though he often still speaks in a monotone, there are times when his tone is conversational, and what he says reflects his growth and increased confidence. Recently, when Steve was visiting Becky and me, I was saying that I had bought him a pair of jeans that he hadn't worn in two weeks. When Steve and I got in the car to drive him home, he seemed upset. A minute later he said, "You embarrassed me." I was astonished. He had never expressed that kind of emotion or self-awareness before. On another recent drive, Steve and I were coming to a small town he wanted to see. I wasn't sure how many exits led into the town, and wanted to check with Steve. I asked, "Steve, is this the exit we want, or is there another one?" He replied, without a pause, "There's always another exit." Of course he was absolutely right, and to get that kind of answer, rather than Steve's usual yes or no, was delightful.

Another satisfaction has been an increased understanding of how to deal with Steve. One insight I've gained is to what degree Steve is like most people. He likes privacy, has trouble understanding the subtle rules of social behavior, dislikes distraction, has a short attention span, and becomes upset when things don't go according to plan. I share every one of those characteristics—though not to the same degree—and I'm sure many other people feel the same. Seeing the similarity between Steve's feelings and mine has changed the way I deal with him. Lately, when Steve has been upset, I've tried to see his side of the problem. If he complains that he has too many things to do, I might say that, yes, that sounds like a lot of work. If he's angry at someone or something, rather than telling him to stop being mad, I'll find out what happened, and most of the time tell Steve that I'm mad about it too. He responds well to this and usually calms down quickly.

I've learned many other important aspects of dealing with Steve. One example is recognizing his slow verbal processing. Often in the past I became impatient when Steve was slow to answer or to respond to a request. At times I thought he was being deliberately contrary. Now I realize that he just needs more time to formulate his response. This may seem simple, like something I should have understood long ago, but I only recently saw this characteristic, and then because it was pointed out by Steve's TEACCH counselor. Sometimes the most obvious facets of Steve's personality, and how to deal with them, have been the hardest for me to recognize.

In general, I've learned to be more understanding, more flexible, to give Steve time to be upset and then to recover. Most important is that I've learned not to expect Steve to change overnight. Interestingly, this is also the way I would hope to deal with any person, autistic or not. Like anyone, Steve expects and deserves a certain amount of sympathy and respect.

As I gradually learn more about Steve's point of view, I see more of it in me. He and I share many fascinations: the restaurants on the Indiana Turnpike, New

York, highways, long trips in the car. My attraction to small, seemingly unimportant things continues to grow. The other day I passed a Yield Ahead sign I had never seen before, and laughed out loud with pleasure. It has been pointed out to me that many of the characters in my short stories are almost obsessively concerned with simple things like dogs, coffee cups, baseball, or eating breakfast.

Steve looks at the elements of the world around him and does not ask that logical connections be made. In Steve's eyes, if a sign in front of a store says, "Sam's Market," that does not necessarily mean that is the name of the store; I imagine he sees the sign and the store as two entirely separate entities. My sense of the world, though not as extreme, is very similar. For instance, in a certain television commercial advertising a radio station, all the actors were dressed in cowboy outfits. It took me weeks to realize the meaning: that the radio station played country music. Like Steve, I just wasn't looking for a logical connection.

Steve's point of view is, in some ways, an artist's point of view. When a painter or photographer looks at a bottle, he sees its shape, its form, not that it contains Italian salad dressing. Steve, like an artist, has his own criteria besides use or meaning for what makes an object worthwhile. (For this reason, he dislikes throwing away candy bar wrappers.) When I write stories, I try to let this point of view overtake me. I try to observe and record; rather than trying to prove a point, I try to let actions or characters speak for themselves. In art and literature, I take pleasure in many things besides meaning, such as color, texture, or the sound of language. I owe a great deal to Steve in this respect. Without him, I may or may not have picked up this point of view, but from the time we were both very young, he has certainly helped me understand and respect it. The view of the world that Steve and I share is a great bond between us, and it is one of the most pleasurable and important experiences in my life.

SUMMARY AND SUGGESTIONS

In going over my life with Steve, I've tried to keep at the back of my mind any advice I might have in light of my experience. One of the strongest suggestions I have with respect to siblings is that they be given some instruction about dealing with their autistic brother or sister, and about autism in general. In our family, and I suspect in many others, we tended to concentrate on daily events, and gave less thought to an overview of our situation. As a result, I was well aware of Steve's characteristics, of his troubles, even of his school program, but I did not have a general understanding of autism, which would in turn have helped me cope with Steve. I wish I had known, to give just one example, that Steve likely would become less hyperactive as he got older. That knowledge would have changed my outlook greatly. And as I said earlier, some simple advice on how to deal with Steve when he was upset would have helped when I took care of him. I might have known when to ignore him, when to sympathize, and when, or if, to punish him. I might have learned that it is better to correct Steve's behavior at a neutral time, rather than while the behavior is occurring. And in general, when Steve behaved badly, I might have been less upset or angry, and more understanding.

This kind of instruction on autism could have come from my parents, or from almost anyone with a knowledge of the subject. At a young age I might have had some difficulty understanding the complexities of autism, but I am convinced that a few pieces of simple advice would have gone a long way toward improving my ability to deal with Steve.

Extending the idea of instruction for the sibling, I would also suggest some kind of informal counseling. I am sure I would have been relieved to have someone to talk to about my relationship with Steve and his effect on our family. As well, our entire family might have benefited from a similar arrangement. The tension in our family—at least my feeling of tension—was compounded by what was left unsaid. I believe that an opportunity, perhaps once a month, for all of us to speak even a part of our minds would have alleviated some of the pressure we felt. I do not mean to give the impression that our family was set to explode and needed a safety valve. However, being able to voice our frustration and fatigue would almost certainly have been at least the beginning of a way to overcome those feelings.

On a different track, I believe that the family should begin as soon as possible to make plans for the autistic child's future, including vocational training and, if and when the time comes, a residence other than the parents' home. I make this suggestion partly with the sibling in mind. My situation with Steve illustrates the difficulties that can arise from a combination of death, minimal planning, and poor local facilities. The possibility of parents' death is probably not as remote as might be imagined, and should certainly be provided for. A will is essential; luckily, my mom had one, and she gave me access to Steve's funds by disinheriting him. Beyond money troubles are questions of a place to live and some kind of occupation or education in lieu of the parents' home and school. In our case, because I was both shocked and ill-prepared to face Steve's problems, it was difficult to meet Steve's best interests. Planning ahead of time could have helped ensure Steve's continued development.

In any case, this kind of planning should help the entire family. After my dad died, my mom used to talk about having the burden of Steve for the rest of her life. As far as she could see, there was no light at the end of the tunnel. She had spent most of her life as a parent refusing to have Steve sent away; when the time and situation arose when both he and she might have been helped by such a move, she had already convinced herself that Steve would be living with her far into the future. Had my parents looked into residential possibilities—a time-consuming and difficult task—they might have had a brighter view of both

Steve's future and their own. In particular, after my dad died, my mom might have felt less of a burden, might have been able to take a more optimistic view of life.

Once, when I was about 12, my mom asked me if I ever wished Steve was different. I told her no, that he was just Steve, and I had never imagined him any other way. That is still true. Growing up with Steve has often been difficult and discouraging, but it has been gratifying too. I've learned a great deal not only about autism but about my own feelings and attitudes. And through all our different situations, through all the growing we've both done, I believe Steve and I are friends. That in itself has made my years with Steve wholly rewarding.

Index